PSYCHOLOGY AND GERIATRICS

PSYCHOLOGY AND GERIATRICS

INTEGRATED CARE FOR AN AGING POPULATION

Edited by

BENJAMIN A. BENSADON
Charles E. Schmidt College of Medicine,
Florida Atlantic University, Boca Raton, Florida, USA

AMSTERDAM • BOSTON • HEIDELBERG • LONDON
NEW YORK • OXFORD • PARIS • SAN DIEGO
SAN FRANCISCO • SINGAPORE • SYDNEY • TOKYO

Academic Press is an imprint of Elsevier

Academic Press is an imprint of Elsevier
125, London Wall, EC2Y 5AS
525 B Street, Suite 1800, San Diego, CA 92101-4495, USA
225 Wyman Street, Waltham, MA 02451, USA
The Boulevard, Langford Lane, Kidlington, Oxford OX5 1GB, UK

Notices
Knowledge and best practice in this field are constantly changing. As new research
and experience broaden our understanding, changes in research methods, professional
practices, or medical treatment may become necessary.

Practitioners and researchers may always rely on their own experience and knowledge in
evaluating and using any information, methods, compounds, or experiments described
herein. In using such information or methods they should be mindful of their own
safety and the safety of others, including parties for whom they have a professional
responsibility.

To the fullest extent of the law, neither the Publisher nor the authors, contributors, or
editors, assume any liability for any injury and/or damage to persons or property as a
matter of products liability, negligence or otherwise, or from any use or operation of any
methods, products, instructions, or ideas contained in the material herein.

ISBN 978-0-12-420123-1

Library of Congress Cataloging-in-Publication Data
A catalog record for this book is available from the Library of Congress

British Library Cataloguing-in-Publication Data
A catalogue record for this book is available from the British Library

For information on all Academic Press publications
visit our website at http://store.elsevier.com

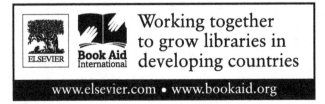

Working together
to grow libraries in
developing countries

www.elsevier.com • www.bookaid.org

Publisher: Nikki Levy
Acquisition Editor: Emily Ekle
Editorial Project Manager: Barbara Makinster
Production Project Manager: Melissa Read
Designer: Maria Ines Cruz

Printed and bound in the United States of America

Contents

4. Communication

TRICIA A. MILLER AND M. ROBIN DiMATTEO

5. Culture of Medicine

WILLIE UNDERWOOD III

6. Psychology Consult: When and Why

ROBERT J. MAIDEN, PETER LICHTENBERG, AND BENJAMIN A. BENSADON

7. Managing Safety and Mobility Needs of Older Drivers

ARNE STINCHCOMBE, GERMAINE L. ODENHEIMER, AND MICHEL BÉDARD

8. Person-Centered Suicide Prevention

PAUL R. DUBERSTEIN AND MARSHA N. WITTINK

9. End-of-Life Care

ELIZABETH C. GUNDERSEN

10. Experiential Learning and "Selling" Geriatrics

JONATHAN M. FLACKER

11. Simulation Education

BENJAMIN A. BENSADON

List of Contributors

Maristela Baruiz Garcia, MD   University of California, Los Angeles, California, USA

Michel Bédard, PhD   Lakehead University, Thunder Bay, Ontario, Canada

Benjamin A. Bensadon, EdM, PhD   Charles E. Schmidt College of Medicine, Florida Atlantic University, Boca Raton, Florida, USA

Susan L. Charette, MD   University of California, Los Angeles, California, USA

M. Robin DiMatteo, PhD   University of California Riverside, Riverside, California, USA

Paul R. Duberstein, PhD   University of Rochester Medical Center, Rochester, New York, USA

Jonathan M. Flacker, MD   Emory University School of Medicine, Atlanta, Georgia, USA

Elizabeth C. Gundersen, MD   Florida Atlantic University, Boca Raton, Florida, USA

Peter Lichtenberg, PhD, ABPP   Wayne State University, Detroit, Michigan, USA

Robert J. Maiden, PhD   Alfred University, Alfred, New York, USA

Tricia A. Miller, MA   University of California Riverside, Riverside, California, USA

Germaine L. Odenheimer, MD   University of Oklahoma Health Sciences Center and Oklahoma City VA Medical Center, Oklahoma City, Oklahoma, USA

David B. Reuben, MD   University of California, Los Angeles, California, USA

Arne Stinchcombe, PhD   University of Ottawa, Ottawa, Ontario, Canada

Willie Underwood III, MD   Roswell Park Cancer Institute, Buffalo, New York, USA

Marsha N. Wittink, MD, MBE   University of Rochester Medical Center, Rochester, New York, USA

Judy M. Zarit, PhD   Center Psychology Group, State College, Pennsylvania, USA

Steven H. Zarit, PhD   The Pennsylvania State University, University Park, Pennsylvania, USA

Foreword

This is a timely and welcome book for the field of geriatric medicine. The importance of integrating psychological knowledge and insights with the care of older patients, their families, caregivers, and the health professionals who care for them, as well as geriatric training and research, cannot be overstated.

While many psychologists are involved in cognitive evaluations and counseling and in various aspects of geriatrics research, the multifaceted role of psychology in geriatrics has not been as integrated or appreciated as it should be. In this groundbreaking work, Benjamin Bensadon confronts this longstanding challenge by clarifying the value of incorporating psychological expertise into a multidisciplinary approach.

Dr. Bensadon brings together here in one place leading geriatric practitioners, educators, and researchers from both psychology and medicine to contribute their extensive knowledge and experience in the care of older patients. By doing so, he models – in type – the integration – in patient care – being proposed here.

I first recognized the importance of psychology in geriatrics when I was a fellow in geriatric medicine providing care on a geropsychiatry unit to older patients with multiple medical problems. The interplay between psychology, physical conditions, and the way they present became very apparent to me. Many symptoms may represent depression, physical illness or both. Often the two exacerbate each other. Chronic pain often causes depression, and depression can in turn exacerbate pain. Many medical conditions, including endocrine, neoplastic, and other diseases present with prominent psychiatric features in geriatric patients.

I have also come to value behavioral psychology in geriatric research. I have had the pleasure of collaborating with a brilliant behavioral psychologist, Dr. John Schnelle, over the last 25 years on clinical research with vulnerable older people in nursing homes. The importance of the psychological aspects of evaluating and managing patients with common geriatric conditions such as urinary incontinence, fall risk, and sleep disruption has been very apparent in our approaches to improving the care of these patients. In addition, behavioral observations have been a critical component of monitoring the fidelity of interventions, and feedback to staff using data from these behavioral observations has been a critical component of the quality improvement interventions we have implemented.

I teach geriatrics using ten basic principles that differentiate geriatric medicine from general internal and family medicine. Psychology is integrated into many of these "Basics in Geriatrics" (or "BIG 10") principles. "Aging is not a disease" implies that impaired cognition and depression are not normal aspects of aging. "Geriatric conditions are multiple and multifactorial" highlights the common presence of mental health disorders in older patients with multiple medical comorbidities. "Function and quality of life are critical" involves teaching students how psychological aspects of patients' conditions impact their overall well-being. "Cognitive and affective disorders are common and often overlooked" speaks for itself in relation to the importance of psychology in geriatrics. "Social history, social supports, and patient preferences are critical" helps students think about the whole patient and the prominent role that psychosocial aspects of care play in patient management. "Ethical issues and end-of-life care are important aspects of geriatrics" helps students understand the importance of psychology in coping with the emotional trauma of facing one's own death or the death of a loved one. And last, but not least, "Geriatric care is multidisciplinary and interdisciplinary" (or as is often said, "Geriatrics is a team sport") helps students understand and respect the roles of various members of the care team, including psychologists. I learned the value of teamwork in geriatrics by working with many respected colleagues in the field, including David Reuben and Jonathan Flacker, who have contributed to this text.

Thus, I believe that psychology must play an integral and prominent role in clinical care, teaching, and research in the field of geriatrics. Integrating psychology and geriatrics will result in improved patient care in innovative comprehensive care programs, will advance interdisciplinary research, and will greatly enhance training of healthcare professionals who will care for our ever-growing older population. Dr. Bensadon's text boldly provides clear, helpful, practical information along with an enlightened perspective on how and why we should make this happen.

Joseph G. Ouslander, M.D.
Professor and Senior Associate Dean for Geriatric Programs
Chair, Department of Integrated Medical Sciences
Charles E. Schmidt College of Medicine
Professor (Courtesy), Christine E. Lynn College of Nursing
Florida Atlantic University

Introduction
Why Integrate?

Benjamin A. Bensadon
Charles E. Schmidt College of Medicine,
Florida Atlantic University, Boca Raton, Florida, USA

In a 1966 issue of the *Journal of the American Medical Association* (*JAMA*), Herman Dickel, M.D., concluded doctoral training in medicine and in clinical psychology were similar, clinicians from both disciplines should work collaboratively to optimize care, and their longstanding inability to do so was harmful to patients (Dickel, 1966). Now, after nearly a half-century, Dr. Dickel's prescient conclusions are more relevant than ever, yet still rarely reflected in practice.

Advancing technology and our nation's decidedly biomedical focus have led to rising life expectancy. As a result, many previously acute health conditions are now chronic. The related demands and lifestyle adjustments caused by incurable chronic illness often exert a powerfully negative psychological impact on quality of life (e.g., Strine et al., 2008), both for patients and their families. Chronic disease is disproportionately fatal (Centers for Disease Control and Prevention, 2014a, 2014b). It follows that some of the more common chronic ailments affecting geriatric patients are depression and anxiety (Byers, Yaffe, Covinsky, Friedman, & Bruce, 2010; Seitz, Purandare, & Conn, 2010), both of which have been shown to improve with psychological intervention (Dobson, 1989; Hendriks, Oude Voshaar, Keijsers, Hoogduin & van Balkom 2008; Hofmann & Smits, 2008; Stanley, 1996; Steuer et al., 1984; Thorp et al., 2009), yet both of which are most frequently managed with medication despite long-term side effects of psychotropic drugs, which are not new and continue to surface (de Gage et al., 2014; Ray, Griffin, Schaffner, Baugh, & Melton III, 1987).

As described later in this publication, incurable chronic disease also impacts informal, familial caregivers. Role-related stressors such as anxiety, strain, and perceived burden often take a dangerous, even fatal, toll (e.g., Bevans & Sternberg, 2012; Rabow, Hauser, & Adams, 2004). And while a Cochrane review of 79 randomized controlled trials has demonstrated benefits of collaborative care models (Archer et al., 2012), psychology training remains peripheral to standard medical education, and standard access to care from clinical psychologists does not exist.

Instead, when these aspects of health and illness are addressed in primary care, management preferences have again emphasized psychotropic medication (Beardsley, Gardocki, Larson, & Hidalgo, 1988; Linden et al., 1999; Sallis & Lichstein, 1982). Less frequently, this has included time-limited, generally sporadic, "counseling" by a nurse, social worker, or at times, clergy/chaplains. Even in geriatric medicine, which explicitly defines itself as a multidisciplinary team-based subspecialty aimed at meeting the biological, social, and psychological needs of the older population, the standard of care erroneously includes coordination only among physicians, nurses, and social workers. Clinical psychologists – the doctors trained in nonpharmacologic management of emotional, cognitive, and behavioral symptoms – are rarely included. As a consequence, all too often, optimal patient management that includes relevant psychological expertise and insight does not occur. Suffice it to say, if there were ever a time to integrate medicine and psychology, it is now.

An exception to the above oversight has been family medicine, a primary care specialty that has recognized for decades the importance of behavior, especially prevention, and clinical psychologists' integrated role via behavioral medicine (Agras, 1982; Pomerleau, 1982). Since the early 1970s (e.g., Birk, 1973) this has included research, teaching (of residents/ medical students), and clinical work. In fact, behavioral medicine constitutes a formal branch of the National Heart, Lung, and Blood Institute (NHLBI) of the National Institutes of Health (NIH). In 1998 a NHLBI task force reported, "It is now widely acknowledged that medicine's concerns extend beyond the biological end points of disease to encompass a wider spectrum of patients' experiences, including their emotional, cognitive, and interpersonal functioning .... With an aging population in the United States (U.S), the prevention and management of chronic illnesses are becoming significant concerns .... Behavioral research is enhancing understanding of the ways patients cope with serious illness and the efficacy of psychosocial and other environmental interventions to ease patients' adjustment to illness, promote their recovery, and prevent the recurrence of disease." Though an encouraging research agenda, it remains unclear who will translate this task force's findings into clinical practice.

Psychiatry is another exception, given the great overlap in training focus and intervention strategy shared with clinical psychology. Clinically, a defining difference between the two is prescriptive authority. As medical doctors, psychiatrists may prescribe, while clinical psychologists may not. However, this may be changing. Currently three states (Louisiana, New Mexico, and Illinois) permit prescriptive authority for clinical psychologists upon completion of state-recognized coursework in psychopharmacology (American Psychological Association, 2014). But not all clinical psychologists want to prescribe. In fact, related debate within the psychologist community led to a change in terminology from prescription *privilege* to prescription *authority*.

It remains unclear how other states will proceed. What is clear, however, is the persistent trend in psychiatry away from behavioral toward pharmacologic intervention (Nordal, 2010; Olfson et al., 2002), even while harm resulting from this shift may be clearer (Tami et al., 2011) than benefit (Kirsch, Moore, Scoboria, & Nicholls, 2002; Moncrieff & Kirsch, 2005). Some have even begun to seek genetic biomarkers for behaviors, including suicide (Guintivano et al., 2014), thanks to a blend of new technology and unwavering insistence on the medicalization of much of American life (Illich, 1976; Postman, 1992). Some psychiatrists, themselves, have suggested this practice behavior may be motivated by economics (Carlat, 2010) more than optimal care. As 73-year-old psychiatrist Michael Taylor (2013) laments in his book *Hippocrates Cried: The Decline of American Psychiatry*, "The decline has occurred in the ability to effectively diagnose and care for patients, and it has been fueled in part by a moral decline, as many in our field sold their souls to the pharmaceutical industry" (ix). This well-documented move away from talking toward medicating may not only lead to suboptimal patient care, it may also explain, in part, the sharp decline in medical graduates opting to specialize in psychiatry. In fact, in 1994 3.2% of U.S. graduates pursued psychiatry, the lowest since 1929 (Sierles & Taylor, 1995). Geriatric psychiatry has experienced a similar decline in physicians seeking fellowship training (Bragg, Warshaw, Cheong, Meganathan, & Brewer, 2012).

The challenge of biopsychosocial integration is something to which the academic medical community is responding. In 2015, the Medical College Admission Test (MCAT) has included content in behavioral and psychological sciences for the first time ever. This formal recognition of psychology's clinical relevance and scientific legitimacy represents an unprecedented milestone. Implicit in this shift is the notion that effective physicians must understand people, not just science (Kirch, 2012a; Rosenthal, 2012). Of course, the professional discipline of psychology, by definition, combines both, and has pursued scientific understanding of human behavior for more than half a century (Berelson & Steiner, 1964; Cronbach, 1957; Skinner, 1953). Darrell Kirch, M.D., Chief Executive Officer of the AAMC, has bravely "defended" the MCAT expansion in *JAMA* by pointing out that the majority of gains in life expectancy over the last 40 years are actually attributable to two health-related *behaviors* – exercise and reduced tobacco consumption (Kirch, 2012b).

Though treating the person rather than the disease is conceptually clear to the sick and those "informally" caring for them, historically, formal integration of physical and psychological care has not been straightforward. Philosopher Rene Descartes separated mind and body in the 1600s, a dichotomy often referred to as Cartesian dualism (Kim, 2000). Care provision has reflected this notion in the ensuing centuries. The concept was challenged in the late 1800s as neurologist Sigmund Freud and physician colleague Josef Breuer published their landmark *Studies on Hysteria*.

This book of clinical cases introduced psychodynamic theory and psychoanalysis as a way to treat patients' physical complaints by targeting physically unobservable mental conflicts and levels of consciousness (Breuer & Freud, 1893). In the 1970s, psychoanalytically trained internist George Engel, M.D., bravely issued a challenge for a new, biopsychosocial medical model (Engel, 1977, 1980) addressing the health-related impact of overlapping biological, psychological, and social factors. Many physicians and some psychologists, occasionally in unison (e.g., Kaplan, Satterfield, & Kington, 2012), have furthered Engel's challenge with similar calls for a "holistic" or "integrative" approach to medical care and training ever since (Bartels, 2004; Bell et al., 2002; deGruy & Etz, 2010; Maizes et al., 2002; Rees & Weil, 2001; Sacks, 1990; Speer & Schneider, 2003).

In fact, the medical literature increasingly includes theoretical terms, concepts, techniques, and measures stemming directly from prominent psychological theory. This is true in both geriatric-specific publications (e.g., *Journal of the American Geriatrics Society*, *Journals of Gerontology*) and the more widely read, general medical journals (e.g., *New England Journal of Medicine*, *JAMA*, *Annals of Internal Medicine*). Recent examples have introduced psychological concepts and behavioral interventions targeting medication adherence (Zullig et al., 2013), caregiver burden (Adelman et al., 2014; Lynn, 2014), mindfulness (Ludwig & Kabat-Zinn, 2008) and self-efficacy to manage chronic disease (Bodenheimer, Lorig, Holman, & Grumbach, 2002). Others have linked personality features ("Type A") to heart disease severity (Frank, Heller, Kornfeld, Sporn, & Weiss, 1978), and clarified anxiety's role in determining whether older patients complaining of dizziness actually fall (Menant et al., 2013).

Medical education and related journals have refocused on defining and measuring professionalism, teaching emotional intelligence (Taylor et al., 2011), and have given significant attention to understanding the correlates of medical student "burnout." This has included its relationship to residency specialty choice (Enoch et al., 2013), psychostimulant drug use (Elnicki, 2013), altruism and cheating behavior (Dyrbye et al., 2010), self-esteem (Dahlin, Joneborg, & Runeson, 2007), suicidal ideation (Dyrbye et al., 2008), a possible protective function of spirituality (Wachholtz & Rogoff, 2013), and use of mental health services (Givens & Tjia, 2002), to name but a few examples. Most recently, Slavin and colleagues (2014) recommended changing curricula in order to explicitly prioritize medical student mental health.

Academic medicine's recognition of the value of psychological insight and experience has not been limited to publications. Curricula are broadening their focus nationally. According to standards set forth in a report by the Liaison Committee on Medical Education (LCME) and AAMC, medical training must include competency in the following areas:

1. Compassionate treatment and respect for patients.
2. Honest interactions with patients' families and colleagues.

3. Understanding and respect for roles of other health care professionals and the need to collaborate.
4. Advocating the interests of one's patients over one's own.
5. Understanding the threats to medical professionalism posed by conflicts of interest.
6. Recognizing limitations in one's knowledge and clinical skills and committing to improving both.
7. Knowledge of nonbiological determinants of poor health and the economic, psychological, social, and cultural factors that contribute to illness.

The report goes on to add that physicians must *"feel obliged to collaborate with other health professionals...promote healthy behaviors through counseling* individual patients and their families...*understand the* economic, *psychological,* occupational, social, and cultural factors that contribute to the development and/or perpetuation of conditions that impair health... be willing both to provide leadership when appropriate and to *defer to the leadership of others* when indicated...." Formal goals for residency training are similar. The Accrediting Council of Graduate Medical Education (ACGME) has synthesized them into six core competencies: patient care, medical knowledge, practice-based learning and improvement, professionalism, interpersonal skills and communication, and systems-based practice. Discrete measurement of these areas is challenged by overlap (Lurie, Mooney, & Lyness, 2009) and a prevailing view among many physicians that there are really only two clinical competencies of importance – medical knowledge and interpersonal skills (Silber et al., 2004), often grossly oversimplified as *science and art*. Recognizing the advantage to integration, Dr. Susan Swing, psychologist and ACGME Vice President for outcome assessment, has been tasked with parceling out these overlapping, but unique, clinically relevant skills.

Precisely how institutions develop such competencies varies. The Philadelphia College of Osteopathic Medicine (PCOM) has paired first-year medical students with psychology doctoral students to co-conduct patient intakes. It has also implemented an "emotional health symposium" into a second-year neuroscience curricular block to "increase understanding and acceptance of those who may have mental illness and reduce stigma associated with mental illness" (PCOM, 2012). The college of medicine at Florida Atlantic University (FAU) has been explicit in naming its clinical department – Integrated Medical Science. As an FAU faculty member myself, I serve on the admissions committee, which fits with the current shift away from relying solely on basic science and test scores in favor of a more "holistic review," as recently discussed in the *New England Journal of Medicine* (Witzburg & Sondheimer, 2013).

Taken together, this "better late than never" response to Dr. Dickel's comments nearly 50 years ago is a dramatic step in the right direction.

Eventual implications, such as whether these changes attract a more diverse array of medical school applicants, are unknown. How (and whether) medical training responds, nationally, is also unknown. But here is what is known:

1. If we are ever to optimize training and care, psychologists and physicians must work together.
2. The primary source of decades-long barriers to integration is also the source of solutions for overcoming them – it is all of us.

PATIENT-CENTERED OUTCOMES RESEARCH INSTITUTE

Not only is academic medicine responding, so is the government. The Patient Protection and Affordable Care Act includes more than $3 billion to be invested in research funding of the Patient-Centered Outcomes Research Institute (PCORI). Unique to the formation and structure of this effort is the prominent decision-making role held by stakeholders *receiving* (not just providing) health care, i.e., patients and informal caregivers. Fittingly, the formal funding announcement published by PCORI board members in the *Annals of Internal Medicine* was titled *Seeing through the Eyes of Patients: The Patient Centered Outcomes Research Institute Funding Announcements* (Krumholz & Selby, 2012). A more recent *JAMA* article coauthored by one of the same PCORI physician board members addressed ways to reduce the trauma (from patients' perspectives) of hospitalization (Detsky & Krumholz, 2014). Again, in principle, understanding and empowering the nation's care recipients to help identify their most urgent and unmet concerns is encouraging. But meeting the biopsychosocial needs of the country's older population poses enormous challenges.

WORKFORCE

While it is premature to predict the eventual impact of recent health care reform (i.e., Obamacare), what is certain is sobering. Primary care medicine itself risks extinction. For economic and other reasons, future physicians are disproportionately choosing specialties in which earnings are high and time spent communicating with patients can be low (e.g., dermatology, radiology, surgery). This does not bode well for geriatric medicine, which, by definition, requires the opposite. Because advanced age is often accompanied by multiple comorbid conditions (multimorbidity), more time is needed to consider the patient's constellation of diseases. Conceptually, this is simple. But taking the necessary time to provide such "comprehensive" care does not currently fit into our nation's acute care medical model and procedure-based reimbursement system (e.g., Avorn, 1984; Siegler, 1984). Thus, it is not surprising that geriatrics is an unpopular career choice.

In medicine, the "reward" for physicians committing the extra time to subspecialty fellowship training in geriatrics is, literally, a pay cut (American Geriatrics Society, 2012). It is reasonable, therefore, that efforts to remedy the shortage of geriatricians have targeted economics. But difficulty attracting people to work with the aged is not new (Papper & Reefe, 1984), and "selling" geriatrics is not limited to financial matters (Leigh, Kravitz, Schembri, Samuels, & Mobley, 2002; Leigh, Tancredi, & Kravitz, 2009). Attitude, stereotypes, and fear are just some of the myriad psychological factors serving as barriers to perceiving elder care as a desirable career choice (Bensadon, Teasdale, & Odenheimer, 2013).

The viability of professional geropsychology practice is perhaps even more perilous. As explained on the Centers for Medicare and Medicaid Services (CMS) website, CMS does reimburse psychotherapy and psychological assessment. The following list indicates the professionals providing covered outpatient "mental" health services under Medicare Part B: *Psychiatrist or other doctor* [this "doctor" should read "physician," since clinical psychologists are also doctors]; *clinical psychologist, clinical social worker, clinical nurse specialist, nurse practitioner, physician assistant, and licensed alcohol or drug counselor.* The reason for the distinction between doctor of medicine and doctor of clinical psychology is unclear. But considering the fact that the CMS "physician definition" (1861r of the Social Security Act) also includes other nonphysician doctors – dentists, podiatrists, optometrists, and chiropractors – this distinction does not seem rational. Currently, clinical psychologists remain the only doctoral-level health care practitioners who are not included in this definition. Advocacy groups have attempted to change this but so far to no avail. Change may be imminent, however. Two members of congress have proposed related legislation (Brown and Schakowsky Bill) to include psychologists in the CMS definition of physicians (American Psychological Association, 2014).

The codes, themselves, are determined by several medically oriented organizations, including American Medical Association (AMA) and CMS. Not surprisingly, "mental" health reimbursement rates are systematically lower than their "physical" health counterparts. While behavioral science evidence continues to show this mental–physical health distinction may be artificial, the difference in payment is unmistakably real. Even when billing codes are the same, doctors of psychology are reimbursed at lower rates than are doctors of medicine. This might not be the case if health care clinicians of all stripes formally recognized that the process of managing an actively suicidal patient can be as "life and death" or "vital" as coronary artery bypass grafting. More important than these clinician payment disparities, those who suffer most from this mistaken mental–physical health dichotomy are patients and their families.

A grave consequence of dualism is that psychology services are consistently the first target of "cost containment." Aside from Medicare, many private insurance companies also cover psychology services. However, these are frequently time-limited (e.g., 12 outpatient visits per year), based on stipulations created by the insurers, themselves. Their rationale, more economic than theoretical, is motivated by profit margin, not therapeutic efficacy. But this trend continues to shape health care in general. As with all medical care in the U.S., third-party payers, whose very existence relies on limiting payouts, dictate how many therapy sessions are clinically adequate. In response, both psychologists and physicians are increasingly choosing not to accept Medicare, and among some clinical psychologists, to not accept any insurance at all. This decision invariably reduces access for many who cannot afford to pay "out of pocket."

Nevertheless, system- and societal-level bias and stigma continue to reinforce the message that psychological or behavioral care is optional, whereas medical services are essential. Of course, suffering patients and families rarely make this distinction. Their focus is simpler – they seek relief.

POLITICS OF "EVIDENCE"

Perhaps more than anywhere else, U.S. health care is a business (e.g., Brill, 2013). As resources shrink and the population grows, member-supported professional organizations often compete, rather than cooperate, to protect and advocate for their own interests. Where patient care fits on their agendas varies. A plethora of national groups represent disciplines, e.g., American Psychological Association (APA) and AMA; specialty board organizations, e.g., American Board of Internal Medicine (ABIM) and Society of Behavioral Medicine (SBM); and subspecialty organizations, e.g., American Geriatrics Society (AGS). While each works feverishly to show its uniqueness, in many ways they are all very similar.

As the number of "relevant" stakeholders increases, their competitiveness intensifies. A common response is reliance on evidence. Evidence-based medicine is national in scope and politically contentious. While objective reliance on science to guide clinical decision-making seems a prudent model, it is also aspirational in nature. One can find "evidence" for most things. And generally those with enough power can choose to believe or "buy" the evidence they prefer.

Unfortunately for older patients and families, all evidence is not created equal. Many physicians find psychological aspects of medical illness uncomfortable or hard to comprehend, which can lead to doubting or even ignoring related evidence. For example, in a leading geriatrician's 90-minute presentation on barriers to exercise among frail elders, fear of falling was never mentioned. This "oversight" should not be surprising even though several diagnostic tools exist to measure this common if not inseparable psychological dimension of frailty (Jorstad, Hauer, Becker, & Lamb, 2005; Morley et al., 2013). For decades psychologists have described perceptions and their influence on "reality." Humans view life through their own lens and see what they know. Physicians are no different. But as evidence in this publication's chapter on geriatric suicide shows, missing psychological insight can be dangerous, and consistent with this text's overall premise, it can also be avoided, but only when both disciplines integrate.

COMMON FACTORS

Psychology and geriatrics have much in common. Both advocate and emphasize care of the whole (complex) person, including illness-related function and psychosocial needs, each essential to quality of life. Both also share an enduring image problem. Disclosing you are a psychologist often leaves people puzzled as to what you actually do. Or, it arouses fearful suspicion that you a) constantly analyze everyone, b) work with "crazy" people, c) are "crazy" yourself, or some combination of the above. Similarly, very few people, including physicians, know what geriatricians are. Nearly a century ago, Edward Steiglitz, M.D., warned against conflating geriatricians (physicians who care for elderly patients) and gerontologists (mostly researchers and other professionals interested in the study of aging). He wrote, "The aged are people; aging is a process" (Steiglitz, 1941). More recently, Leipzig and colleagues have fleshed out specific professional activities that define the geriatrician's scope and expertise (Leipzig et al., 2014). Among those recognizing geriatrics as the care of the aged, many assume it is therefore boring, depressing, and defined by death, or by patients for whom care is futile.

Fortunately, the above "reputations" are based on misconceptions. Yet correcting these negative perceptions and educating professionals, patients, and the general public, alike, remains a daunting task. There does appear to be reason for optimism, however. Both the American Geriatrics Society and American Psychological Association are targeting more effective communication via rebranding and marketing efforts to better educate the nation about what each discipline does.

Beyond geriatrics, psychologists have struggled for decades to articulate their value and occupy a role in standard health care. Skepticism and mind-body dualism remain major barriers. It is not uncommon to hear neurologists base the "legitimacy" of patients' symptoms on whether their etiology is "psychogenic" or "neurogenic" (e.g., Macleod, 2010). Often, similar debate can morph into interspecialty (e.g., neurology vs. psychiatry) or interdisciplinary (e.g., orthopaedic surgery vs. physical therapy) turf battles. This is a longstanding problem in medicine, and sadly shifts focus away from patients to professionals. Iatrogenic consequences of medicine's one-upmanship culture are pervasive. Time and effort spent proving one's superiority have major implications for patients, their families, and trainees. In standard health care, the prefix "psycho" often equates to less, not only in terms of pay but also seriousness. Patients presenting with psychological symptoms, even if acutely severe, may be minimized, redirected, or even ignored. In medicine, psychosomatic complaints often elicit a formal diagnostic thought process of exclusion, a diagnostic approach that has both positive and negative implications.

As mentioned earlier, geriatricians have faced their own struggles articulating their value and finding a stable niche in the world of medicine. Despite official recognition as a board certifiable subspecialty (American Board of Physician Specialties, 2014), attempts to convince health care financiers that geriatric care requires more expertise (and time) than other types of care has achieved mixed success. More importantly, and analogous to psychologists' challenges integrating with medicine, geriatricians have not convinced their (nongeriatrician) physician colleagues of their unique expertise. Many, if not most, physicians assume that merely caring for older patients within their practice adequately prepares them to manage the complex, biopsychosocial issues facing the geriatric population (Diachun, Van Bussel, Hansen, Charise & Rieder 2010). Similarly, many physicians and other health care workers place comparatively little value on nonbiomedical, often psychological and behavioral aspects of care. Even those who "buy" the theoretical value and importance of empathic communication, active listening, and related skills tend to assume they themselves are as "expert" about behavior as anyone else (including psychologists) and are, therefore, qualified to handle these facets of care, often referred to by physicians as the "art" of medicine (Charon et al., 1995; Rosenbaum, 2011).

PERCEPTION

While some of this intimates a common struggle for respect and legitimacy, there is a fundamental yet subtle difference. While the public and even some physicians may not know exactly what a geriatrician is, geriatricians are physicians. Clinical psychologists are not physicians. They are, however, doctors. Or are they? This is a crucial question where perception matters more than reality. While not everyone views physicians positively, the credibility of medicine remains strong. Psychologically, white coats and medical jargon can create an intimidating image of expertise, powerful enough to literally raise one's otherwise normal blood pressure (Pickering et al., 1988). Understandably, much of the public equates "doctor" with medical doctor (M.D.). Conversely, psychologists may work in medicine but they are not medical. Or are they? This gray area has been confusing for decades (Harms, 1966). And physicians often only trust, and choose to discuss certain issues with, other physicians (Kane & West, 2005).

As mentioned, the enduring stigma associated with the prefix *psycho* remains strong. So is the evidence, demonstrated nearly 40 years ago (by psychologists), that human decision-making and causal attributions are subjective (e.g., Larson, 1977). How does this apply to the above distinction? Consider the following:

1. When patients have a suboptimal experience with a physician, they may recognize this but will likely *blame the individual physician* rather than the legitimacy of medicine.
2. When patients have a suboptimal experience with a psychologist, they may recognize this but will likely *blame the discipline of psychology* rather than the individual clinician.

While this subtlety may seem trivial in the context of complex illness, suicide, and death, it is not. Careful review of the medical literature reveals consistent recognition of the relevance of and need for psychological insight described throughout this publication. This recognition spans the entire gamut of medicine, from general practice and primary care (e.g., Cooper et al., 2003) to surgical (e.g., Karimi, McKneally, & Adamson, 2012) and nonsurgical specialties (e.g., Mayer, 2011; Samuels, 2007). Yet while clinical psychologists, by definition, have the longest, most focused and comprehensive behavioral training, whether they are best equipped to provide this care somehow remains an open question. Of course, without their inclusion in standard care, the objective criteria upon which this is based remains unclear and logistically difficult to test. Three particular obstacles stand out:

1. Many physicians are skeptical about psychologists' value.
2. Psychologists have not been successful in articulating their role.
3. Payment.

By including both physicians and psychologists as chapter contributors, this book provides a model for interdisciplinary collaboration and elucidates how such integration yields better outcomes for clinicians, older patients and their families, and, as demonstrated by our national health care crisis, shows why neither discipline can provide optimal care alone.

To some physicians, the notion that psychologists are, by definition, the most highly trained experts in understanding and managing behavior is often met with questions regarding data and evidence. Such questions are legitimate. The following chapters offer answers.

References

Adelman, R. D., Tmanova, L. L., Delgado, D., Dion, S., & Lachs, M. S. (2014). Caregiver burden: A clinical review. *Journal of the American Medical Association, 311*(10), 1052–1060.

Agras, W. S. (1982). Behavioral medicine in the 1980s: Nonrandom connections. *Journal of Consulting & Clinical Psychology, 50*(6), 797–803.

American Board of Physician Specialties (2014). Geriatric medicine. Available at: <http://www.abpsus.org/geriatric-medicine>. Accessed 16.02.14.

American Geriatrics Society (2012). Loan debt and salary statistics for geriatrics health care providers. Available from: <http://www.americangeriatrics.org/files/documents/Adv_Resources/loan_debt.pdf>. American Geriatrics Society website. Accessed 20.07.14.

American Psychological Association (2014). APA applauds landmark Illinois law allowing psychologists to prescribe medications. Available from: <http://www.apa.org/news/press/releases/2014/06/prescribe-medications.aspx>. Accessed 20.07.14.

Archer, J., Bower, P., Gilbody, S., Lovell, K., Richards, D., Gask, L., et al. (2012). Collaborative care for depression and anxiety problems. *Cochrane Database System Review, 10.*

Avorn, J. (1984). Benefit and cost analysis in geriatric care – Turning age discrimination into health policy. *New England Journal of Medicine, 310*, 1294–1301.

Bartels, S. J. (2004). Caring for the whole person: Integrated health care for older adults with severe mental illness and medical comorbidity. *Journal of the American Geriatrics Society, 52*(s12), s249–s257.

Beardsley, R. S., Gardocki, G. J., Larson, D. B., & Hidalgo, J. (1988). Prescribing of psychotropic medication by primary care physicians and psychiatrists. *Archives of General Psychiatry, 45*(12), 1117–1119.

Bell, I. R., Caspi, O., Schwartz, G. E., Grant, K. L., Gaudet, T. W., Rychener, D., et al. (2002). Integrative medicine and systemic outcomes research: issues in the emergence of a new model for primary health care. *Archives of Internal Medicine, 162*(2), 133–140.

Bensadon, B. A., Teasdale, T. A., & Odenheimer, G. L. (2013). Attitude adjustment: Shaping medical students' perceptions of older patients with a geriatrics curriculum. *Academic Medicine, 88*(11), 1630–1634.

Berelson, B., & Steiner, G. A. (1964). *Human behavior: An inventory of scientific findings.* Harcourt Brace & World.

Bevans, M., & Sternberg, E. M. (2012). Caregiving burden, stress, and health effects among family caregivers of adult cancer patients. *Journal of the American Medical Association, 307*(4), 398–403.

Birk, L. (1973). *Biofeedback: Behavioral medicine.* New York: Grune & Stratton.

Bodenheimer, T., Lorig, K., Holman, H., & Grumbach, K. (2002). Patient self-management of chronic disease in primary care. *Journal of the American Medical Association, 288*(19), 2469–2475.

Bragg, E. J., Warshaw, G. A., Cheong, J., Meganathan, K., & Brewer, D. E. (2012). National survey of geriatric psychiatry fellowship programs: Comparing findings in 2006/07 and 2001/02 from the American Geriatrics Society and Association of Directors of Geriatric Academic Programs' Geriatrics Workforce Policy Studies Center. *The American Journal of Geriatric Psychiatry, 20*(2), 169–178.

Breuer, J., & Freud, S. (*1893*). 1895, 'Studies on hysteria'. The standard edition of the complete psychological works of Sigmund Freud, 2.

Brill, S. (2013). Bitter pill: Why medical bills are killing us. Time, March 4, 2013.

Byers, A. L., Yaffe, K., Covinsky, K. E., Friedman, M. B., & Bruce, M. L. (2010). High occurrence of mood and anxiety disorders among older adults: The national comorbidity survey replication. *Archives of General Psychiatry, 67*(5), 489–496.

Carlat, D. (2010). *Unhinged: The trouble with psychiatry: A doctor's revelations about a profession in crisis.* Simon and Schuster.

Centers for Disease Control and Prevention. (2014a). Death and Mortality. NCHS Fast Stats Web site. Available at: <http://www.cdc.gov/nchs/fastats/deaths.htm>. Accessed 15.09.14.

Centers for Disease Control and Prevention. (2014b). Death rates for suicide, by sex, race, Hispanic origin, and age: United States, selected years 1950–2010. Available at: <http://www.cdc.gov/nchs/data/hus/2012/035.pdf>. Accessed 16.02.14.

Charon, R., Banks, J. T., Connelly, J. E., Hawkins, A. H., Hunter, K. M., Jones, A. H., et al. (1995). Literature and medicine: Contributions to clinical practice. *Annals of Internal Medicine, 122*(8), 599–606.

Cooper, L. A., Gonzales, J. J., Gallo, J. J., Rost, K. M., Meredith, L. S., Rubenstein, L. V., et al. (2003). The acceptability of treatment for depression among African-American, Hispanic, and white primary care patients. *Medical Care, 41*(4), 479–489.

Cronbach, L. J. (1957). The two disciplines of scientific psychology. *American Psychologist, 12*(11), 671–684.

Dahlin, M., Joneborg, N., & Runeson, B. (2007). Performance-based self-esteem and burnout in a cross sectional study of medical students. *Medical Teacher, 29*(1), 43–48.

de Gage, S. B., Moride, Y., Ducruet, T., Kurth, T., Verdoux, H., Tournier, M., et al. (2014). Benzodiazepine use and risk of Alzheimer's disease: Case-control study. *BMJ, 349,* g5205.

deGruy, F. V., & Etz, R. S. (2010). Attending to the whole person in the patient centered medical home: The case for incorporating mental healthcare, substance abuse care, and health behavior change. *Families, Systems, & Health, 28*(4), 298–307.

Detsky, A. S., & Krumholz, H. M. (2014). Reducing the trauma of hospitalization. *Journal of the American Medical Association, 311*(21), E1–E2.

Diachun, L., Van Bussel, L., Hansen, K. T., Charise, A., & Rieder, M. J. (2010). But I see old people everywhere: Dispelling the myth that eldercare is learned in nongeriatric clerkships. *Academic Medicine, 85*(7), 1221–1228.

Dickel, H. A. (1966). The physician and the clinical psychologist: A comparison of their education and their interrelationship. *Journal of the American Medical Association (JAMA), 195*(5), 365–370.

Dobson, K. S. (1989). A meta-analysis of the efficacy of cognitive therapy for depression. *Journal of Consulting and Clinical Psychology, 57*(3), 414–419.

Dyrbye, L. N., Thomas, M. R., Massie, F. S., Power, D. V., Eacker, A., Harper, W., et al. (2008). Burnout and suicidal ideation among us medical students. *Annals of Internal Medicine, 149*(5), 334–341.

Dyrbye, L. N., Massie, F. S., Eacker, A., Harper, W., Power, D., Durning, S. J., et al. (2010). Relationship between burnout and professional conduct and attitudes among US medical students. *Journal of the American Medical Association, 304*(11), 1173–1180.

Elnicki, D. M. (2013). Cognitive enhancement drug use among medical students and concerns about medical student well-being. *Journal of General Internal Medicine, 28*(8), 984–985.

Engel, G. L. (1977). The need for a new medical model: A challenge for biomedicine. *Science, 196,* 129–136.

Engel, G. L. (1980). The clinical application of the biopsychosocial model. *American Journal of Psychiatry, 137,* 535–544.

Enoch, L., Chibnall, J. T., Schindler, D. L., & Slavin, S. J. (2013). Association of medical student burnout with residency specialty choice. *Medical Education, 47*(2), 173–181.

Frank, K. A., Heller, S. S., Kornfeld, D. S., Sporn, A. A., & Weiss, M. B. (1978). *Journal of the American Medical Association, 240*(8), 761–763.

Givens, J. L., & Tjia, J. (2002). Depressed medical students' use of mental health services and barriers to use. *Academic Medicine, 77*(9), 918–921.

Guintivano, J., Brown, T., Newcomer, A., Jones, M., Cox, O., Maher, B. S., et al. (2014). Identification and replication of a combined epigenetic and genetic biomarker predicting suicide and suicidal behaviors. *American Journal of Psychiatry* <http://dx.doi.org/10.1176/appi.ajp.2014.14010008>. [Epub ahead of print].

Harms, E. (1966). The acceptance of clinical psychology. *Journal of the American Medical Association, 196*(8) 742-742.

Hendriks, G. J., Oude Voshaar, R. C., Keijsers, G. P., Hoogduin, C. A., & van Balkom, A. J. (2008). Cognitive-behavioural therapy for late-life anxiety disorders: A systematic review and meta-analysis. *Acta Psychiatrica Scandinavica, 117*(6), 403–411.

Hofmann, S. G., & Smits, J. A. J. (2008). Cognitive-behavioral therapy for adult anxiety disorders: A meta-analysis of randomized placebo-controlled trials. *Journal of Clinical Psychiatry, 69*(4), 621–632.

Illich, I. (1976). *Medical nemesis: The expropriation of health.* Pantheon.

Jorstad, E. C., Hauer, K., Becker, C., & Lamb, S. E. (2005). Measuring the psychological outcomes of falling: A systematic review. *Journal of the American Geriatrics Society, 53*(3), 501–510.

Kane, R. L., & West, J. C. (2005). *It shouldn't be this way: The failure of long-term care.* Nashville, TN: Vanderbilt University Press.

Kaplan, R. M., Satterfield, J. M., & Kington, R. S. (2012). Building a better physician – The case for the new MCAT. *New England Journal of Medicine, 366*, 1265–1268.

Karimi, K., McKneally, M. F., & Adamson, P. A. (2012). Ethical considerations in aesthetic rhinoplasty – A survey, critical analysis, and review. *Archives of Facial Plastic Surgery, 14*(6), 442–450.

Kim, J. (2000). *Mind in a physical world: An essay on the mind-body problem and mental causation.* Cambridge: The MIT Press.

Kirch, D. (2012a). A Word from the President: MCAT 2015: An Open Letter to Pre-Med Students. Retrieved from: <https://www.aamc.org/newsroom/reporter/march2012/276772/word.html>.

Kirch, D. (2012b). Transforming admissions: The gateway to medicine. *JAMA, 308*(21), 2250–2251.

Kirsch, I., Moore, T. J., Scoboria, A., & Nicholls, S. S. (2002). The Emperor's new drugs: An analysis of antidepressant medication data submitted to the U.S. Food and Drug Administration. *Prevention & Treatment, 5*(1), 23a.

Krumholz, H. M., & Selby, J. V. (2012). Seeing through the eyes of patients: The Patient-Centered Outcomes Research Institute funding announcements. *Annals of Internal Medicine, 157*(6), 446–447.

Larson, J. R. (1977). Evidence for a self-serving bias in the attribution of causality. *Journal of Personality, 45*(3), 430–441.

Leigh, J. P., Kravitz, R. L., Schembri, M., Samuels, S. J., & Mobley, S. (2002). Physician career satisfaction across specialties. *Archives of Internal Medicine, 162*, 1577–1584.

Leigh, J. P., Tancredi, D. J., & Kravitz, R. L. (2009). Physician career satisfaction within specialties. *BMC Health Services Research., 9*, 166.

Leipzig, R. M., Sauvigne, K., Granville, L. J., Harper, G. M., Kirk, L. M., Levine, S. A., et al. (2014). What is a geriatrician? American Geriatrics Society and Association of Directors of Geriatric Academic Programs end-of-training entrustable professional activities for geriatric medicine. *Journal of the American Geriatrics Society, 62*, 924–929.

Linden, M., Lecrubier, Y., Bellantuono, C., Benkert, O., Kisely, S., & Simon, G. (1999). The prescribing of psychotropic drugs by primary care physicians: An international collaborative study. *Journal of Clinical Psychopharmacology, 19*(2), 132–140.

Ludwig, D. S., & Kabat-Zinn, J. (2008). Mindfulness in medicine. *Journal of the American Medical Association, 300*(11), 1350–1352.

Lurie, S. J., Mooney, C. J., & Lyness, J. M. (2009). Measurement of the general competencies of the Accreditation Council for Graduate Medical Education: A systematic review. *Academic Medicine, 84*, 301–309.

Lynn, J. (2014). Strategies to ease the burden of family caregivers. *Journal of the American Medical Association, 311*(10), 1021–1022.

Macleod, S. (2010). Post concussion syndrome: The attraction of the psychological by the organic. *Medical Hypotheses, 74*(6), 1033–1035.

Mayer, E. A. (2011). Gut feelings: The emerging biology of gut–brain communication. *Nature Reviews Neuroscience, 12*(8), 453–466.

Menant, J. C., Menant, J. C., Wong, A., Sturnieks, D. L., Close, J. C., Delbaere, K., et al. (2013). Pain and anxiety mediate the relationship between dizziness and falls in older people. *Journal of the American Geriatrics Society, 61*(3), 423–428.

Moncrieff, J., & Kirsch, I. (2005). Efficacy of antidepressants in adults. *BMJ, 331*, 155.

Morley, J. E., Vellas, B., van Kan, G. A., Anker, S. D., Bauer, J. M., Bernabei, R., et al. (2013). *Journal of the American Medical Directors Association, 14*(6), 392–397.

Nordal, K. C. (2010). Where has all the psychotherapy gone? American Psychological Association, available at: <http://www.apa.org/monitor/2010/11/perspectives.aspx>. Accessed 20.07.14.

Olfson, M., Marcus, S. C., Druss, B., Elinson, L., Tanielian, T., & Pincus, H. A. (2002). National trends in the outpatient treatment of depression. *Journal of the American Medical Association, 287*(2), 203–209.

Papper, S., & Reefe, W. E. (1984). The future of geriatrics. *Archives of Internal Medicine, 144*(11), 2241–2242.

Philadelphia College of Osteopathic Medicine, (2012). Retrieved at < http://digitalcommons.pcom.edu/posters/2/>.

Pickering, T. G., James, G. D., Boddie, C., Harshfield, G. A., Blank, S., & Laragh, J. H. (1988). How common Is white coat hypertension? *Journal of the American Medical Association, 259*(2), 225–228.

Pomerleau, O. F. (1982). A discourse on behavioral medicine: Current status and future trends. *Journal of Consulting and Clinical Psychology, 50*(6), 1030.

Postman, N. (1992). *Technopoly: The surrender of culture to technology.* Random House LLC.

Rabow, M. W., Hauser, J. M., & Adams, J. (2004). Supporting family caregivers at the end of life: They don't know what they don't know. *Journal of the American Medical Association, 291*(4), 483–491.

Ray, W. A., Griffin, M. R., Schaffner, W., Baugh, D. K., & Melton, L. J., III (1987). Psychotropic drug use and the risk of hip fracture. *New England Journal of Medicine, 316*, 363–369.

Rees, L., & Weil, A. (2001). Integrated medicine: Imbues orthodox medicine with the values of complementary medicine. *British Medical Journal, 322*(7279), 119–120.

Rosenbaum, L. (2011). The art of doing nothing. *New England Journal of Medicine, 365*, 782–785.

Rosenthal, E. (2012). Pre-med's new priorities. Heart and soul and social science. *New York Times* website. Available from: <http://www.nytimes.com/2012/04/15/education/edlife/pre-meds-new-priorities-heart-and-soul-and-social-science.html?_r=2&src=me&ref=education&>. Accessed 01.06.14.

Sacks, O. (1990). Neurology and the soul. *The New York Review of Books.* November 20, 1990.

Sallis, J. F., & Lichstein, K. L. (1982). Analysis and management of geriatric anxiety. *The International Journal of Aging and Human Development, 15*(3), 197–211.

Samuels, M. A. (2007). The brain–heart connection. *Circulation, 116*(1), 77–84.

Seitz, D., Purandare, N., & Conn, D. (2010). Prevalence of psychiatric disorders among older adults in long-term care homes: A systematic review. *International Psychogeriatrics, 22*(7), 1025–1039.

Siegler, M. (1984). Should age be a criterion in health care? *The Hastings Center Report, 14*(5), 24–27.

Sierles, F. S., & Taylor, M. D. (1995). Decline of U.S. medical student career choice of psychiatry and what to do about it. *American Journal of Psychiatry, 152,* 1416–1426.

Silber, C. G., Nasca, T. J., Paskin, D. L., Eiger, G., Robeson, M., & Veloski, J. J. (2004). Do global rating forms enable program directors to assess the ACGME competencies? *Academic Medicine, 79*(6), 549–556.

Skinner, B. F. (1953). *Science and human behavior.* New York: Simon and Schuster.

Slavin, S. J., Schindler, D. L., & Chibnall, J. T. (2014). Medical student mental health 3.0: Improving student wellness through curricular changes. *Academic Medicine, 89*(4), 573–577.

Speer, D. C., & Schneider, M. G. (2003). Mental health needs of older adults and primary care: Opportunity for interdisciplinary geriatric team practice. *Clinical Psychology: Science & Practice, 10*(1), 85–101.

Stanley, M. A. (1996). Treatment of generalized anxiety in older adults: A preliminary comparison of cognitive-behavioral and supportive approaches. *Behavior Therapy, 27*(4), 565–581.

Steiglitz, E. J. (1941). The potentialities of preventive geriatrics. *New England Journal of Medicine, 225*(7), 247–254.

Steuer, J. L., Mintz, J., Hammen, C. L., Hill, M. A., Jarvik, L. F., McCarley, T., et al. (1984). Cognitive-behavioral and psychodynamic group psychotherapy in treatment of geriatric depression. *Journal of Consulting and Clinical Psychology, 52*(2), 180–189.

Strine, T. W., Mokdad, A. H., Balluz, L. S., Gonzalez, O., Crider, R., & Berry, J. T. (2008). Depression and anxiety in the United States: Findings from the 2006 Behavioral Risk Factor Surveillance System. *Psychiatric Services, 59*(12), 1383–1390.

Tami, M. L., Joish, V. N., Hay, J. W., Sheehan, D. V., Johnston, S. S., & Cao, Z. (2011). Antidepressant use in geriatric populations: The burden of side effects and interactions and their impact on adherence and costs. *American Journal of Geriatric Psychiatry, 19,* 2117–2221.

Taylor, M. A. (2013). *Hippocrates cried: The decline of American psychiatry.* Oxford: Oxford University Press.

Taylor, C., Farver, C., & Stoller, J. K. (2011). Perspective: Can emotional intelligence training serve as an alternative approach to teaching professionalism to residents? *Academic Medicine, 86*(12), 1551–1554.

Thorp, S. R., Ayers, C. R., Nuevo, R., Stoddard, J. A., Sorrell, J. T., & Wetherell, J. L. (2009). Meta-analysis comparing different behavioral treatments for late-life anxiety. *American Journal of Geriatric Psychiatry, 17*(2), 105–115.

Wachholtz, A., & Rogoff, M. (2013). The relationship between spirituality and burnout among medical students. *Journal of Contemporary Medical Education, 1*(2), 83–91.

Witzburg, R. A., & Sondheimer, H. M. (2013). Holistic review – Shaping the medical profession one applicant at a time. *New England Journal of Medicine, 368,* 1565–1567.

Zullig, L. L., Peterson, E. D., & Bosworth, H. B. (2013). Ingredients of successful interventions to improve medication adherence. *Journal of the American Medical Association, 310*(24), 2611–2612.

1

Goal-Oriented Care

Susan L. Charette, Maristela Baruiz Garcia, and David B. Reuben

University of California, Los Angeles, California, USA

INTRODUCTION

As a result of better public health and nutrition and improved treatment of disease, Americans are living longer with more chronic conditions. Although many older persons have aged with few illnesses and good functional status, over 70% have two or more chronic conditions (Anderson, 2010). The term "multimorbidity" has been coined to describe this trend, which is associated with higher rates of death, disability, adverse effects, institutionalization, use of health care resources, and poorer quality of life (American Geriatrics Society Expert Panel on the Care of Older Adults with Multimorbidity, 2012). These patients are also at increased risk of adverse effects of medical therapy (Fried, Tinetti, Agostini, Iannone, & Towle, 2011).

Although clinical practice guidelines (CPCs) have been developed to guide the care of specific individual diseases, this management approach may be problematic when several conditions with competing guidelines are present (Boyd & Fortin, 2011; Tinetti, Fried, & Boyd, 2012). Nevertheless, to date, the Centers for Medicare and Medicaid Services (CMS) have focused on evaluating preventive measures (e.g., bone mineral density) and quality indicators for specific disease management (e.g., frequency of measurement of glycohemoglobin and blood glucose control). It has been suggested, however, that quality of care goes much further than just meeting individualized disease quality metrics.

In its 2001 report *Crossing the Quality Chasm: A New Health System for the 21st Century*, the Institute of Medicine (IOM) recommended a shift to patient-centered medical care. At its core, this approach is respectful of and responsive to individual patient preferences, needs and values, and ensures that patient values guide all clinical decisions. Meeting this challenge requires that health providers are cognizant of the patient's values

B. Bensadon (Ed): Psychology and Geriatrics.
DOI: http://dx.doi.org/10.1016/B978-0-12-420123-1.00001-0

as they determine preferences and goals in the face of changes in health status. This shifts the framework of treating illnesses as purely biomedical processes to approaching them in the context of psychosocial factors that have a dynamic influence on the individual's personal health goals.

Patient-centered care can be disease-specific by incorporating the principles above into treatment decisions for the disease. With multimorbidity, however, it is more difficult to provide disease-specific patient care without considering the context of other illnesses. Hence, the disease paradigm is an insufficient model to guide treatment. The practice of prioritizing patients' health goals and moving away from disease-directed care is foreign territory for most physicians. Thus patient-centered care requires physicians to use a skill set and approach with which they may be both unfamiliar and uncomfortable.

Goal-setting is a useful alternative to the traditional disease-focused approach in the care of older adults and is more likely to achieve patient-centeredness in medical encounters (Reuben & Tinetti, 2012). Far from a new concept, the important link between motivation and goal-setting has been discussed in the field of psychology for half a century (Locke & Latham, 2002).

Since the 1960s, psychology and several other health care disciplines, most notably physical rehabilitation and palliative care, have described and incorporated a different paradigm to guide decision-making through goal-oriented care. Goal-setting stems from the theory of self-efficacy, which refers to peoples' beliefs in their ability to achieve a goal; that is, the more they believe they will be successful (high self-efficacy), the more likely they will do what is necessary to achieve their goal (Bandura, 1977).

In physical rehabilitation programs, goal-setting is integral to the collaborative development between the patient and the rehabilitation team of individualized, realistically attainable treatment goals. Perception is a key to success. Patients are more likely to participate in the rehabilitation process if they perceive the treatment goals as being personally relevant. Similarly, goal-directed psychotherapy involves the sequential identification of first, the foci of treatment (i.e., problems) derived from the diagnoses; second, the development of actionable goals and objectives and the selection of the treatment plan; third, an estimate of the time required to attain the goals using available resources, and fourth, the subsequent monitoring mechanisms to evaluate treatment effectiveness until the treatment is terminated (Nurcombe, 2008). Goal-directed therapy in this setting has the advantage of providing a useful framework within which effectiveness of treatment plans or lack thereof can be assessed.

Another example of goal-setting that has become widely accepted is known as goals-of-care discussion, when a patient has a terminal or advanced illness, and decisions are being made whether to continue treatment or consider palliative care and hospice. This process can be incorporated into the care of multimorbid patients, who are often faced with making decisions among many options while weighing the pros and cons of various choices. The goals-of-care discussion should be part of routine care and should address basic patient preferences, including goals for their health, physical function, and life. These conversations can serve as a map that enables patients and practitioners to collaboratively navigate the health care journey.

Incorporating patient-centered goal-setting in the care of older adults involves considerations that go well beyond evidence-based management of specific diseases. It recognizes the current limits of medical science, including prognostic uncertainties, tradeoffs, and the lack of evidence-based data to guide treatment of multimorbidities. More importantly, patient-centered goal-setting restores emphasis on the patient's values and preferences as a guide to care and responds to the individual's ability to adapt to changes in health status as they arise. Individualized goal-setting acknowledges that perceptions of "quality of life" (QoL) may vary among different individuals. Moreover, it recognizes that a person's QoL standard may change over time as that person's health trajectory unfolds and as he or she copes with the experience of new disease or health states.

In goal-oriented care, an outcome may not be a cancer remission or cure of an infection, but rather the reaching of a milestone (e.g., attending a graduation or celebrating an anniversary), improving symptoms (e.g., reduced pain or shortness of breath), or achieving the ability to complete an activity with less effort or help.

GOAL-ORIENTED CARE: A PRACTICAL APPROACH

A patient-centered approach that focuses on the individual's personal health goals requires a fundamental understanding of the older adult's values, objectives, and health-related expectations. It also necessitates clarifying which of multiple medical conditions to address and how these comorbidities and their respective treatments affect one another. This approach considers what "quality" and "beneficial" care mean to the individual, and aligns treatment plans that will most likely contribute positively towards the patient's desired outcomes. To be effective, clinicians must set aside their personal preferences and interests and listen actively to identify those of their patients. This is a trainable skill set.

Preparation for goal-oriented visits may include a review of the results of recent studies and the recommendations of specialists. This information is helpful in assessing the patient's current health status and determining prognosis. Predicting an older adult's health trajectory involves drawing upon clinical experience and epidemiologic data on life expectancy. Life expectancy tables include a wide range for individuals 65 years and older.

The clinician's assessment of the patient's overall health status as being above (75th percentile), at (50th percentile), or below (25th percentile) average for age and sex is an important consideration. Overall health status is largely influenced by the presence of comorbidities and functional status (Arias, 2012; Reuben et al., 2012). Additionally, life expectancy is consistently associated with sociocultural factors such as race, education level, and economic status (Reuben et al., 2012). This background knowledge enables the health care provider to better frame decisions for treatment of existing diseases and for disease prevention strategies.

To provide goal-oriented care, clinicians should start each visit by exploring the patient's priorities and concerns. Discussions can begin with patient-generated lists, which identify the main problems and priorities, according to the patient. Knowledge of the patient's agenda saves time and energy for the physician and may have the psychological benefit of communicating the physician's caring and concern for the patient. Explicit recognition of patient preparation and reference to the list during the visit reinforce the importance of the patient's role and set the tone for the visit.

The next step is to assess what the patient knows about his or her medical conditions and health status. This assessment may include a discussion of the patient's understanding of the diagnoses, prognosis and clinical options, as well as tradeoffs involved in choosing to undergo or forgo therapies (Billings & Bernacki, 2014). This is also the time to explore what else is important to the patient, including wishes for the future, goals for function, and activities the patient wants to do. Some patients will not want to participate in such a discussion and will defer to the physician while others will be able to share their priorities and preferences – both what they want and what they don't want. Patients may have trouble predicting preferences for the future, and may not fully understand the implications, even when it appears that they do (Weeks et al., 2012). Again, clinicians must listen closely to what the patient tells them, explain what is possible and what is not, and ultimately negotiate a plan that is agreeable to both.

Though extremely challenging, a patient-centered approach requires physicians to move away from traditional disease-centered assessment and planning. Within the context of predicted life expectancy, goals for an older adult with a longer life expectancy can be arbitrarily subcategorized as short-term (e.g., return to baseline functional status following a hospitalization for pneumonia), mid-range (e.g., maintain physical ability to continue caregiving role for spouse in the next few years), and long-range (e.g., disability-free survival) (Reuben, 2009). Identifying the goal that is of highest priority to the patient and facilitating a frank, transparent, jargon-free discussion of the potential tradeoffs are important steps in the goal-setting process. Categories of goals to consider include symptom control, physical function, ability to engage in social activities, and the ability to fulfill a role (Reuben & Tinetti, 2012).

When framing long-term goals with patients, it is important to recognize that *actual survival* may deviate significantly from *predicted survival* and may require revisiting established goals. In contrast, temporal goals for an older adult with a shorter life expectancy or life-limiting illness can be framed differently and may be more qualitative; short-term goals may involve better control of pain and dyspnea within the next 24 hours, mid-range goals may involve avoidance of rehospitalization in the next several weeks, and a longer-range goal may involve living long enough to attend a family wedding. Sometimes, those who are frail have a goal of simply not being a burden to others.

The goals that are discussed need to be realistic and achievable. The discussion should emphasize the health outcome of greatest interest to the patient (Reuben & Tinetti, 2012). For some patients, the desired goal will not be attainable (e.g., the patient with a dense right hemiparesis after a stroke who wants to drive but will never be able to do so). For others, there will be competing issues, such as whether to take an aspirin after a recent myocardial infarction vs. gastrointestinal bleeding. Prioritization should take into account the preferences of the patient and the assessment of the physician and health care team. Patients' preferences need to be explored beyond one-dimensional requests such as "cure my cancer" and "prevent another stroke" to the broader category of health outcomes, including function, symptom management, QoL, and survival.

Goals-of-care discussions are most useful when addressing a patient's current medical conditions and state of health. For example, advance care planning can be very difficult to do when patients are healthy and doing well, as they will often choose more aggressive interventions (e.g., full code, dialysis), while these preferences may change with advanced age and severe illness (Billings & Bernacki, 2014). Some older patients will not want to participate in these conversations and prefer a family-directed or physician-directed approach to decision-making (Levinson, Kao, Kuby, & Thisted, 2005). In these cases, the approach should be modified to the patient's level of comfort.

There are established models from clinical practice that offer a structure for these discussions: for example, Buckman's six-step protocol for breaking bad news, also known as the SPIKES method, where S is for setting, P is for patient perception, I is an invitation from the patient to the practitioner to participate in a discussion, K is sharing of knowledge, E is responding to emotion with empathy, and S is strategizing and summarizing (Baile et al., 2000). Although this method was developed for breaking bad news, the format is useful for goals-of-care discussions as well. The SPIKES protocol provides the clinician with a clear structure for gathering information from the patient, transmitting the medical information, providing support to the patient, and eliciting the patient's collaboration in developing a strategy or treatment plan for the future (Baile et al., 2000). Utilizing a structured format ensures a consistent approach that includes all of the essential components of the discussion, which may cover many topics.

Older patients often come to medical appointments with another person. Typically these individuals are spouses or children, but they may include hired caregivers, siblings, extended family members, friends, and conservators. Generally, the presence of a family member or friend is in the best interest of the patient. These persons can bear witness to the discussion and provide moral support when topics are difficult. Research has shown that family members may have more influence on patient choices than the evidence-based information presented by the clinician (Siminoff, 2013).

The quandary is when the significant others "take over" the discussion or the surrogate overtly disagrees with the patient's wishes. These behaviors distract from the task at hand – listening to and helping the patient make decisions about his or her medical care. Based on the ethical principle of autonomy, the patient remains his or her own decision-maker unless there is a loss of capacity, as determined following a formal assessment by trained clinicians such as psychiatrists or clinical psychologists. Patients may lack capacity for some decisions (e.g., consent for anesthesia), but not for others (e.g., need for pain medication). When a patient loses decision-making capacity, his or her durable power of attorney for health care or other legally recognized decision-maker (e.g., spouse, conservator) becomes responsible for carrying out the patient's wishes.

The family member or friend who attends a visit with a patient may not be the legal decision maker. If a physician or other health care provider determines that the legal surrogate decision-maker is not acting in the best interest of the patient, the issue must be addressed. Related disagreement can be extremely challenging for physicians to manage. Qualified clinical psychologists, as part of integrated care teams, could occupy a much needed "moderator" role in managing these complex behavioral dynamics that often require time and skills physicians may not have.

Goal attainment scaling (GAS) is a method of individualized goal-setting and assessment that is used in both clinical and research settings. Also originally developed in the field of psychology, goal attainment scaling (Kiresuk & Sherman, 1968) consists of an individualized GAS guide that includes specific goals and associated scales with points assigned reflecting the degree of attainment of the goal. Future assessments use the individualized GAS guide to measure the degree of goal attainment. This system for goal-setting has been widely used in rehabilitation settings and has been implemented in clinical research with the geriatric population (e.g., Hurn, Kneebone, & Cropley, 2006; Rockwood et al., 2003;

Rockwood, Fay, Song, MacKnight, & Gorman, 2006; Stolee et al., 2012). GAS is a potentially useful method to develop, document and assess goal attainment in patients with multiple health problems.

Researchers have tried to develop tools to assist with the determination of goals and treatment preferences among older patients with multiple medical problems. "Health outcome prioritization" is the process by which persons are asked to think about potential outcomes in domains such as physical and cognitive functioning and survival, and decide which are most important to them, both currently and in the future. The "Attitude Scale" requires patients to rate the strength of their preferences regarding tradeoffs in areas of health care outcomes and current versus future health. The "Now vs. Later" tool rates the relative importance of quality of life now versus at one year and at five years in the future on a visual analogue scale. While the use of decision aids has been shown to help some patients clarify their preferences among alternate treatment options, these tools also have their limitations. Shortcomings have included fair to poor test–retest reliability, variability in patients' preferred tool and perceptions of difficulty (Case, Fried, & O'Leary, 2013; Fried, Tinetti, Agostini et al., 2011).

Patient preferences and goals for care need to be documented and reassessed over time. Documentation in the health record provides a synopsis of the discussion as well as a means for communicating and sharing information with other members of the health care team. Time-sensitive requests or specific changes in care should be communicated directly to the appropriate health care personnel to ensure care continues in line with the patient's preferences. Goals-of-care discussions should address end-of-life (EoL) preferences, particularly in patients with advanced and terminal illness. When a patient has a change in status – such as an admission to the hospital or a newly diagnosed life-threatening illness – goals of care should be addressed, preferences should be reassessed and the advance directive should be updated (Billings & Bernacki, 2014). Some patients are more likely to accept treatments with limited benefit as their medical condition worsens and their options decrease (Fried et al., 2006). Tradeoffs may change – what is acceptable now may not be later.

BARRIERS/CHALLENGES TO GOAL-SETTING IN CLINICAL PRACTICE

Goal-setting has become an important tool in primary care practice for the management of certain chronic health problems such as obesity, diabetes, and smoking. However, the implementation of the goal-setting approach in the overall management of the older adult with multiple medical problems is encumbered by a number of factors, discussed in the following sections.

System Level Barriers

Inadequate Resource Allocation

Experts believe that the most important challenge to goal-oriented care in the management of older adults with comorbidities is a health system that currently supports and incentivizes disease-oriented practice of medicine (Reuben & Tinetti, 2012). Unless health policies are refined to acknowledge that care processes that focus on society's older, sicker members are as important as those that focus on the younger and healthier population, health providers will continue to emphasize adherence to disease-specific guidelines and the achievement of individual disease quality metrics in clinical care. Additionally, the Resource Based Relative Value Scale (RBRVS) historically used by CMS in calculating payment to clinicians does not adequately capture the complexity involved in the quality care of frail, multimorbid older adults (Resnick & Radulovich, 2014). Specifically, it does not recognize the importance of eliciting patients' values and goals of care, counseling, conducting family meetings, and care coordination among various agencies and specialties. Recently, however, CMS did add the Transitional Care Management (TCM) codes to the physician fee schedule allowing primary care physicians to be reimbursed for such time spent coordinating care for patients discharged from hospitals and skilled nursing facilities back to the community (Centers for Medicare & Medicaid Services, 2012).

Public health resources directed at advancing the science of multimorbidity management and supporting alternative care approaches are vital to the delivery of patient-centered, clinically sound health care for the growing older adult population.

Time-Constrained Patient-Clinician Encounters

A study of the national trends of health care delivery from 1997–2010 showed that the mean visit length for visits to generalists was 19.3 minutes (Edwards, Mafi, & Landon, 2014). Many health systems allow providers even less time for a follow-up visit. Moreover, in the past two decades, the number of clinical items addressed during a primary care visit has increased from 5.4 to 7.1, significantly decreasing the amount of time spent for each problem (Abbo, Zhang, Zelder, & Huang, 2008). Health providers report they are particularly challenged when balancing an array of disease-specific guidelines in the overall treatment of older adults with multiple chronic conditions (Fried, Tinetti, & Iannone, 2011). Medicare patients in particular tend to have more clinical items managed per visit, the longest visit times, and the shortest time per clinical item (Abbo et al., 2008). If the chronic conditions are poorly controlled, the time available for the health care provider to address each condition thoroughly becomes more limited. Additionally, most primary care office appointments are currently designed in a *one-size-fits-all* manner, leaving little flexibility to accommodate older adults with a longer list of chronic conditions, hearing and speech difficulty, mood-related concerns, and cognitive impairment. These factors, by necessity, prolong the length of routine medical encounters. Patient-physician interactions required in goal-setting and goal-attainment planning may involve a longer time investment if the magnitude of the health issues and the number and complexity of potential interventions are substantial.

Care Fragmentation

Another major barrier to the effective use of the goal-setting approach for older adults is the lack of continuity of care across various health settings and the involvement of multiple specialists. A Gallup Serious Chronic Illness survey showed that more than half of patients with serious chronic conditions receive care from three or more physicians, with 11% being treated by 6 or more (Anderson, 2010). The typical Medicare patient sees a median of 7 physicians per year. Adults with chronic conditions are likely, therefore, to receive conflicting health advice and are more likely to receive drug prescriptions that interact with each other.

To be effective, goal-setting requires a treatment team with a unified approach to care and with whom the patient has developed a trusting relationship. Older adults with multimorbidity are especially at risk of not having their primary care physicians be directly involved in their care when their health status changes. This often happens during ER visits, hospitalizations (including ICU stays), and post-acute care in skilled nursing facilities and acute rehabilitation units. At these times, important reexamination of goals must occur. Frequently, these discussions will need to be led by clinicians who are unfamiliar with these patients' personal and medical histories and values prior to their acute illness.

Reductionism and Jurisdiction

Primary care clinicians who embark on the goal-setting approach in their practices must successfully navigate the pressures of reductionism and jurisdiction when caring for older adults who see multiple specialists. Reductionism is an approach whereby the patient's complaints are compartmentalized by organ system leading to a narrowly focused organ-based therapeutic plan and a limited consideration of the overall effects of both disease and treatment (Federoff & Gostin, 2009). The modern era of evidence-based medicine has unintentionally legitimized this reductionist view in the management of the individual patient. Simply combining the application of each disease-specific treatment guideline in the management of the older adult with multiple clinical conditions has led to the erroneous belief that such a strategy is the appropriate adherence to standards of care in the management of the whole patient. Jurisdiction is the notion that specialists or certain care settings are superior in treating certain diseases, conditions, or parts of the body, regardless of the individual's circumstances (Levenson, 2010). In fact, an expert in the management of heart failure may not be the best-qualified person to manage this disease in an older adult who not only has heart failure, but also has recurrent falls, malnutrition, gait and balance problems, and cognitive impairment. Likewise, an acute care hospital may not be the optimal setting to treat pneumonia in a patient with advanced dementia who has adequate support at home. Effective goal-setting in the care of multimorbid older adults aligns the important contributions of various disciplines and care settings to best achieve the patient's preferred outcome.

Clinician Level Barriers

Lack of Emphasis in the Academic Curricula

Medical education is ingrained in the scientific approach that begins with the systematic study of human organs, and leads to organ-based exploration of the biological mechanisms underlying disease processes as well as their corresponding remedies. However, this compartmentalization often continues through the clinical years, with training programs offering variable amounts of curricular instruction addressing the complex interactions between biomedical processes and nonbiomedical factors such as the psychological, socio-cultural, environmental, and economic conditions that influence the art and science of healing.

Significant efforts to transform graduate medical education over the past decade include the development of core competencies aimed at identifying skills and knowledge that will predictably lead to quality-care physicians. While patient-centeredness is implied in all the competency domains, the focus of "patient care" as a competency remains the ability to deliver care that is "…effective for the treatment of health problems" (Accreditation Council of Graduate Medical Education, 2014). In geriatrics, this means achieving the outcomes that older patients care about most.

Core competency evaluation for physician-trainees who will be caring for older adults in their future practices must explicitly include an assessment of the ability not only to diagnose and effectively treat health problems but to accurately identify the values and preferences of the individual patient whom they seek to treat. This requires understanding of *patients as people*: understanding their priorities and life circumstances outside of the biomedical domain and most relevant to the patient's preferred health goals. Clinical geropsychologists with experience in graduate medical education can be extremely helpful in complementing the role of attending physicians in providing medical trainees with the necessary proficiency in the nonbiomedical aspects of patient care.

Failure to Contextualize

Patient-centered care has been characterized as applying the best scientific evidence to the care of the individual patient. Individualizing care and contextualization involve the deliberate consideration of the patient's circumstances that affect biomedical processes, treatment recommendations, and goal-setting. Physicians are notably prone to contextual errors. In a study of more than 100 board-certified internists involving unannounced visits by standardized patients, appropriate care was provided 73% of the time when adherence to guidelines and best-practice recommendations was all that was required. However, when contextual factors were added that needed to be considered to avoid ineffective or potentially harmful care, appropriate care was delivered only 22% of the time (Weiner et al., 2010). Inattention to the relevant contextual factors that affect patient preference and influence treatment options can be a significant barrier to effective goal-setting and care.

Weiner (2004) suggests a number of contextual factors to consider for each patient. Importantly, the elements that tend to be overlooked are generally nonbiomedical in nature. These include the following:

- Cognition (e.g., does the patient have the cognitive ability required to accurately manage a more complex regimen for his heart failure?)
- Emotional state (e.g., is the patient currently too distraught to think about the treatment options?)
- Cultural beliefs (e.g., how does the patient's culture regard disability?)
- Spiritual beliefs (e.g., does the patient have beliefs that will help cope with loss?)
- Access to care (e.g., does the patient have transportation for appointments?)
- Social support (e.g., does the patient have family who could provide care at home if the patient decides to undergo chemotherapy?)
- Caregiver responsibilities (e.g., are caregiving responsibilities limiting patients' ability to show up for their own appointments?)
- Attitude to illness/treatment (e.g., what is the patient's understanding of what surgery can do?)
- Economic situation (e.g., would the patient be able to afford this medication?)
- Relationship to other health providers (e.g., will the patient believe the primary care physician who informs him or her of a poor prognosis if the oncologist is still offering treatment?)

Paternalism, Lack of Introspection, and Difficulty Dealing with Uncertainty

The practice of medicine has long been deeply entrenched in paternalism. Physicians decide what is best for patients and patients generally embrace the physicians' recommendations. The goal-setting approach is not intended to diminish the value that the physician's skills and medical knowledge bring to the decision-making process, nor is it proposed to relieve health providers of the burden that complex clinical situations create. The goal-setting process starts with the recognition that in some instances the evidence supporting the benefits of treatment may be quite clear, and the clinician's recommendations are straightforward. However, it also acknowledges that in some health states, the best science available is insufficient to guide the care of the patient.

The goal-setting approach presupposes that in the presence of tradeoffs and competing outcomes, the *patient* is the better evaluator in determining the health outcome that he cares about most, with the health provider identifying the clinical strategy that will most likely achieve it (Reuben, 2009; Reuben & Tinetti, 2012). A paternalistic attitude that assumes knowledge of the patient's preferred outcomes can often close the door to any meaningful goal-setting discussion.

If not sufficiently mindful of their own biases, beliefs and expectations, clinicians may inadvertently undermine the patient-centered goal-setting process. Many physicians receive inadequate or no training in introspection and in developing personal awareness of how their life circumstances and core beliefs can inadvertently shift the focus of their caregiving from the patient's values and priorities to their own (Novack et al., 1997). In order to remain effective advocates for their patients, health providers must periodically perform the necessary self-reflection to maintain a clear patient focus. Consultation with clinical psychologist team members can facilitate this process.

Another difficulty clinicians may face in the goal-setting process is the patient's need to understand his or her prognosis. Accurate prognostication is often an enormous, emotionally challenging task. Acknowledgment of uncertainty when predicting outcomes and prognosis, likely to be raised during the goal-setting discussion, may be psychologically uncomfortable for many physicians and patients alike. Avoidance of such discussions may seem easier, and in some instances, physician recommendations for additional testing, specialist referrals and alternative treatment strategies are inappropriately used to "substitute."

Cultural Competence

The demographic shift of the aging population in the United States obliges clinicians to better understand cultural backgrounds that may influence an individual patient's health beliefs. It is projected that by 2030, roughly 40% of the US population will be composed of racial minority groups (Pratt & Apple, 2007). The physician's insight into a patient's cultural beliefs provides an essential framework for goal-setting efforts. Beliefs about disease causation and the merits of Western medicine may affect a patient's adherence to disease screening programs and treatment preferences that are key considerations in any goal-setting and goal-attainment discussion. For example, an awareness of AIDS-related conspiracy theories (e.g., Bogart & Thorburn, 2005) and the historical roots of mistrust in government may help a clinician understand the HIV testing behavior of older black men and develop strategies to more effectively promote advocacy in this group (Ford, Wallace, Newman, Lee, & Cunningham, 2013).

Failure to Recognize Response Shifts

Patients with chronic illness and changing health experiences are confronted with the need to adapt to their illness. This adaptation process or "response shift" involves adjusting internal standards, values, and the conceptualization of QoL when patients experience changes in their health (Schwartz et al., 2006). In clinical practice, this is a commonly recognized phenomenon. The capacity to accept burdens of treatment resulting in diminished states of health may increase over time for some patients (Fried et al., 2006) Timely reevaluation of previously set goals assures that patient-centered care is maintained across the health care continuum. Failure or delay in recognizing response shifts may result in care that is no longer contextually appropriate nor an accurate reflection of the patient's changing values.

Patient Level Barriers

Difficulty in Making Decisions

Studies with time tradeoff (TTO) (e.g., Burström, Johannesson, & Diderichsen, 2006) and standard gamble (e.g., Gafni, 1994) have demonstrated the difficult nature of clinical decision-making. When faced with treatment choices and numerous potential outcomes, some individuals may have difficulty envisioning future scenarios. A large study on health valuations using the TTO method noted that, generally, individuals are able to differentiate between health states that involve a range of severity. However, it has also been shown that the measures of dispersion were much higher than predicted, which may reflect the inherent difficulty people face when imagining themselves in certain hypothetical states of health (Dolan, Gudex, Kind, & Williams, 1996).

Level of Patient Engagement in the Goal-Setting Process

The process of goal-setting involves active patient engagement. However, it is recognized that some patients may not want to be active participants. A population-based survey involving a representative sample of the US population demonstrated that people vary considerably in their preferences regarding participation in decision-making. While 96% of respondents preferred to be offered choices and to be asked their opinions, 52% preferred to leave the final decision to their physicians (Levinson et al., 2005). Nevertheless, the IOM report encourages physicians to engage patients in the clinical decision-making process. (Institute of Medicine, 2001)

Variability in Degree of Health Literacy

Goal-setting in its most ideal application facilitates care that embraces patient-centeredness. However, goal-setting also involves making choices that depend on the patient's ability to understand information, something physicians may tend to overestimate (e.g., Kelly & Haidet, 2007). In fact the IOM estimates that nearly half of all American adults have difficulty understanding and acting upon health information (Nielsen-Bohlman, Panzer, & Kindig, 2004). Patients with limited health literacy and education are inherently more vulnerable when presented with treatment options that involve processing of complex health information, and may experience more difficulty making choices and comprehending hypothetical tradeoffs. For example, the TTO, an important tool for determining health valuations and quality adjusted life years (QALYs), may be influenced by the patients' level of education; respondents with less than 10 years of education are more prone to misunderstanding tradeoff scenarios (Edelaar-Peeters, Stiggelbout, & Van Den Hout, 2014). This may partly explain consistent trends toward more aggressive EoL care among ethnic and racial minority patients (e.g., Barnato, Anthony, Skinner, Gallagher, & Fisher, 2009; Cohen, 2008; Connolly, Sampson, & Purandare, 2012; Kwak & Haley, 2005).

Unrealistic Goals

The clinician's understanding of the older adult's beliefs about his illness, preferences and expectations are foundational elements in the development of treatment strategies that will best attain the patient's desired outcome. However, there are instances when the patient's expectations and health goals are not realistically achievable. A candid dialogue regarding what is not possible, exploring what goals may be more achievable with available treatments, ongoing advocacy and encouragement, and empathically conveying openness to readdress the issues if conditions change are all vital elements to the provision of care in this challenging area (e.g., Reuben, 2009).

Heterogeneity Among Older Adults

Biomedical heterogeneity exists in the older adult population in terms of degree of frailty, functional status, disease severity, and tolerance to adverse treatment effects. For example, an 85-year-old person may be living independently in the community, while another 85-year-old person may be living in a nursing home, totally dependent on others for self-care activities. Although frailty is associated with "age-related declines in physiologic reserve across neuromuscular, metabolic, and immune systems" (Walston et al., 2006), the onset of frailty among older adults varies across the age spectrum. Screening tools to identify frailty in older adults include the Cardiovascular Health Study Frailty Screening Scale and the simple FRAIL Questionnaire Screening Tool. In the former, developed by Fried and colleagues (2001), the presence of three or more of the following indicates frailty: unintentional weight loss of >10 lbs in the prior year, weak grip strength, poor endurance, low gait speed, and low physical activity (Fried et al., 2001). When using the FRAIL Questionnaire Screening Tool, deficits in three or more of the following domains suggests frailty: Fatigue, Resistance (inability to walk up a flight of stairs), Aerobic (inability to walk a block), Illnesses (having more than five illnesses), and Loss of Weight (weight loss greater than 5% in the past 6 months) (Abellan van Kan, Rolland, Morley, & Vellas, 2008; Lopez, Flicker, & Dobson, 2012).

Detection of frailty is important because of associated vulnerability to adverse outcomes of both illness and treatment interventions. Goal-setting discussions may need to occur more frequently to respond to sometimes dramatic changes in health status.

Older adults may also vary in terms of their risk of death for a given health condition. For instance, a population-based study showed that the overall mortality rate of hip fractures, an important cause of death among older adults, is 24% at 12 months after the fracture (Lu-Yao, Baron, Barrett, & Fisher, 1994). An observational, multisite cohort study showed that the *young-old* (less than 75 years old) had a mortality rate of only 6.3% at 6 months. Among the 75- to 84-year-olds, those with greater walking and activities of daily living (ADL) independence prefracture had a 9% mortality rate at 6 months, compared to a 23% mortality rate among the same age group that had a higher prevalence of dementia and need for assistance with ambulation prefracture (Penrod et al., 2007). Goal-setting discussions must be grounded on more finely tuned prognostic indicators that reflect the individual patient's overall status, whenever they are available.

CONCLUSION

Given the inadequacies of the traditional disease-specific model of care, particularly the limitations of meaningful outcomes for those with multiple morbidities and/or short life expectancy, goal-setting will become an increasingly important part of medical care in the future. There will not only be more older adults, but older adults will live longer with more chronic conditions. Medical science continues to advance and the options for treatment are expanding. It is medicine's responsibility to ensure that treatment achieves patient-centered goals. While a goal-oriented approach may be most appropriate for our older, multimorbid patients, there are barriers to implementation at multiple levels – system, clinician and patient.

The move away from the traditional disease-oriented approach to truly patient-centered care requires a dramatic paradigm shift. Changes will need to occur at multiple levels from health policy to education to patient expectations. Medical school curricula are often centered on problem-based learning. Educating future physicians to expand their approach will require institutional and cultural change. Trainees need modeling and instruction – this is not an inherent skill. Medical education and training will need to embrace this approach, integrate it into an already full curriculum, and compete with medical advances and work hours restrictions (in residency training). For practicing physicians, a lack of adherence to disease-specific guidelines in favor of goal-oriented care may negatively affect their performance on quality metrics within their health care organization, and there may be insufficient time for goal-directed discussions during routine visits.

There must be an ongoing dialogue between patients and health care providers and documentation of these discussions. Perhaps most importantly, goal-setting is a process – not a one-time event. The above changes may demand practice redesign and payment reform. An interdisciplinary approach would be most advantageous and has a long history of success in geriatric patient care. Clinical psychologists must be included in such an approach to both medical education and interdisciplinary care, as goal-setting has long been integral to their clinical practice. In view of the potential barriers and competing interests, the move from a disease-specific to a patient-centered care approach presents a formidable but worthwhile challenge. Patient-centered care offers a comprehensive model that may best address the health care needs and goals of our diverse, rapidly aging population.

References

Abbo, E. D., Zhang, Q., Zelder, M., & Huang, E. S. (2008). The increasing number of clinical items addressed during the time of adult primary care visits. *Journal of General Internal Medicine, 23*(12), 2058–2065.

Abellan van Kan, G., Rolland, Y. M., Morley, J. E., & Vellas, B. (2008). Frailty: Toward a clinical definition. *Journal of the American Medical Directors Association, 9*(2), 71–72.

Accreditation Council of Graduate Medical Education (2014). *Common program requirements.* Available from: <www.acgme.org/acgmeweb/tabid/429/ProgramandInstitutional Accreditation/CommonProgramRequirements.aspx>. Accessed 06.04.14.

American Geriatrics Society Expert Panel on the Care of Older Adults with Multimorbidity, (2012). Patient-centered care for older adults with multiple chronic conditions: a stepwise approach from the American Geriatrics Society: American Geriatrics Society Expert Panel on the Care of Older Adults with Multimorbidity. *Journal of the American Geriatrics Society, 60*(10), 1957–1968.

Anderson, G. (2010). *Chronic care: Making the case for ongoing care.* Robert Wood Johnson Foundation. Available from: <www.rwjf.org/en/research-publications/find-rwjf-research/2010/01/chronic-care.html>. Accessed 17.02.14.

Arias, E. (2012). United states life tables, 2008. *National Vital Statistics Reports, 61*, 3.

Baile, W. F., Buckman, R., Lenzi, R., Glober, G., Beale, E. A., & Kudelka, A. P. (2000). SPIKES – A six-step protocol for delivering bad news: Application to the patient with cancer. *Oncologist, 5*(4), 302–311.

Bandura, A. (1977). Self-efficacy: Toward a unifying theory of behavioral change. *Psychological Review, 84*(2), 191–215.

Barnato, A. E., Anthony, D. L., Skinner, J., Gallagher, P. M., & Fisher, E. S. (2009). Racial and ethnic differences in preferences for end-of-life treatment. *Journal of General Internal Medicine, 24*(6), 695–701.

Billings, J. A., & Bernacki, R. (2014). Strategic targeting of advance care planning interventions: The Goldilocks phenomenon. *JAMA Internal Medicine, 174*(4), 620–624.

Bogart, L. M., & Thorburn, S. (2005). Are HIV/AIDS conspiracy beliefs a barrier to HIV prevention among African Americans? *Journal of Acquired Immune Deficiency Syndromes, 38*(2), 213–8.

Boyd, C. M., & Fortin, M. (2011). Future of multimorbidity research: How should understanding of multimorbidity inform health system design? *Public Health Review, 32*, 451–474.

Burström, K., Johannesson, M., & Diderichsen, F. (2006). A comparison of individual and social time- trade-off values for health states in the general population. *Health Policy, 76*(3), 359–370.

Case, S. M., Fried, T. R., & O'Leary, J. (2013). How to ask: Older adults' preferred tools in health outcome prioritization. *Patient Education & Counseling, 91*, 29–36.

Centers for Medicare and Medicaid Services, (2012). Medicare Program; Revisions to payment policies under the physician fee schedule, DME face-to-face encounters, elimination for the requirement for termination of non-random prepayment complex medical review and other revisions to Part B for CY 2013. Final Rule with Comment Period. *Federal Registry, 77*, 68891–69373.

Cohen, L. L. (2008). Racial/ethnic disparities in hospice care: A systematic review. *Journal of Palliative Medicine, 11*(5), 763–768.

Connolly, A., Sampson, E. L., & Purandare, N. (2012). End-of-life care for people with dementia from ethnic minority groups: A systematic review. *Journal of the American Geriatrics Society, 60*(2), 351–360.

Dolan, P., Gudex, C., Kind, P., & Williams, A. (1996). The time trade-off method: Results from a general population study. *Health Economics, 5*(2), 141–154.

Edelaar-Peeters, Y., Stiggelbout, A. M., & Van Den Hout, W. B. (2014). Qualitative and quantitative analysis of interviewer help answering the time tradeoff. *Medical Decision Making, 34*(5), 655–665.

Edwards, S. T., Mafi, J. N., & Landon, B. E. (2014). Trends and quality of care in outpatient visits to generalist and specialist physicians delivering primary care in the United States, 1997–2010. *Journal of General Internal Medicine, 29*(6), 947–955.

Federoff, H. J., & Gostin, L. O. (2009). Evolving from reductionism to holism: Is there a future for systems medicine? *Journal of the American Medical Association, 302*(9), 994–996.

Ford, C. L., Wallace, S. P., Newman, P. A., Lee, S. J., & Cunningham, W. E. (2013). Belief in AIDS-related conspiracy theories and mistrust in the government: Relationship with HIV testing among at-risk older adults. *The Gerontologist, 53*(6), 973–984.

Fried, L. P., Tangen, C. M., Walston, J., Newman, A. B., Hirsch, C., Gottdiener, J., et al. (2001). Frailty in older adults: Evidence for a phenotype. *The Journals of Gerontology Series A, Biological Sciences & Medical Sciences, 56*(3), M146–M156.

Fried, T. R., Byers, A. L., Gallo, W. T., Van Ness, P. H., Towle, V. R., O'Leary, J. R., et al. (2006). Prospective study of health status preferences and changes in preferences over time in older adults. *Archives of Internal Medicine, 166,* 890–895.

Fried, T. R., Tinetti, M., Agostini, J., Iannone, L., & Towle, V. (2011). Health outcome prioritization to elicit preferences of older persons with multiple health conditions. *Patient Education & Counseling, 83,* 278–282.

Fried, T. R., Tinetti, M. E., & Iannone, L. (2011). Primary care clinicians' experiences with treatment decision making for older persons with multiple conditions. *Archives of Internal Medicine, 171*(1), 75–80.

Gafni, A. (1994). The standard gamble method: What is being measured and how it is interpreted. *Health Services Research, 29,* 207–224.

Hurn, J., Kneebone, I., & Cropley, M. (2006). Goal setting as an outcome measure: a systematic review. *Clinical Rehabilitation, 20,* 756–772.

Institute of Medicine, (2001). *Crossing the quality chasm: A new health system for the 21st century.* Washington, DC: National Academy Press.

Kelly, P. A., & Haidet, P. (2007). Physician overestimation of patient literacy: A potential source of healthcare disparities. *Patient Education and Counseling, 66*(1), 119–122.

Kiresuk, T. J., & Sherman, R. E. (1968). Goal attainment scaling: A general method for evaluating community mental health problems. *Community Mental Health Journal, 4,* 443–453.

Kwak, J., & Haley, W. E. (2005). Current research findings on end-of-life decision making among racially or ethnically diverse groups. *The Gerontologist, 45*(5), 634–641.

Levenson, S. A. (2010). The basis for improving and reforming long-term care. Part 4: Identifying meaningful improvement approaches (segment 2). *Journal of the American Medical Directors Association, 11*(3), 161–170.

Levinson, W., Kao, A., Kuby, A., & Thisted, R. A. (2005). Not all patients want to participate in decision making. A national study of public preferences. *Journal of General Internal Medicine, 20,* 531–535.

Locke, E. A., & Latham, G. P. (2002). Building a practically useful theory of goal setting and task motivation. A 35-year odyssey. *American Psychologist, 57*(9), 705–717.

Lopez, D., Flicker, L., & Dobson, A. (2012). Validation of the frail scale in a cohort of older Australian women. *Journal of the American Geriatrics Society, 60*(1), 171–173.

Lu-Yao, G. L., Baron, J. A., Barrett, J. A., & Fisher, E. S. (1994). Treatment and survival among elderly Americans with hip fractures: A population-based study. *American Journal of Public Health, 84*(8), 1287–1291.

Nielsen-Bohlman, L., Panzer, A. M., & Kindig, D. A. (Eds.), (2004). *Health literacy: A prescription to end confusion.* Washington, DC: Institute of Medicine. Available from: <www.iom.edu/Reports/2004/health-literacy-a-prescription-to-end-confusion.aspx>. Accessed 13.04.14.

Novack, D. H., Suchman, A. L., Clark, W., Epstein, R. M., Najberg, E., & Kaplan, C. (1997). Calibrating the physician. Personal awareness and effective patient care. Working Group on Promoting Physician Personal Awareness, American Academy on Physician and Patient. *Journal of the American Medical Association, 278*(6), 502–509.

Nurcombe, B. (2008). Diagnostic formulation, treatment planning, and modes of treatment in children and adolescents. In M. H. Ebert, P. T. Loosen, B. Nurcombe, & J. F. Leckman (Eds.), *Current diagnosis & treatment: Psychiatry* (2nd ed.). New York, NY: McGraw-Hill.

Penrod, J. D., Litke, A., Hawkes, W. G., Magaziner, J., Koval, K. J., Doucette, J. T., et al. (2007). Heterogeneity in hip fracture patients: Age, functional status, and comorbidity. *Journal of the American Geriatrics Society, 55*(3), 407–413.

Pratt, H. D., & Apple, R. W. (2007). Cross-cultural assessment and management in primary care. *Primary Care, 34*(2), 227–242.

Resnick, N. M., & Radulovich, N. (2014). The Relative Value Unit in academic geriatrics: Incentive or impediment? *Journal of the American Geriatrics Society, 62*(3), 553–557.

Reuben, D. B. (2009). Medical care for the final years of life: "When you're 83, it's not going to be 20 years". *Journal of the American Medical Association, 302*(24), 2686–2694.

Reuben, D. B., Herr, K. A., Pacala, J. T., Pollock, B. G., Potter, J. F., & Semla, T. P. (2012). *Geriatrics at Your Fingertips* (14th ed.). New York, NY: The American Geriatrics Society. (p. 8).

Reuben, D. B., & Tinetti, M. E. (2012). Goal-oriented patient care – an alternative health outcomes paradigm. *New England Journal of Medicine, 366*, 777–779.

Rockwood, K., Fay, S., Song, X., MacKnight, C., & Gorman, M. (2006). Attainment of treatment goals by people with Alzheimer's disease receiving galantamine: A randomized controlled trial. *Canadian Medical Association Journal, 174*(8), 1099–1105.

Rockwood, K., Howlett, S., Stadnyk, K., Carver, D., Powell, C., & Stolee, P. (2003). Responsiveness of goal attainment scaling in a randomized controlled trial of comprehensive geriatric assessment. *Journal of Clinical Epidemiology, 56*, 736–743.

Schwartz, C. E., Bode, R., Repucci, N., Becker, J., Sprangers, M. A., & Fayers, P. M. (2006). The clinical significance of adaptation to changing health: A meta-analysis of response shift. *Quality of Life Research, 15*(9), 1533–1550.

Siminoff, L. (2013). Incorporating patient and family preferences into evidence-based medicine. *Medical Informatics and Decision Making, 13*(Suppl 3), S6.

Stolee, P., Awad, M., Byrne, K., Deforge, R., Clements, S., Glenny, C., & Day Hospital Goal Attainment Scaling Interest Group of the Regional Geriatric Programs of Ontario, (2012). A multi-site study of the feasibility and clinical utility of Goal Attainment Scaling in geriatric day hospitals. *Disability & Rehabilitation, 34*(20), 1716–1726.

Tinetti, M. E., Fried, T. R., & Boyd, C. M. (2012). Designing health care for the most common chronic condition – multimorbidity. *Journal of the American Medical Association, 307*(23), 2493–2494.

Walston, J., Hadley, E. C., Ferrucci, L., Guralnik, J. M., Newman, A. B., Studenski, S. A., et al. (2006). Research agenda for frailty in older adults: Toward a better understanding of physiology and etiology: Summary from the American Geriatrics Society/National Institute on Aging Research Conference on Frailty in Older Adults. *Journal of the American Geriatrics Society, 54*(6), 991–1001.

Weeks, J. C., Catalano, P. J., Cronin, A., Finkelman, M. D., Mack, J. W., Keating, N. L., et al. (2012). Patients' expectations about effects of chemotherapy for advanced cancer. *New England Journal of Medicine, 367*, 1616–1625.

Weiner, S. J. (2004). Contextualizing medical decisions to individualize care: Lessons from the qualitative sciences. *Journal of General Internal Medicine, 19*(3), 281–285.

Weiner, S. J., Schwartz, A., Weaver, F., Goldberg, J., Yudkowsky, R., Sharma, G., et al. (2010). Contextual errors and failures in individualizing patient care: A multicenter study. *Annals of Internal Medicine, 153*(2), 69–75.

2

Family Caregiving

Steven H. Zarit[1], and Judy M. Zarit[2]

[1]The Pennsylvania State University, University Park, Pennsylvania, USA;
[2]Center Psychology Group, State College, Pennsylvania, USA

INTRODUCTION

Families have always provided care for children, parents, and other relatives with health problems. But family caregiving in contemporary society has become a more frequent and complex endeavor as the result of medical advances that have increased both the number and lifespan of those with chronic disabilities. Complicating matters today is the fact that the majority of adults now work full-time, reducing the ability of family members to provide all the care that is needed.

It has been estimated that in the United States more than 1 in 4 adults over the age of 18 – nearly 66 million people – provide assistance to an adult or child in their family each year (National Alliance for Caregiving and AARP, 2009). While caregivers may derive satisfaction from their caregiving role, many encounter high levels of stress that lead to adverse changes in their health and well-being (Aneshensel, Pearlin, Mullen, Zarit & Whitlatch, 1995). Specifically, caregivers vs. noncaregivers have higher rates of health problems (Cuijpers, 2005), including cardiovascular risk factors such as inflammation and high blood pressure (Haley, Roth, Howard, & Safford, 2010; Mausbach et al., 2011). What's more, caregivers experiencing strain in their role have been found to have higher rates of mortality than age-matched groups of noncaregivers (Lazzarino, Hamer, Stamatakis, & Steptoe, 2013).

Given the large number of people providing care, many patients seen by physicians and psychologists are likely to be caregivers or care receivers, and at least some of the health concerns of caregivers may be related to stress from the caregiving role. Sometimes, caregivers are essential to the planning and implementation of a relative's treatment. In fact, family caregivers often make a critical difference in the care receiver's ability and

B. Bensadon (Ed): Psychology and Geriatrics.
DOI: http://dx.doi.org/10.1016/B978-0-12-420123-1.00002-2

willingness to follow through on treatment recommendations. Caregivers also provide help in meeting patients' basic needs, including *instrumental activities of daily living* (IADL) such as preparing meals or managing finances, and basic *activities of daily living* (ADLs), such as bathing, dressing and toileting. They may also assure that the care recipient is safe living at home. Thus, physicians and psychologists share a common responsibility to identify who among their patients is receiving care, who provides the care, and what impact this has on patients' lives.

In describing the consequences of family caregiving on health and well-being, this chapter will identify factors that contribute to caregiver stress, and explore why some caregivers manage these stressors well while others are overwhelmed by them. Supportive behavioral treatments to help caregivers manage their challenges more effectively will be presented, as will a variety of tools and information to aid clinical decision-making. Although providing health care to caregivers and recipients can be complicated and challenging, it is highly rewarding, particularly when treatment leads to significant improvement.

THE SCOPE OF CAREGIVING IN CONTEMPORARY SOCIETY

The social philosopher Christopher Lasch described contemporary families as "a haven in a heartless world" (Lasch, 1995). Indeed, family members often exchange help and emotional support; parents care for their young children and frequently play a supportive role for older parents. In turn, many older parents, often viewed as recipients of help, may actually continue providing assistance to their grown offspring and grandchildren (Bangerter, Kim, Zarit, Birditt, & Fingerman, 2014).

Caregiving grows out from and expands these everyday exchanges of help and support. It can generally be defined as providing regular assistance to people with health problems. Furthermore, caregiving encompasses situations where one family member assists another who needs help with ADL or IADL and/or needs to be regularly monitored for safety.

Caregivers may be young or old, and they may be helping someone who is young or old. A recent national survey of caregivers (National Alliance for Caregiving and AARP, 2009) found 14% were assisting children under 18 with special needs, such as autism spectrum disorder, and another 14% were assisting adults between the ages of 18 and 49. The largest percentage, however, was assisting older adults: 28% were helping someone aged 50 to 74 and 44% were assisting someone aged 75 and older. Conditions requiring such care are typically chronic. Thus, 65% of people who identify themselves as caregivers have been providing care for more than one year and 31% for more than 5 years. More than half of all caregivers give 9 or more hours of help a week, and 13% report providing 40 hours of help per week. Nearly all those caring for adults assist with instrumental activities of daily living (IADL). Somewhat more than half of those caring for adults (56%) help with basic ADL. Caregivers frequently manage care recipients' behavioral and psychological problems. Additionally, many caregivers work outside the home and/or have other family responsibilities in addition to providing care. Not surprisingly, 31% of caregivers report they are highly stressed (National Alliance for Caregiving and AARP, 2009).

Most caregivers (66%) receive at least some help from family or friends (National Alliance for Caregiving and AARP, 2009). Ironically, these additional helpers can at times be a source of stress. Nevertheless, they may provide the primary helper with regular relief that enables him or her to continue in the primary caregiving role.

IDENTIFYING AND WORKING WITH CAREGIVERS IN CLINICAL SETTINGS

As a first step in identifying caregivers and beginning discussions with them, clinicians must become sensitized to caregiving as a clinical issue. Physicians, and at times psychologists, are not always aware that their patients are caregivers. These are the *hidden* caregivers.

Recent implementation of the U.S. Affordable Care Act is resulting in many Americans seeking out new physicians. This increased incidence of first-time physician–patient encounters underscores the need for a careful family and social history, including identifying who, if anyone, is occupying caregiver and care receiver roles.

For new patients, two simple questions are recommended as part of the initial screening process: (1) Who lives in your household? and (2) Are you providing care for someone in the household or for a family member or friend living somewhere else? These questions can be asked verbally or can be added to the standard health risks screening patients must generally complete at their initial visit.

For continuing patients, these questions can be included in annually administered questionnaires to determine if there have been any changes in a patient's health. Importantly, becoming a caregiver entails health risks that warrant discussion in the same way that a patient's new medical symptoms demand a physician's workup. Though psychologists, for their part, are often more aware of family dynamics, they also would do well to review regularly whether caregiving situations have emerged with existing patients.

Including Caregivers in Patient Discussions

The flip side of determining who is a caregiver is identifying those patients who, because of their health conditions and associated disabilities, are receiving care from a family member. Figure 2.1 shows a clinical decision tree that can be useful for physicians and psychologists in identifying whether a new or current patient is receiving care from someone at home, and how to effectively include that caregiver in relevant discussions addressing the patient's chief complaint, presenting symptoms, and history of present illness.

Caregiver presence during a patient visit may improve treatment adherence, but can conflict with the need to protect the patient's confidentiality. This is especially difficult with patients suffering from dementia. Many patients with moderate dementia are able to hide their symptoms from physicians and use adequate social presentation. In these cases, physicians may not know what problems their patients are experiencing without the input of a caregiver.

Patients, even those living with dementia, should be asked to give consent for caregivers to be included. Individuals with early and middle stage dementia can usually understand the consent process. In many

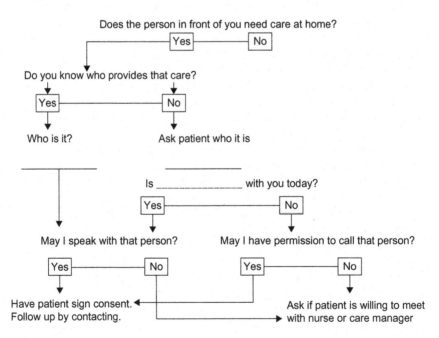

FIGURE 2.1 Clinical decision tree useful in identifying whether a new or current patient is receiving care from someone at home, and how to include that caregiver in relevant discussions.

states, next of kin can be included in medical decisions when the patient is unable to consent (American Bar Association Commission on Law and Aging and American Psychological Association, 2008). Generally, patients with dementia rarely refuse to allow the caregiver to participate in discussions. When including caregivers in discussions with patients, it is always important to do so in a nonthreatening way.

The utility of including relatives in discussions with patients is not limited to the dementia population. In general it can be challenging for older patients to remember details about a diagnosis or treatment plan, so a caregiver may be useful in recording the details. The physician may see the person is having trouble remembering and may be unable to follow through on medical treatment. A simple task to assess this problem is to ask the person to repeat instructions in their own words – for example, about when and how to take a medication. Though inconsistently used (Jager & Wynia, 2012; Schillinger et al., 2003), this interactive "teach back method" has been associated with positive outcomes (e.g., Esquivel, White, Carroll, & Brinker, 2011; Kripalani, Jackson, Schnipper, & Coleman, 2007; Rothman et al., 2004). Based on patient performance, clinicians can then decide whether to bring the caregiver in to help. As part of integrated care initiatives, clinical psychologists, who are trained to recognize subtle behavioral cues and gauge levels of comprehension, can assist physicians with this task or provide physicians with related communications training.

Family involvement is particularly important to assure adequate follow-up and care when a patient is discharged from the hospital. Currently, many hospitals give patients discharge documents that are incomprehensible. Instead, there should be a discussion with the caregiver regarding how to manage the patient's condition because the patient is less likely to remember instructions, especially following surgery. The primary care physician can also follow up with patients and caregivers after discharge. In fact, recent studies document that follow-up with patients after hospital discharge effectively reduces rates of rehospitalization, and probably leads to better care as well (Bowles et al., 2011).

Memory Concerns and Dementia

Deciding to involve caregivers depends on the patient's cognitive abilities to process and retain information. Detecting dementia and other causes of cognitive problems can be difficult, especially with one's ongoing patients. As noted, many patients with moderate dementia are able to hide their symptoms in front of physicians and use adequate social presentation. In these cases, physicians are often unaware of the problems patients are experiencing. Furthermore, some physicians will minimize their patients' memory problems. It is the old story – the patient goes to the physician and complains about memory, and the physician replies, "It's no worse than mine." Some physicians take the view that memory gets worse with aging so it is normal to have problems, and there is nothing that can be done anyway. While dealing with a memory problem this way may keep the communication between physician and patient comfortable, it may be devastating for the patient's caregiver, who may well be at his or her wit's end because of the patient's memory loss and related behavioral and emotional problems. Even if the physician recognizes the problem, patients with dementia often minimize the disability, which puts the physician in an awkward position about bringing a caregiver into the discussion. Managing such situations is an area in which training can help physicians feel more comfortable and help them recognize when and how to refer patients for neuropsychological assessment or psychotherapeutic services.

Case Example

The patient was a woman in her early 80s in moderately good health, diagnosed with mild to moderate dementia. She had good social presentation so her significant memory and word-finding difficulties were not obvious. Her longtime primary care physician did not think she had dementia and did not assess for it. The physician was in her early 60s, and she herself had an unrecognized reluctance to see dementia in her patients. Yet she wanted the patient's daughter to be present when she talked with the patient, because while she did not think the patient had dementia, at some level she recognized how devoid of content the patient's answers were and knew she needed the daughter involved to get accurate information and to assure that treatment was implemented.

In such situations, the clinician identifies with the patient and joins in the patient's denial. Further fueling the physician's denial is the recognition that available medical treatments for dementia have only limited benefit. Unfortunately, this denial leads to two negative outcomes: First, because the physician wants to help the patient, he or she may order unnecessary tests in the hope that something will turn up. Second, by not identifying the dementia, the clinician overlooks the things that can make an immediate difference for the caregiver. Specifically, by helping the caregiver understand that this is not just ordinary forgetfulness, the physician can help the caregiver begin to seek information useful in caring for the patient.

Evaluating Memory Concerns

Consultation is advisable when patients report memory complaints to primary care physicians or when there are other reasons to suspect dementia. Neuropsychological testing at this point is useful in both (1) determining if the patient's complaints are due to a dementing illness or simply reflective of normal age-related memory changes and (2) providing a baseline against which future changes can be assessed.

Alzheimer's disease and related disorders are insidious in onset and progressive in their course, so repeated testing (at yearly or biannual intervals) is the best way to accurately differentiate a neurodegenerative or dementing process from normal age changes or from other disorders from normal age changes or from other disorders.

It is also important to recognize that memory complaints can reflect many different problems (see Zarit & Zarit, 2007, for a review). Older people frequently report memory complaints, but in most cases these problems reflect normal lapses that can occur at any age. While frequency of such lapses may increase with age, subjective memory complaints are particularly common correlates of three psychological conditions: depression, anxiety and personality disorders.

Depression

Depressed patients often complain of memory problems, which reflect, in part, a pattern of negative beliefs characteristic of depressive disorders (Zarit & Zarit, 2007). The most beneficial step a physician can take when older patients present with both depression and memory concerns is to focus on the depression. While depression and dementia can coexist, depression alone can present like dementia (e.g., pseudodementia). When a patient seems concomitantly depressed and demented, is treated for depression, and then returns to normal, albeit with age-related memory problems, it is illuminating: The depression exacerbates age-related memory problems, making the person's overall functioning and appearance worse. Studies now document that cognition improves with treatment of depression in older patients (Mackin et al., 2014).

Anxiety

Highly anxious people may also be concerned about their memory and the possibility of dementia. In fact, fears of dementia are not uncommon, and extensive publicity about Alzheimer's disease has increased some anxious individuals' focus on their memory problems. Anxious persons continually monitor themselves and are therefore likely to fixate on memory difficulties and even become convinced they have dementia. Physicians and psychologists must avoid exacerbating such fears among their patients.

Personality Disorders

Personality disorders are a significant source of memory complaints. Individuals with longstanding difficulties in adjustment, particularly in their relationships with others, or those who have narcissistic tendencies, will sometimes focus on their memory as they get older. The ongoing crises in their lives suggest the kind of decompensation that can occur with dementia, but a careful history can reveal that they have always lurched from crisis to crisis. Of course, people with lifelong personality disorders can also develop dementia. Only careful, comprehensive neuropsychological examination can differentiate the two.

Difficulties Determining Who Is the Caregiver

There are situations in which it is unclear who the caregiver is, or where there is family conflict over who should provide the care. These are often complicated, emotionally charged situations, where collaborative, physician–psychologist partnerships can be especially helpful. The psychologist can meet with the involved individuals, clarify the older person's need for care and capacity for making decisions, and help the family formulate a workable plan. The care receiver's preferences should be honored, of course, except when he or she does not have the capacity to evaluate the choices.

Clinicians are faced with a different dilemma when the patient clearly needs help, but no caregiver is involved or available. Such situations may involve people estranged from family or without close relatives, individuals with paranoid beliefs and afraid to seek help, or true isolates who are secretive about their life's details and have no close ties to anyone. Often the primary care physician is the only person who sees these individuals. By definition it is difficult to estimate just how many people might fall into this category, but social isolation is not uncommon in the geriatric population and evidence linking it with deleterious health consequences, including death, is strong (Berkman & Krishna, 2014).

Quality care for such patients requires that clinicians first recognize that the patient belongs to this group. This may be especially difficult, since these patients often prefer to minimize symptoms and disabilities. In some instances, it may be possible to refer such a patient to a clinical psychologist, but often there will be resistance to such a referral because of the stigma perceived by the patient. If the physician suspects cognitive impairment, a referral for a neuropsychological evaluation may provide a needed bridge between physician and clinical psychologist that will allow them to work together in the future. Psychologists can be particularly helpful in dealing with isolated patients who are ambivalent about needing help, by effectively building trust, generally a slow process, and then using this alliance to help patients address emerging problems.

A confounding factor in some couples is that both members of the dyad have significant impairment. Although one may be trying to help the other, both may have limited ability to function independently at home.

Case Example

An older couple were referred for counseling by a primary care physician. The woman had become depressed following her diabetes diagnosis. She also had macular degeneration and could no longer drive. Her husband had dementia, significant hearing loss and paranoia. They helped each other in the house, but that was clearly inadequate. As in many such cases, the husband refused to let helpers come to the home to assist with their daily needs. Although the couple had a son who lived in the area, they shielded him from knowing the extent of their need for help. Through family therapy discussions that included both couple and son, the decision was made to move the couple to a continuing care retirement community where they could maintain some independence, with additional care available if needed. Though the husband's paranoia made the transition difficult, it was nevertheless successful. The facility arranged for needed health care, and the wife was no longer isolated and developed relationships with other residents. The husband, however, remained isolated in their apartment.

TYPES OF STRESS: CHALLENGES AND RESOURCES

Understanding the burden caregivers experience begins with identifying the various types of help they provide. The "primary stressors," as they are sometimes called, place demands on the caregiver's time and require physical exertion and mental effort to perform. Caregivers respond to these stressors in very different ways, and what is stressful for one person may not be stressful for another (e.g., Aneshensel et al., 1995; Zarit, Todd, & Zarit, 1986). Thus, the burden of care is a *subjective* experience. It is not a *one-size-fits-all* phenomenon. The clinical psychologist can help in identifying the type and frequency of stressors the caregiver faces (e.g., the relative's agitation, nighttime insomnia), identify which of these problems the caregiver finds most stressful, and determine how to most efficiently intervene. It is worth repeating that it is not the objective number or type of problems that matter in determining a caregiver's overall burden, but rather how much each problem bothers the caregiver.

Caregivers differ considerably from one another in what problems are present in their situation and which problems they find stressful (Zarit, Femia, Kim, & Whitlatch, 2010). Differences in caregiving arrangements and resources are further accentuated across various ethnic, cultural and racial groups, although recent research suggests similar feelings of obligation and emotional attachment are found across groups (Friedemann, Buckwalter, Newman, & Mauro, 2013).

Several comprehensive tools are available to guide discussions of primary stressors with caregivers. In cases of dementia, the Revised Memory and Behavior Problems Checklist (Teri et al., 1992) effectively assesses the occurrence of typical problems and how much each problem disturbs the caregiver. It is also important to identify the tasks the caregiver helps with: ADL and/or IADL. Furthermore, how the patient responds to help is paramount in evaluating stress. The patient may struggle with, resist, or refuse help with bathing, dressing or other activities. Generally, these responses are likely to be experienced by caregivers as stressful.

Once it is determined *which* care-related problems are most stressful for the caregiver, one must determine *why*, which can then contribute to developing appropriate intervention strategies. Although the reasons vary from one caregiver to another, four broad categories can be identified: (1) the meaning of the problem to the caregiver; (2) the caregiver's problem-solving skills; (3) the support the caregiver receives; and (4) the history of the relationship between caregiver and patient.

(1) The meaning of the problem to the caregiver.

Problems are experienced as stressful in part because of the meaning that caregivers ascribe to them. For example, consider how caregivers of people with dementia react to their relatives' memory problems: Many caregivers find repetitive questions very stressful because they assume their relative is not paying attention, is "just lazy," or is trying to get attention or even annoy the caregiver. In such situations, helping caregivers understand that this behavior is not intentional but rather a disease-related symptom can enhance tolerance. Recommending other adaptive strategies, such as distracting the care receiver or involving him or her in an activity, can also be helpful.

(2) The caregiver's problem-solving skills.

Problem-solving and the ability to regulate one's emotions often go hand-in-hand. The better one is at these functions, the better one is at providing care. Some people are natural caregivers. They have always been called upon to solve family problems, and they do so without becoming emotionally overwhelmed. For others, however, everything is overwhelming and dramatic, and their response style paralyzes them when faced with a problem. People with obsessive tendencies may be poor problem-solvers because they have difficulty making choices about how to adjust to the care receiver when a change in response is necessary. But fortunately, problem-solving can be taught, as discussed later.

(3) The support the caregiver receives.

People with a good social network are able to spread the stress of care across several individuals. They are not as easily overwhelmed because they are able to get timely help. Sometimes, it is not a specific problem that bothers caregivers most, but rather the lack of respite or feeling "on call" all the time, something that should resonate with medical clinicians, given their own training. The knowledge that help is on the horizon – for example, a planned break or even a scheduled phone call – may be critical in helping a caregiver manage daily problems without getting overwhelmed. In addition to family, friends or other volunteers, paid help can play an important role in lowering caregivers' subjective burden (S. Zarit et al., 2013) and will be discussed later.

Physicians and psychologists, together, can have a major impact on stress reduction. When caregivers appear overwhelmed during office visits, clinicians should empathically communicate understanding of the caregiver's difficulty. At the same time, providers can let caregivers know there are resources, such as home care providers, for temporary relief. Psychologically, this conveys something crucial, namely the encouragement and confidence that caregiving is a problem that can be solved.

During medical visits, when care receivers seem overwhelmed yet resist practical suggestions that might improve their situation, it is common for physicians to respond by advising caregivers to place the patient in a nursing home. Regardless of the appropriateness of such advice, it can inadvertently reinforce the caregiver's hopelessness. Instead, the physician should remain objective and refer the caregiver to a psychologist who can provide solutions. Additionally, physicians should check in regularly with their patients' caregivers since caregivers often ignore their own health and/or feel too guilty to make an appointment for themselves, even when they experience symptoms.

(4) History of the relationship.

All human relationships contain unresolved issues. A caregiving situation in which one person is dependent on another can reveal latent tensions that have been dormant for years. For example, care receivers will do things reminiscent of their earlier, premorbid behaviors, which can trigger caregiver stress. The new challenge for caregivers is to recognize why they are upset and realize that only they can make appropriate changes, because longstanding family conflict cannot be resolved without both parties' participation and care receivers may no longer have the insight or ability to inhibit their behavior (Marková et al., 2014).

The shift in the balance of power between caregiver and care receiver that occurs with increasing dependency can also exacerbate longstanding tensions in a relationship. Some care receivers accept the changing relationship, while others fight against it. As addressed elsewhere in this publication, driving ability is among the most emotionally volatile sources of related conflict, particularly when the patient may be cognitively or otherwise unfit to drive (Byszewski et al., 2013; Carr & Ott, 2010).

In parent-child dyads, each relationship is unique. The child who is serving as caregiver is likely to have had a different relationship with his or her parent than other siblings have had. When providing day-to-day care, caregivers may see things they never saw before in their relationship with a parent, and may be unpleasantly surprised and unprepared to cope. It is common for caregivers to feel they are meeting a completely different person (e.g., "he's not himself"). An adult child's decision to institutionalize a parent can be traumatic (Buhr, Kuchibhatla, & Clipp, 2006), so adult children may instead opt for their parent to move back in with them. While there are many advantages to this approach, including cost savings and an increased sense of control, there are disadvantages too, including insufficient space, both physical and psychological, to allow each person to manage his or her emotions and minimize unpleasant experiences. What often defines the success of this arrangement is the degree to which caregivers take personally the parent's criticism, anger or other disagreeable behavior.

Secondary Stressors

In addition to the stressors caregivers experience in providing daily care, the time and effort they spend in caregiving may interfere with other areas of their life. These "secondary" stressors, though often subtle, can have as much impact on the caregiver's subjective burden as the patient's behavioral or emotional problems (Aneshensel et al., 1995). Clinicians must note which of these challenges may be facing caregivers, and which is experienced as stressful. Secondary stressors include the following:

- Employment Outside the Home. A caregiver who balances work with caregiving responsibilities faces unique, subjective challenges. Among them are the need to find a substitute caregiver if the patient cannot safely stay at home alone; the need to take time off work for medical appointments and emergencies; interruptions at work by calls from the patient; and worry while at work about the care receiver's well-being. Conversely, these challenges can be balanced by positive experiences at work. For example, some caregivers describe work as the only time when they feel in control of their lives and feel able to get things done (Edwards, Zarit, Stephens, & Townsend, 2002). This duality of the work experience was confirmed in a 2013 study reported by S. Zarit and colleagues. Work days introduced additional stressors but also added positive experiences to the caregiver's day.

- Family Conflict. Problems arise when family members are unsupportive, critical and unhelpful. Aneshensel and colleagues (1995) identified three common sources of conflict: the medical and related care the patient receives, the type and amount of patient care other family members provide, and the help the family provides (or does not provide) the caregiver.
- Financial Resources. Of course, one of the most quantifiable impacts of caregiving is economic. Costs associated with providing care often strain the caregiver's budget, particularly when caregivers leave the workplace altogether to help a parent or spouse. These costs include substantial amounts of lost wages and lost contributions to pensions and social security (MetLife Mature Market Institute, 2011). When a child is providing care to a parent, conflict with siblings may arise over how the parent's money is being spent. Siblings may accuse the caregiver of siphoning off the parent's money for his or her own use, a charge that is accurate in only a minority of cases. For spousal caregivers, medical and long-term care expenses can reduce the couple's joint assets up to a maximum amount as determined by state-specific Medicaid regulations. It is critical that spousal caregivers get responsible financial advice to avoid depleting their assets more than necessary when paying for a nursing home or other care. Area Agencies on Aging or other state offices can provide appropriate guidance. Lawyers with elder law training can be helpful as well.
- Leisure and Social Activities. The time and effort involved in providing care can make it difficult for caregivers to engage in leisure activities. In addition, caregivers may cut themselves off from friends and family because of embarrassment about the patient's condition, especially when that person is suffering from dementia or other stigmatized mental health problems. In other cases, it is the family and friends themselves who avoid the care receiver. As described earlier, caregivers may not feel they "deserve" to engage in leisure activities and may feel guilty for even considering them. Skaff and Pearlin (1992) describe the feeling expressed by caregivers that caregiving has completely taken over their lives, leaving them nothing they enjoy or that gives meaning to their life.

"Persistent" Stressors

A particular challenge of caregiving is its indeterminate length. When individuals face a challenging situation that will run its course in six months or a year, they may feel equipped to control and manage it. But generally, a relative's chronic health problems have no predictable end in sight, leaving the duration and scope of caregiving unknown. Pearlin,

Nguyen, Schieman, and Milkie (2007) have described how these "stubbornly persistent" stressors erode a sense of mastery in one's life and cause caregivers to feel a loss of control. These sequelae are robustly associated with depression as well as declining physical health (Infurna, Gerstorf, & Zarit, 2012; Martire & Schulz, 2012). In particular, studies have found increased risk of cardiovascular disease and stroke among caregivers (Haley et al., 2010; Mausbach et al., 2011; von Känel et al., 2012).

Often caregivers have two conflicting emotions. The first is feeling a positive obligation to care for a parent, spouse, or child. Caring helps build self-esteem. But, second, when caregivers find they must do things they had not anticipated or are no longer able to do things that are important to them, they may resent having taken on the caregiving role. This is one of the major obstacles that must be addressed during caregiving interventions. Anger and accompanying guilt can exacerbate the relationship with the care receiver and drive away family and friends who might otherwise help.

INTERVENTION STRATEGIES

Summarized below are key components and characteristics of treatments that have been evaluated in controlled trials and have been found to lower subjective burden and emotional distress, and, in a few cases, to reduce the risk of medical illness among caregivers.

As previously noted, recommending institutionalization of the patient may be the easiest and quickest response to an overwhelmed caregiver, but it is not what most families want. It is not financially possible for many families and it is not the preference of most care receivers. For clinicians to be seen as a resource for solutions, they must remain neutral about such a choice. It is important that placement be considered along with other alternatives, allowing the family to come to that conclusion themselves. For physicians, it is helpful to offer a psychology referral to help families consider all available options. Clinical psychologists are well positioned to provide strategies that help caregivers manage this decision-making process and related challenges most effectively.

It is also important for clinicians to recognize caregiver stress can be reduced even when the care recipient has a chronic and/or degenerative disease. For example, treatment with behavioral interventions enables caregivers to think about the patient's problems in new ways, learn new skills, and feel it is acceptable to seek assistance. This treatment can reduce perceived stress and burden, improve the care receiver's quality of life, and keep the care receiver at home for as long as appropriate.

Structural Characteristics of Treatment

Effective treatments have been found to be structured in specific ways (Coon, Thompson, Steffen, Sorocco, & Gallagher-Thompson, 2003; Sörensen, Pinquart, & Duberstein, 2002; Zarit & Femia, 2008b). First, they actively involve caregivers in learning and implementing new skills, in contrast with interventions that only provide educational information.

Second, because caregivers experience multiple types of stressors, they respond best to interventions that incorporate multiple treatment components.

Third, treatments that flexibly address a caregiver's most pressing problems, rather than follow a strict manual, have better outcomes. For example, Mittelman, Roth, Coon, and Haley (2004) developed an intervention for families of persons with dementia in which sessions target the most pressing problems caregivers experience at the moment. Similarly, Belle and colleagues (2006) set individualized treatment goals collaboratively with caregivers, and then tailored treatment to those goals. These adaptive interventions are best suited to caregivers, given the heterogeneity among the problems they find stressful and in their values and resources (Zarit et al., 2010).

Fourth, treatment must be provided in adequate doses. In psychoeducational interventions, caregivers require sufficient time and repetition to learn and apply new skills. Similarly, with respite services such as adult day care, caregivers need to receive adequate amounts on a regular basis before they show positive effects (Zarit, Stephens, Townsend, & Greene, 1998).

Finally, the challenges that caregivers and care receivers experience constitute an evolving process that may span several years. Time-limited intervention can help caregivers in the short run, but no short-term treatment is likely to prepare them for every problem they face in the future. The Mittelman intervention is unique in providing long-term access to ongoing support groups. Not surprisingly, this project has demonstrated long-term improvements in caregiver health and emotional well-being, as well as significant economic benefits associated with reduced nursing home placement (Long, Moriarty, Mittelman, & Foldes, 2014). Respite services can also provide caregivers support over the long haul (Kim, Zarit, Femia, & Savla, 2012).

Empirically validated psychoeducational approaches have included both individual and group interventions. Some caregivers are more uncomfortable in groups, and some will not get adequate attention in a group to make a difference. Facilitators must have sufficient training in group process to create a therapeutic environment in which caregivers feel supported and can learn new skills. The Savvy Caregiver is a group intervention that has shown considerable promise and is offered in several regions of the country (Hepburn, Lewis, Tonatore, Sherman, & Bremer, 2007; Hepburn, Tornatore, Center, & Ostwald, 2001).

Treatment Components

Effective treatment components include:

1. Provision of information about the care receiver's disease and its implications.

    The first step for any clinician aiming to support caregivers is the provision of disease-related information, such as its likely course, treatment options, and available resources. This communication should come first from physicians, followed by psychologists who expand the discussion to include behavioral aspects of the disease and management resources. Equipped with this information, caregivers will likely feel less isolated and more effective as they adjust to their caregiver role.

2. Changing caregivers' perceptions.

    As previously discussed, the meaning caregivers attribute to the care receiver's behaviors and emotions is a major source of stress. Interventions that help caregivers modify these perceptions are effective (e.g., Hepburn et al., 2001, 2007; Livingston et al., 2013; Whitlatch, Zarit, & von Eye, 1991). These interventions help caregivers learn to look at problems as originating in the illness rather than taking frustrating behaviors personally. The patient's "annoying" behavior may be out of the caregiver's control, but feeling aggravated or frustrated is not. With effective behavioral intervention, beliefs can be adjusted, tolerance built, and more adaptive responses modeled.

    The above challenges are not limited to dementing illness. Caregivers of patients suffering from other types of brain dysfunction or post-traumatic stress disorder (PTSD) face similar issues.

    Caregivers must also recognize when it is necessary to take over decision-making for individuals with dementia or similar conditions that compromise capacity (Hepburn et al., 2001, 2007). Emotionally, this can be particularly difficult for adult children who have relied on their parents as a source of clarity and stability since birth.

    Logistics, such as motivating and mobilizing a parent with dementia to attend a medical appointment, also present challenges. For example, patients may resist going to the physician when asked directly if they want to go. It is more effective for caregivers to simply say "We are going out." Caregivers should avoid asking yes-no questions. It is generally more effective to give the care receiver a choice of two alternatives (e.g., "Do you want to eat now or later?"). These strategies reduce the potential for struggles over issues of independence or control, thereby removing a major source of tension in the caregiver–care receiver relationship.

3. Improving problem-solving skills.

Growing evidence has shown that caregivers can learn simple behavioral management techniques to manage behavioral and emotional problems that accompany many chronic illnesses (Belle et al., 2006; Livingston et al., 2013; Teri et al., 2003; Teri, Logsdon, Uomoto, & McCurry, 1997; Whitlatch et al., 1991). As previously discussed, problem-solving for behavioral and emotional difficulties begins by helping caregivers identify which behaviors, among many, they find most stressful and want to change. Caregivers are then shown how to gather information about when the problem occurs and what events precede and follow the problem. This approach has been characterized by Teri and her colleagues (1997) as the A-B-C model: Antecedents–Behavior–Consequences. Antecedents may trigger the behavior and consequences may provide reinforcement. Through psychotherapy, caregiver and clinician can collaboratively brainstorm possible strategies to reduce the behavior problem and develop plans for implementing that strategy. This approach has been successful in reducing the frequency of many of the more troubling behaviors associated with dementia (McCurry, Gibbons, Logsdon, Vitiello, & Teri, 2005; Teri et al., 1997, 2003).

This collaborative problem-solving approach can also be effective in addressing practical and psychological problems when caregivers are considering the use of paid help, e.g., home health care aides or adult day care facilities, as discussed below (Zarit & Zarit, 2007). Another problem-solving tool is helping caregivers find time for activities they enjoy. Sometimes the barriers are *practical*, e.g., no one is available to stay with the patient, and sometimes *psychological*, e.g., believing it is not appropriate to take time for one's self. A recent study showed that a six-week program designed to increase caregivers' engagement in pleasant activities reduced depression and also reduced two biological markers of cardiovascular risk, Interleukin-6 and D-dimer (Moore et al., 2013).

4. Stress reduction strategies.

The growing scientific interest in efficacy of mindfulness-based stress reduction has included studies examining effects among family caregivers. These studies have found immediate benefits on subjective stress and depressive symptoms (Hou et al., 2014; Whitebird et al., 2012), as well as on cognition and biomarkers of stress (Lavretsky et al., 2013). Apart from such immediate benefits, these approaches can help caregivers develop deeper awareness of how they react to the care receiver's behavior, and allow them to develop the emotional distance needed to make more adaptive responses.

5. Improving family support.

Family interventions are designed to increase the support that caregivers receive while reducing care-related conflict. These approaches have consistently demonstrated benefit in reducing subjective burden and emotional distress (Marriott, Donaldson, Tarrier, & Burns, 2000; Mittelman et al., 2004; Whitlatch et al., 1991). Family members can help by giving caregivers breaks from providing care, assisting them with practical tasks, and simply giving emotional support. However, family members may not know what help caregivers need, and many caregivers are reluctant to ask for help. Therefore, family interventions can be particularly useful by clarifying and identifying what care may benefit the caregivers themselves – medical and nonmedical – and who should provide this help (Zarit, Orr, & Zarit, 1985; Zarit & Zarit, 2007).

Family meetings should be led by clinical psychologists with family therapy training. Communication patterns among family members can be complicated and reflect old relationship tensions mixed with concerns about the patient. An effective clinician maintains focus on caregiving issues and steers a neutral course, not siding with any individual (Zarit & Zarit, 2007). Anything else leads to disaster. Once families understand the caregiver's dilemmas, they are often able to engage in solving the problems and coming up with a plan to give ongoing help. Even families that are deeply divided on other issues can nevertheless come together and agree on a plan for helping the caregiver.

6. Reducing burden by using paid help.

As mentioned, one of the most direct ways to reduce stress is the use of regular paid services. Turning care over to someone else for part of the time reduces the caregiver's exposure to stress. However, there are both practical and psychological obstacles to retaining paid services.

Practical barriers include the cost and availability of services. The psychological barriers are typically more difficult to overcome. Caregivers may be reluctant to turn the care receiver over to someone else or may believe that the care receiver will not accept help from someone else. They may believe they should provide all the help, or that no one else can provide the same level of personalized care that they do. What's more, care receivers' difficulty accepting help can be extremely challenging to overcome. This is an area where caregivers can benefit from consulting with a clinical psychologist who can help them examine the pros and cons of using paid help and identify how best to approach a care receiver who is reluctant to do so (S. Zarit & J. Zarit, 2007). It can be useful to have caregivers devise a list of the types of care they can easily, and happily, provide, along with another list of care that would be either too physically taxing (such as physically transferring someone who is overweight) or emotionally challenging (bathing or changing adult diapers). Then it can be pointed out that hiring someone to handle the second list will free them up to retain a pleasurable relationship with their family member.

The challenge is how to arrange such care at the right time, without care receivers asking for it, since they are unlikely to acknowledge their need for help. As illustrated in the following case example, negotiation is an important, learnable skill.

Case Example

A previously independent elderly mother faces increasing difficulty with ADL and recently moved in with her daughter. Mother and daughter mutually agreed on the move because of the mother's problems with ADL. Her daughter wanted to have someone continuously present to provide help with housekeeping tasks and errands, as well as companionship. The mother only wanted someone to stay with her at night. After several discussions in therapy, mother and daughter reached a compromise, arranging for someone to come in the evening when the daughter was away. Though this solution was not "perfect" from the daughter's point of view, it was acceptable to her mother, and thus opened the door to expanding the use of paid help if necessary.

Adult day services (ADS) programs provide respite while also giving care receivers cognitive, physical and social stimulation (Zarit et al., 2011). Some programs also provide rehabilitation services and daily ADL support. Related research has shown that caregivers experience a 40% reduction in care-related stressors on days they use ADS, compared with days they provide most or all of the care themselves (Zarit et al., 2011). In turn, decreased stressor exposure on ADS days leads to lower emotional distress (Zarit et al., 1998; Zarit, Kim, Femia, Almeida, & Klein, 2013). Reducing daily stressor exposure through ADS use also was found to improve regulation of two stress hormones, cortisol and DHEA-S (Klein et al., 2014, in press; Zarit et al., 2014, in press). When not using ADS, caregivers' levels of these hormones were in ranges associated with increased risk of health problems including depression. ADS use, however, brought these levels into more normal ranges.

Follow-up with Caregivers

Many care receivers will spend some time before the end of their life in a nursing home or assisted living facility. A common misconception is that institutionalization will relieve the stress caregivers are experiencing. Data suggest that it may not, and that placement simply shifts the types of stressors caregivers face (Zarit & Whitlatch, 1992). Often, following placement, the acute daily burden of providing care morphs into frequent or even daily nursing home visits motivated by concern about quality of care. Caregivers often feel guilty about their decision to institutionalize their relatives and in some cases feel lonely or isolated since the care receiver no longer lives with them.

The death of care receivers can be experienced with caregiver relief because the patient is no longer suffering, or can trigger caregiver depression that may continue for a long time (Aneshensel, Botticello, & Yamamoto-Mitani, 2004). It is important to follow up with caregivers who have experienced these transitions to make sure they are managing well. Placement or death exerts a psychological toll even on those caregivers who appear most resilient.

CONCLUSIONS

Just as partnerships between primary care physicians and psychologists have been effective in the treatment of patients with mental health problems (e.g., Arean, Hegel, Vannoy, Fam, & Unuzter, 2008), they are also likely to be helpful for caregivers. Caregiving can be challenging and overwhelming, leading to increased risk of illness. But research now shows that targeted interventions can lower caregiver stress and burden, improving their lives and the lives of the patients they care for. Further integration is needed, and can likely maximize these outcomes.

References

American Bar Association Commission on Law and Aging and American Psychological Association, (2008). *Assessment of older adults with diminished capacity: A handbook for psychologists.* Washington, DC: American Bar Association and American Psychological Association.

Aneshensel, C., Pearlin, L. I., Mullan, J. T., Zarit, S. H., & Whitlatch, C. J. (1995). *Profiles in caregiving: The unexpected career.* New York: Academic Press.

Aneshensel, C. S., Botticello, A. L., & Yamamoto-Mitani, N. (2004). When caregiving ends: The course of depressive symptoms after bereavement. *Journal of Health and Social Behavior, 45,* 422–440.

Arean, P., Hegel, M., Vannoy, S., Fam, M. -Y., & Unuzter, J. (2008). Effectiveness of problem-solving therapy for older, primary care patients with depression: Results from the IMPACT project. *Gerontologist, 48,* 311–323.

Bangerter, L., Kim, K., Zarit, S. H., Birditt, K., & Fingerman, K. (2014). Perceptions of giving support and depressive symptoms in late life. *Gerontologist* http://dx.doi.org/10.1093/geront/gnt210 [Epub ahead of print].

Belle, S. H., Burgio, L., Burns, R., Coon, D., Czaja, S. J., Gallagher-Thompson, D., et al. (2006). Enhancing the quality of life of dementia caregivers from different ethnic or racial groups. *Annals of Internal Medicine, 145,* 727–738.

Berkman, L. F., & Krishna, A. (2014). Social network epidemiology. In L. F. Berkman, I. Kawachi, & M. M. Glymour (Eds.), *Social epidemiology* (pp. 234–281). New York, NY: Oxford.

Bowles, K. H., Hanlon, A. L., Glick, H. A., Naylor, M. D., O'Connor, M., Riegel, B., et al. (2011). Clinical effectiveness, access to, and satisfaction with care using a telehomecare substitution intervention: A randomized controlled trial. *International Journal of Telemedicine and Applications, 2011,* 1–13.

Buhr, G. T., Kuchibhatla, M., & Clipp, E. C. (2006). Caregivers' reasons for nursing home placement: Clues for improving discussions with families prior to the transition. *The Gerontologist, 46*(1), 52–61.

Byszewski, A., Aminzadeh, F., Robinson, K., Molnar, F., Dalziel, W., Man Son Hing, M., et al. (2013). When is it time to hang up the keys: The driving and dementia toolkit – for persons with dementia (PWD) and caregivers – a practical resource. *BMC Geriatrics, 13,* 117.

Carr, D. B., & Ott, B. R. (2010). The older adult driver with cognitive impairment: It's a very frustrating life. *Journal of the American Medical Association, 303,* 1633–1641.

Coon, D. W., Thompson, L., Steffen, A., Sorocco, K., & Gallagher-Thompson, D. (2003). Anger and depression management: Psychoeducational skill training intervention for women caregivers of a relative with dementia. *Gerontologist, 43,* 678–689.

Cuijpers, P. (2005). Depressive disorders in caregivers of dementia patients: A systematic review. *Aging and Mental Health, 9,* 325–330.

Edwards, A. B., Zarit, S. H., Stephens, M. A. P., & Townsend, A. (2002). Employed family caregivers of cognitively impaired elderly: An examination of role strain and depressive symptoms. *Aging and Mental Health, 6,* 55–61.

Esquivel, J., White, M., Carroll, M., & Brinker, E. (2011). Teach-back is an effective strategy for educating older heart failure patients. *Circulation, 124*(21 Supplement), A10786.

Friedemann, M. -L., Buckwalter, K. C., Newman, F. L., & Mauro, A. C. (2013). Patterns of caregiving of Cuban, other Hispanic, Caribbean black and white elders in South Florida. *Journal of Cross Cultural Gerontology, 28,* 137–152.

Haley, W. E., Roth, D. L., Howard, G., & Safford, M. M. (2010). Caregiving strain and estimated risk for stroke and coronary heart disease among spouse caregivers: Differential effects by race and sex. *Stroke, 41,* 331–336.

Hepburn, K., Lewis, M., Tornatore, J., Sherman, C. W., & Bremer, K. L. (2007). The Savvy Caregiver program: The demonstrated effectiveness of a transportable dementia caregiver psychoeducation program. *Journal of Gerontological Nursing, 33,* 30–36.

Hepburn, K. W., Tornatore, J., Center, B., & Ostwald, S. W. (2001). Dementia family caregiver training: Affecting beliefs about caregiving and caregiver outcomes. *Journal of the American Geriatrics Society, 49,* 450–457.

Infurna, F. J., Gerstorf, D., & Zarit, S. H. (2012). Substantial changes in mastery perceptions of dementia caregivers with the placement of a care recipient. *Journal of Gerontology: Psychological Sciences, 68,* 202–214.

Jager, A. J., & Wynia, M. K. (2012). Who gets a teach-back? Patient-reported incidence of experiencing a teach-back. *Journal of Health Communication: International Perspectives, 17*(3), 294–302.

Kim, K., Zarit, S. H., Femia, E. E., & Savla, J. (2012). Kin relationship of caregivers and people with dementia: Stress and response to intervention. *International Journal of Geriatric Psychiatry, 27,* 59–66.

Klein, L. C., Kim, K., Almeida, D. M., Femia, E. E., Rovine, M. L., & Zarit, S. H. (2014). Anticipating an easier day: Effects of adult day services on daily cortisol and stress. *The Gerontologist* http://dx.doi.org/10.1083/geront/gne060 [Epub ahead of print].

Kripalani, S., Jackson, A. T., Schnipper, J. L., & Coleman, E. A. (2007). Promoting effective transitions of care at hospital discharger: A review of key issues for hospitalists. *Journal of Hospital Medicine, 2,* 314–323.

Lasch, C. (1995). *Haven in a heartless world: The family besieged* (Reprint ed.). New York, NY: Basic Books.

Lazzarino, A. I., Hamer, M., Stamatakis, E., & Steptoe, A. (2013). The combined association of psychological distress and socioeconomic status with all-cause mortality: A national cohort study. *JAMA Internal Medicine, 173,* 22–27.

Livingston, G., Barber, J., Rapaport, P., Knapp, M., Griffin, M., King, D., et al. (2013). Clinical effectiveness of a manual based coping strategy programme (START, STrAtegies for RelaTives) in promoting the mental health of carers of family members with dementia: Pragmatic randomized controlled trial. *British Medical Journal.*, 347, 6342.

Long, K. H., Moriatry, J. P., Mittelman, M. S., & Foldes, S. S. (2014). Estimating the potential cost savings from the New York University caregiver intervention in Minnesota. *Health Affairs*, 33, 596–604.

Marková, I. S., Clare, L., Whitaker, C. J., Roth, I., Nelis, S. M., Martyr, A., et al. (2014). Phenomena of awareness in dementia: Heterogeneity and its implications. *Consciousness and Cognition*, 25 17–16.

Marriott, A., Donaldson, C., Tarrier, N., & Burns, A. (2000). Effectiveness of cognitive-behavioral family intervention in reducing the burden of care in carers of patients with Alzheimer's disease. *British Journal of Psychiatry*, 176, 557–562.

Martire, L., & Schulz, R. (2012). Caregiving and care receiving in later life. In A. Baum, T. A. Revenson, & J. Singer (Eds.), *Handbook of Health Psychology* (pp. 293–307). New York, NY: Psychology Press, Taylor & Francis Group.

Mausbach, B. T., von Känel, R., Roepke, S. K., Moore, R., Patterson, T. L., Mills, P. J., et al. (2011). Self-efficacy buffers the relationship between dementia caregiving stress and circulating concentrations of the proinflammatory cytokine Interleukin-6. *American Journal of Geriatric Psychiatry*, 19, 64–71.

McCurry, S. M., Gibbons, L. E., Logsdon, R. G., Vitiello, M. V., & Teri, L. (2005). Nighttime insomnia treatment and education for Alzheimer's disease: A randomized controlled trial. *Journal of the American Geriatric Society*, 53(5), 793–802.

MetLife Mature Market Institute, (2011). The MetLife study of caregiving costs to working caregivers: Double jeopardy for baby boomers caring for their parents. Availale from: <www.caregiving.org/research/impact-of-caregiving>. Accessed 16.06.14.

Mittelman, M. S., Roth, D. L., Coon, D. W., & Haley, W. E. (2004). Sustained benefit of supportive intervention for depressive symptoms in caregivers of patients with Alzheimer's disease. *American Journal of Psychiatry*, 161(5), 850–856.

Moore, R. C., Chattillion, E. A., Ceglowski, J., Ho, J., von Känel, R., Mills, P. J., et al. (2013). A randomized clinical trial of Behavioral Activation (BA) therapy for improving psychological and physical health in dementia caregivers: Results of the Pleasant Events Program (PEP). *Behaviour Research and Therapy*, 51, 623–632.

National Alliance for Caregiving and AARP, (2009). *Caregiving in the U.S.: A focused look at those caring for someone age 50 or older*. Bethesda, MD: National Alliance for Caregiving, Washington, DC.

Pearlin, L. I., Nguyen, K. B., Schieman, S., & Milkie, M. A. (2007). The life-course origins of mastery among older people. *Journal of Health and Social Behavior*, 48, 164–179.

Rothman, R. L., DeWalt, D. A., Malone, R., Bryant, B., Shintani, A., Crigler, B., et al. (2004). Influence of patient literacy on the effectiveness of a primary care-based diabetes disease management program. *Journal of the American Medical Association*, 292(14), 1711–1716.

Schillinger, D., Piette, J., Grumbach, K., Wang, F., Daher, C., Leong-Grotz, K., et al. (2003). Closing the loop: Physician communication with diabetic patients who have low health literacy. *Archives of Internal Medicine*, 163(1), 83–90.

Skaff, M. M., & Pearlin, L. I. (1992). Caregiving: Role engulfment and the loss of self. *Gerontologist*, 32, 656–664.

Sörensen, S., Pinquart, M., & Duberstein, P. (2002). How effective are interventions with caregivers? An updated meta-analysis. *Gerontologist*, 42, 356–372.

Teri, L., Gibbons, L. E., McCurry, S. M., Logsdon, R. G., Buchner, D. M., Barlow, W. E., et al. (2003). Exercise plus behavioral management in patients with Alzheimer disease: A randomized control trial. *Journal of the American Medical Association*, 290, 2015–2022.

Teri, L., Logsdon, R. G., Uomoto, J., & McCurry, S. M. (1997). Behavioral treatment of depression in dementia patients: A controlled clinical trial. *Journals of Gerontology Series B-Psychological Sciences and Social Sciences, 52B*(4), 159–P166.

Teri, L., Truax, P., Logsdon, R., Uomoto, J., Zarit, S. H., & Vitaliano, P. P. (1992). Assessment of behavioral problems in dementia: The revised memory and behavior problems checklist. *Psychology and Aging, 7*, 622–631.

von Känel, R., Mills, P. J., Mausbach, B. T., Dimsdale, J. E., Patterson, T. L., Ziegler, M. G., et al. (2012). Effect of Alzheimer caregiving on circulating levels of C-reactive protein and other biomarkers relevant to cardiovascular disease risk: A longitudinal study. *Gerontology, 58*, 354–365.

Whitlatch, C. J., Zarit, S. H., & von Eye, A. (1991). Efficacy of interventions with caregivers: A reanalysis. *Gerontologist, 31*, 9–14.

Zarit, S. H., & Femia, E. E. (2008a). A future for family care and dementia intervention research? Challenges and strategies. *Aging and Mental Health, 12*(1), 5–13.

Zarit, S. H., & Femia, E. E. (2008b). Behavioral and psychosocial interventions for family caregivers. *American Journal of Nursing, 108*(9, supp.), 47–53.

Zarit, S. H., & Whitlatch, C. (1992). Institutional placement: Phases of the transition. *The Gerontologist, 32*, 665–672.

Zarit, S. H., & Zarit, J. M. (2007). *Mental disorders in older adults* (2nd ed.). New York, NY: Guilford Press.

Zarit, S. H., Orr, N. K., & Zarit, J. M. (1985). *The hidden victims of Alzheimer's Disease: Families under stress*. New York: NYU Press.

Zarit, S. H., Todd, P. A., & Zarit, J. M. (1986). Subjective burden of husbands and wives as caregivers: A longitudinal study. *The Gerontologist, 26*, 260–270.

Zarit, S. H., Stephens, M. A. P., Townsend, A., & Greene, R. (1998). Stress reduction for family caregivers: Effects of day care use. *Journal of Gerontology: Social Sciences, 53B*, S267–S277.

Zarit, S. H., Femia, E. E., Kim, K., & Whitlatch, C. J. (2010). The structure of risk factors and outcomes for family caregivers: Implications for assessment and treatment. *Aging and Mental Health, 14*, 220–231.

Zarit, S. H., Kim, K., Femia, E. E., Almeida, D. M., Savla, J., & Molenaar, P. C. M. (2011). Effects of adult day care on daily stress of caregivers: A within person approach. *Journal of Gerontology: Psychological Sciences, 66B*, 538–547.

Zarit, S. H., Kim, K., Femia, E. E., Almeida, D. M., & Klein, L. C. (2013). The effects of adult day services on family caregivers' daily stress, affect and health: Outcomes from the DaSH Study. *The Gerontologist, 54*(4), 570–579.

Zarit, S. H., Whetzel, C. A., Kim, K., Femia, E. E., Almeida, D. M., Rovine, M. J., et al. (2014). Daily stressors and adult day service use by family caregivers: Effects on depressive symptoms, positive mood and DHEA-S. *American Journal of Geriatric Psychiatry* http://dx.doi.org/10.1016/j.jagp.2014.01.013.

Attitudes, Beliefs, and Behavior

Benjamin A. Bensadon

Charles E. Schmidt College of Medicine, Florida Atlantic University,
Boca Raton, Florida, USA

INTRODUCTION

Robust empirical evidence linking beliefs and behavior has been accumulating for several decades. Underpinning this research are psychological concepts including Bandura's theory of self-efficacy (Bandura, 1997), perhaps the most widely referenced and empirically supported. Central to this theory is that individuals' perceived competence (i.e., confidence, or self-efficacy) correlates directly and uniquely with their actual behavior. The greater a person's self-efficacy, the more apt he or she is to view novel tasks as challenging rather than threatening, and the more likely he or she is to persevere in the face of setbacks. Conversely, those who do not feel self-efficacious in a particular domain tend to avoid related tasks out of fear. Simply put, self-efficacy represents the bridge between beliefs and behavior.

Stereotypes constitute another type of belief shown to influence behavior. In 1954, Harvard psychologist Gordon Allport dedicated an entire text to the inherently human nature of prejudice (Allport, 1954). Fifteen years later geriatric physician Robert Butler applied these concepts to the elderly by coining the term ageism (Butler, 1969). He later expanded this in a seminal critique aptly titled *Why Survive? Being Old in America* (Butler, 1975) and was appointed director of the National Institute on Aging (NIA) of the National Institutes of Health (NIH) before going on to establish the first academic department of geriatric medicine in 1982 at New York's Mt. Sinai School of Medicine.

Research psychologists have since devised and tested several theories of stereotype impact. Two prominent examples within the geriatric population are self-stereotyping (e.g., Levy, 1996; Levy, 2000) and stereotype threat (e.g., Steele & Aronson, 1995; Steele, 1997). Although challenging

B. Bensadon (Ed): Psychology and Geriatrics.
DOI: http://dx.doi.org/10.1016/B978-0-12-420123-1.00003-4

to simulate in a laboratory setting, emerging evidence has shown that aging stereotypes can directly impact behavior. Generally, published results have demonstrated behavior-enhancing effects of positive aging stereotypes and inhibitory effects, both direct and indirect (via anxiety), of negative aging stereotypes. Measured behavioral outcomes have included gait speed, handwriting quality, and even will to live (Levy, 2003).

The above evidence has largely involved research with community-dwelling (aka nonclinical) samples of the older population. While these findings are valuable in their own right, as shown below, they are just as relevant to geriatric medicine, though common professional silos and lack of integration make this less obvious.

CLINICAL RELEVANCE

Levy and colleagues (2014) recently found older people who hold more negative aging self-stereotypes had a 50% higher chance of being hospitalized over a 10-year period than those holding more positive self-stereotypes. Their earlier study with the same sample, published in *Journal of the American Medical Association* (*JAMA*), found older people holding more positive age stereotypes were 44% more likely to fully recover from disability (Levy, Slade, Murphy, & Gill, 2012). Analogously, an earlier study by Levy and colleagues reported positive age stereotypes can help reduce cardiovascular stress (Levy, Hausdorff, Hencke, & Wei, 2000). This is particularly important in light of her more recent work, which, along with geriatrician and NIA Scientific Director Luigi Ferrucci, found that negative age stereotypes held early in life actually predicted cardiovascular events up to 38 years later (Levy, Zonderman, Slade, & Ferrucci, 2009). This link between beliefs and cardiovascular health has been demonstrated for many decades. Cardiologists in the 1950s posited, tested, and demonstrated links between "type A" behavior and cardiac risk (Friedman & Rosenman, 1959). In fact, findings were convincing enough for the authors to write an entire book 15 years later titled *Type A Behavior and Your Heart* (Friedman & Rosenman, 1974). As noted earlier in this publication, psychologists and cardiologists may collaborate for research purposes (e.g., National Heart, Lung, & Blood Institute), but rarely is their clinical care integrated.

MEMORY

The belief–behavior link and benefit of integration are particularly relevant to cognitive aging. Scientific terms such as "demented" and "senile" are commonly used colloquially, mainly to describe older people unfavorably. The content of most aging-based stereotypes pertains to memory and cognition. Not surprisingly, these beliefs are often internalized by elders themselves, and can directly influence their self-evaluations of aging (Kotter-Gruhn, & Hess, 2012). In fact, some older adults rely on their perceived memory function to gauge their overall (not just cognitive) health, and the memory domain holds increasing salience as people age (Dark-Freudeman, West, & Viverito, 2006). This trend becomes more critical when considering the decades of evidence linking subjective self-report measures of health and subsequent mortality (e.g., DeSalvo, Bloser, Reynolds, He, & Muntner, 2006; Idler & Benyamini, 1997; Mossey & Shapiro, 1982). Notably, Desalvo and Muntner (2011) analyzed related data on nearly 15,000 Americans and found not only did people's perceived health differ from their physicians' perceptions, but those who believed their health was worse than their physicians believed actually experienced higher rates of mortality.

Memory-related self-efficacy (MSE) has been measured in different ways, but the Memory Self-Efficacy Questionnaire (MSEQ; Berry, West, & Dennehy, 1989) is most closely aligned with the theory. This tool uses 10-point Likert scales to assess an individual's confidence in performing specific tasks of varying difficulty. These include remembering names of faces, locations of objects, excerpts from a short story, and items from a shopping list. Over several decades, psychologist and MSEQ co-author Dr. Robin West and colleagues have empirically tested the MSE-memory performance relationship (e.g., West, Bagwell, & Dark-Freudeman, 2005, 2008; West, Crook, & Barron, 1992; West, Dark-Freudeman, & Bagwell, 2009; West, Dennehy-Basile, & Norris, 1996; West, Thorn, & Bagwell, 2003; West, Welch, & Knabb, 2002; West, Welch, & Thorn, 2001; West & Yassuda, 2004). Two consistent trends have emerged from this research: 1) Memory self-efficacy and memory performance tend to decline with age, and 2) actual memory performance tends to improve as memory self-efficacy increases.

Importantly, negative aging-related stereotypes can harm memory self-efficacy, especially because stereotype content is often cognition or memory-specific. Levy's early work demonstrated the direct impact of aging self-stereotypes on memory performance (e.g., Levy & Langer, 1994). Psychologist Tom Hess and colleagues (2003, 2004, 2006, 2009) have also measured the "threat" to cognition induced by these stereotypes. Comparatively few studies (e.g., Bensadon, 2010) have examined the impact of both mechanisms – age stereotypes and MSE – on each other and older adult memory performance. What is clear, however, based on the preponderance of evidence, is that aging-related beliefs and perceptions do influence health and behavior, and memory is particularly susceptible.

"Anti-Dementia" Therapy

At the same time, a proliferation of medical research has focused on neurocognitive disorders such as Alzheimer's disease, now the sixth leading cause of death nationwide and fifth among those aged 65 years and older (Centers for Disease Control and Prevention). Unfortunately, decades of costly drug trials targeting beta amyloid protein have yielded very limited evidence of benefit (Friedrich, 2012). Similarly, effectiveness of pharmacotherapy with acetylcholinesterase inhibitors (AChEI) or N-methyl-D-aspartate (NMDA) antagonists for those with Alzheimer's and related dementias (ADRD) is also limited. Literature reviews of other drugs, such as statins, have demonstrated no cognitive benefit (e.g., McGuinness et al., 2013) and some disturbing side effects (Bruckert, Hayem, Dejager, Yau, & Begaud, 2005; Golomb, McGraw, Evans, & Dimsdale, 2007). Interestingly, some of these side effects have been cognitive in nature and discontinuation of statin therapy has even led to reported reversal of dementia or Alzheimer's diagnosis (Evans & Golomb, 2009). Furthermore, efficacy of "anti-dementia" drugs is generally defined by statistically significant improvements on measures of cognitive status, such as the widely used Mini Mental State Examination (Folstein, Folstein, & McHugh, 1975). Their clinical significance, and relevance to daily life, is unclear. Thus, the most modifiable aspects of these devastating illnesses may actually be psychosocial.

Based on this evidence, some physicians have recommended abandoning the focus on amyloid entirely in order to explore new options, including more immediately available nonpharmacologic, behavioral approaches (e.g., George & Whitehouse, 2014). While such interventions have shown promise, particularly in terms of supporting family caregivers (Chien et al., 2011; Thompson et al., 2007), their integration with standard dementia care remains suboptimal, and community-based advocacy groups struggle to fill this gap (Reuben et al., 2009). Importantly, related insight is not routine in medical practice, though some physicians (e.g., Reuben et al., 2010) have openly recognized this, referring to "inadequate knowledge of physicians about community resources and behavioral management needed for optimal care for patients with dementia. ... Moreover, there is little time during the office visit for physicians to provide counseling and support for caregivers" (pp. 324–5).

Resistance to a change in course regarding the amyloid cascade hypothesis is not surprising given the enormous financial and human resources already invested. In fact, it was psychologists Amos Tversky and Daniel Kahneman (1974) whose seminal article in the journal *Science*, "Judgment under Uncertainty: Heuristics and Biases," established a cognitive basis for common human errors in judgment and decision-making. Kahneman was awarded a Nobel Prize for his work and the above article has been cited more than 29,000 times. Inspired by this research, other psychologists (e.g., Arkes & Blumer, 1985) have more explicitly defined and measured the "sunk cost effect," or tendency for people to continue an endeavor once significant investments have been made, even if, objectively, desired results are unlikely to be achieved without a change. While medicine and science emphasize rationality, human decision-making remains inherently subjective, an admission directly addressed by Cain and Detsky (2008) in a *JAMA* commentary titled "Everyone's a Little Bit Biased (Even Physicians)."

Caregiver Burden

In the absence of effective pharmacotherapy and with the help of psychology-geriatrics integration (Dunkin & Anderson-Hanley, 1998), physicians have begun to recognize the clinically relevant and susceptible nature of caregiver health. This extends beyond dementia, as evidenced by a recent *JAMA* clinical review of caregiver burden (Adelman, Tmanova, Delgado, Dion, & Lachs, 2014). These authors' stated objectives were: "to outline the epidemiology of caregiver burden; to provide strategies to diagnose, assess, and intervene for caregiver burden in clinical practice; and to evaluate evidence on interventions intended to avert or mitigate caregiver burden and related caregiver distress" (p. 1052). Notably, the team of authors represented an array of educational backgrounds – two physicians, one veterinarian, one library scientist, and one holding a bachelor's degree. Interestingly and significantly, it did not include a psychologist. Encouragingly though, the authors identified depression, social isolation, and lack of choice in being a caregiver as risk factors for burden. They also quantified comparable "mild to modest efficacy" for both psychosocial and pharmacologic interventions. But perhaps most informative was their final result:

> "Many studies showed improvements in caregiver burden-associated symptoms (e.g., mood, coping, self-efficacy), even when caregiver burden itself was minimally improved."

This crucial distinction between objective vs. subjective burden fits precisely with the core tenets of Bandura's and other psychologists' long-standing theories. While the "objective" situation matters, so too does an individual's perceived (i.e., "subjective") ability to respond, which then contributes to the actual behavioral response that follows. Many people will be burdened with the caregiving role, but not all will experience that role as "burden." Related health correlates (physical and mental) and perceived coping ability will vary by individual. Intrusiveness, be it of caregiving duties or of one's own illness, pertains to beliefs (e.g., Hundt et al., 2013). Most importantly, from an intervention standpoint, these authors' meta-analysis showed that associated beliefs can be modified (by psychosocial and psychoeducational interventions) even when the situation cannot.

As elucidated in this publication's caregiving chapter, perceived caregiver burden and subsequent decisions to institutionalize care recipients do not necessarily correlate with severity of dementia-related behavioral problems (e.g., Zarit, Reever, & Bach-Peterson, 1980; Zarit, Todd, & Zarit, 1986). Unfortunately, this concept was not emphasized in the *JAMA* review. Instead, the authors concluded that physicians must recognize and assess burden, and offered specific questions ("discussion catalysts") by which to do so.

Taken together, the above examples demonstrate that for patients, family members, and their providers, especially with regard to cognitive aging, subjective beliefs and perceptions matter. Unfortunately, many medical experts in neurology, psychiatry, and geriatrics, along with "stakeholders" from diagnostic imaging and pharmaceutical industries, appear unaware of this scientific evidence. Instead, their attention has focused on identifying disease markers via earlier screening and diagnosis, regardless of the absence of evidence to support their value. A plethora of diagnostic equipment (e.g., Beta-Amyloid Positron Emission Tomography) and terminology such as cognitive impairment no dementia (CIND), age-associated memory impairment (AAMI), and mild cognitive impairment (MCI), have followed.

Mild Cognitive Impairment

The term MCI, popularized by Mayo Clinic neurologist Ronald Petersen and colleagues in the 1990s (Petersen, Smith, Ivnik, Tangalos, & Kokmen, 1994; Petersen, Smith, Waring, et al., 1999; Smith, et al., 1996), is increasingly *believed*, though not proven, to be a "prodromal" form of dementia, an intermediate stage between normal cognition and eventual dementia (see review by Bensadon & Odenheimer, 2013). Those favoring this classification emphasize the prudence of earlier identification of those at risk for developing Alzheimer's disease and related disorders (e.g., Gauthier et al., 2006; Petersen et al., 2009). This label remains controversial, however, as data from population-based studies have consistently shown that many individuals diagnosed with MCI do not progress to dementia and may even revert back to premorbid, baseline (aka "normal") functioning (Perri, Carlesimo, Serra, & Caltagirone, 2009; Perri, Serra, Carlesimo, & Caltagirone, 2007). Data revealing similar prognostic uncertainty have been published by Petersen and colleagues (2014) themselves, yet they continue to believe that MCI always has prognostic value (e.g., Roberts,

Knopman, Mielke, Cha, Pankratz, et al., 2014). Despite the evidence, or absence thereof, very few physicians have concluded that MCI, as currently measured, is not a clinical entity and therefore should not be treated (e.g., Gauthier & Touchon, 2005).

A notable exception is the Food and Drug Administration (FDA). Given the lack of diagnostic clarity, there is currently no FDA-approved medication to prevent or treat MCI symptoms or progression, and both medical and psychological research have shown limited to no relationship between subjective memory complaint and objective memory performance. Instead, such complaints are more likely evidence of depression and low MSE mentioned earlier, than impaired cognition. This insight has led some to advocate removing subjective complaint from MCI diagnostic criteria (Lenehan, Klekociuk, & Summers, 2012). Nonetheless, in medical practice, "anti-dementia" drugs such as statins, AchEI, or Memantine, an NMDA antagonist – each of which has shown limited efficacy (e.g., Raschetti, Albanese, Vanacore, & Maggini, 2007) but consistent adverse side effects – continue to be prescribed "off label" for MCI management (Weinstein, Barton, Ross, Kramer, & Yaffe, 2009). In contrast, potentially beneficial behavioral interventions targeting self-efficacy enhancement or cognitive rehabilitation – shown to improve confidence and quality of life (Greenaway, Duncan, & Smith, 2013; Kurz, Pohl, Ramsenthaler, & Sorg, 2009; Regan & Varanelli, 2013) while posing little to no risk of harm – remain rare.

The potential harm of this failure to integrate medical and behavioral approaches is not limited to geriatric patients and their families. In fact, a recent *JAMA* article promoted future trials of pharmacologic therapeutics aimed at "cognitively healthy but at-risk populations" (Friedrich, 2014). Because the number one known risk factor for Alzheimer's disease is advanced age, the above description of "at-risk" includes us all. Should the entire nation really receive pharmacotherapy "just in case?" Physicians are not likely to become familiar with the aforementioned impact of psychological variables on cognition, including memory-related anxiety, confidence (self-efficacy), and even stereotypes. Collaboration with psychologists, on the other hand, might well enable a more comprehensive understanding and ability to differentiate between clinical (i.e., pathological) and nonclinical (normative) patterns of cognitive aging.

BEYOND COGNITION

The relevance of patient beliefs to behavior extends well beyond cognition. Nearly 30 years ago psychologist Ann O'Leary reviewed the literature identifying self-efficacy's role as mediator between health behavior interventions and their subsequent benefits (O'Leary, 1985). Interventions targeted smoking cessation relapse, pain management, eating and weight control, and recovery from myocardial infarction. Recently investigators have targeted self-management of chronic diseases such as hypertension, diabetes mellitus, heart disease, and arthritis. In a 2001 study, nurse Kate Lorig and colleagues (including Dr. Bandura himself) followed for 2 years a sample of 831 participants with history of heart disease, arthritis, or lung disease. Compared to a control group, participants trained in a chronic disease self-management program (CDSMP) showed significant increases in perceived self-efficacy and reductions in health distress, fewer visits to physicians or emergency rooms.

Primary care medicine has also taken notice. A year later physicians joined Lorig in publishing a *JAMA* article that articulated the insepa-rable relationship between patient self-efficacy and chronic disease self-management (Bodenheimer, Lorig, Holman, & Grumbach, 2002). In the 12 years since its publication, the article has been cited nearly 2000 times. CDC psychologist Teresa Brady and colleagues meta-analyzed 23 CDSMP studies and found program participants showed significant improve-ments in aerobic exercise, cognitive symptom management, stretching/strengthening exercise, and psychological health up to 1 year after base-line, compared to nonparticipants (Brady et al., 2013).

ADHERENCE

A vital and challenging concern likely to benefit from integrating behavioral and biomedical approaches to care is medication nonad-herence, a prevalent behavior of epidemic proportions. Recent pub-lications of the American Medical Association and American College of Physicians have acknowledged the associated costs – in terms of both health and economics (e.g., Butterfield, 2014; Zullig, Peterson, & Bosworth, 2013). While complex and multifactorial in nature, adherence is a *behavior*. Consistent with the above examples, beliefs and adherence go hand in hand. Examples of relevant patient and physician beliefs are listed in Boxes 3.1 and 3.2.

As referenced earlier in this chapter, Zullig and colleagues recognized the clinical relevance of patient self-efficacy, referring to it by name in a recent *JAMA* article on successful ingredients for improving medica-tion adherence. Yet nationally, the clinicians depended upon to translate these concepts and related theories into practice continue unfortunately to exclude psychologists, and include physicians, nurse practitioners (NP), and more recently, pharmacists. Below is a letter to the editor several col-leagues and I submitted in response.

BOX 3.1

COMMON PATIENT BELIEFS AFFECTING ADHERENCE

About Physician

- Prescribing physician is (not) an expert.
- Prescribing physician cares about me.
- Prescribing physician wants me to get better.
- Prescribing physician knows why I am sick.
- Prescribing physician knows how I can get better.
- Prescribing physician is someone I can trust.
- Prescribing physician is someone I should trust.
- Prescribing physician trusts me.
- Prescribing physician likes me.
- Prescribing physician will (not) become angry if I do not take medication properly.

About Self

- I am (not) capable of understanding what to do to get better.
- I am (not) motivated to do what is necessary to get better.
- I (don't) deserve to get better.
- I want to get better and don't want to be sick.
- Eventually I will get better.
- I may never get better.

About Illness/Medication

- Even if I don't feel symptoms, I am still sick.
- Taking medication as directed will (not) help me.
- Benefits of medication (don't) outweigh the side-effects.
- If I (don't) take medication I will be worse off.
- No one really understands my illness-related pain.
- No one really knows what is wrong with me.
- Long-term side effects of medication are (not) dangerous.

BOX 3.2

COMMON PHYSICIAN BELIEFS AFFECTING ADHERENCE

About Patient

- Patient needs and wants my expertise.
- Patient knows and feels I care about him/her.
- Patient wants help to get better.
- Patient does (not) know why he/she is sick.
- Patient will trust that I know how he/she can get better.
- Patient will listen and respect me.
- Patient must and will adhere to my recommendations.
- Patient needs me in order to get better.
- Patient must automatically trust me.
- Patient does trust me to help.
- Patient can (not) afford and access medication.
- Patient can (not) follow directions appropriately.
- Patient likes me.
- If patient does not take medication as prescribed, this shows he/she doesn't want to get better.
- If patient does adhere to my directions, he/she will improve.
- If patient wants to get better, he/she will follow my advice.
- Patients always lie and cannot be trusted to take medication appropriately.

About Self

- I should be respected.
- I am empathic when trying to help patients.
- I am capable of helping most patients.
- I care equally about all patients.
- Patient background and sociocultural factors do not influence how I see the patient.
- My decisions about medication are objective.
- Once I've prescribed medication and educated the patient, I have done my job.
- I cannot control whether patients take their medication.
- I should not have to control whether patients take their medication.
- I am unlikely to change a patient's behavior.
- My role in supporting adherence is vital.

continued

BOX 3.2   *(Cont'd)*

- My clinical behavior will influence whether a patient trusts me and follows my advice.

About Illness/Medication

- Benefits of medication (don't) outweigh the side-effects.
- Medication cannot be effective if it is not taken (appropriately).
- Efficacy of medication can only be trusted if shown in randomized controlled trials.
- It is easier to change medication than lifestyle.
- Adherence difficulty is (not) part of illness.

We commend the authors and journal for providing this much-needed list of "ingredients" for improving medication adherence. The article clearly demonstrates psychological insight into patient behavior, not surprising since the senior author is a psychologist. Adherence strategies and target outcomes are elucidated – "behavioral change and intervention strategies, managing patient perceptions, and supportive counseling" are all made explicit. The role of psychologists, however, is not. In fact, psychologists are never mentioned. Instead, physicians, nurse practitioners, and pharmacists are identified as the clinicians accountable for behavioral health. In terms of access, this makes sense, but in terms of training, it may not.

Cost concerns and other factors continue to impede the delivery of integrated services. Currently, routine care generally includes patient contact with the aforementioned clinicians. Thus, they are, as the authors show, well-positioned to improve adherence. This standard of care does not include patient contact with clinical psychologists, whose precise focus is, in fact, managing behavior (including adherence). But perhaps it should. The authors target patient self-efficacy, an appropriate outcome of supportive counseling, given longstanding evidence linking self-efficacy to health-related behavior. But are physicians, nurse practitioners, and pharmacists adequately informed about this psychological construct theorized by a psychologist? If they are unfamiliar, who will help translate this theory into clinical practice?

Now more than ever, academic medicine has recognized the link between behavior and health. Most notably, the Medical College Admissions Test (MCAT) will expand in 2015 to include psychological and behavioral science content for the first time in history. Though promising, practice implications are unknown. But if clinical psychologists do not provide direct patient care, nor help train those who do, can we truly expect suboptimal adherence rates to improve?

Physician Michel Burnier and colleagues (2013) took quite a different perspective in their published review of drug adherence in resistant hypertension, informed by their belief that patients will never adequately take their medication on their own. They propose as a "solution" the avoidance of medication entirely, and instead, performance by physicians of invasive procedures (baroreflex stimulation and renal denervation). Further, if the procedures prove ineffective (which to date they have), their next recommended step is to perform them earlier. Integration to enhance physician-patient partnerships and implement well-established communication and behavioral management approaches such as motivational interviewing (e.g., Miller, 1982; Knight, McGowan, Dickens, & Bundy, 2006; Madson, Loignon, & Lane, 2009; Smedslund et al., 2011) are not considered. Again, as with the earlier cognitive aging examples, the prevailing attitude among many physicians is an *earlier and/or procedure-based* rather than *integrated* approach. To optimally treat the whole patient, this belief system must change (e.g., Bensadon, 2014).

To be clear, it is extremely encouraging to note the medical profession is beginning to recognize the behavioral and psychosocial (i.e., psychological) impact, needs, and management options associated with medical illness. Geriatric patients in particular, for whom polypharmacy and multimorbidity are common, can benefit greatly from nonpharmacologic options in terms of both safety and quality of life. Yet when it comes to care provision, clinical psychologists are consistently and conspicuously absent. While the above articles are on the right track, calling for nonpsychologists to ask screening questions about mood, translate psychological theory into practice, and recognize the often subtle cues of caregiving-associated psychological burden, are not sufficient to influence physicians' beliefs and practice behavior.

UNCOMFORTABLE DISCUSSIONS

As with adherence, well-intentioned but ineffective management recommendations for physicians surround the frequency and quality of "uncomfortable" discussion about end of life, driving cessation, and suicide. Decades of evidence have shown that in medical practice, each has been and remains suboptimal (Ahluwalia, Levin, Lorenz, & Gordon, 2013; Hofmann et al., 1997; Tulsky, Fischer, Rose, & Arnold, 1998). Nonetheless, while some physicians have advocated for an interdisciplinary approach to address the behavioral aspects of care (e.g., Carr & Ott, 2010), and revealed their own low self-confidence or self-efficacy beliefs in these areas (e.g., Brown & Ott, 2004; Jang et al., 2007), enhanced clinical integration is generally not emphasized. Rather, to address these challenges, the focus continues to be utility and perpetual refinement of decision aids, algorithms, and other research "tools" (e.g., Lee, Brummel-Smith, Meyer, Drew, & London, 2000; Lau, Cloutier-Fisher, Kuziemsky, Black, Downing, Borycki, et al., 2007). Evidence suggests this approach is misguided.

More than a decade has passed since the American Medical Association first published formal guidelines for physician assessment of older drivers in 2003 but a 2013 literature review of such assessment found no evidence of benefit (Martin, Marottoli, O'Neill, 2013). A 1997 review article evaluated 20 "new" suicide assessment instruments (Range & Knott, 1997) but about 10 years later as many as 83% of people completing suicides were seen but apparently neither recognized nor adequately managed as suicidal by a primary care physician within the same year of their death and 66% within the same month (Mann et al., 2005). A 2007 review of measures of end-of-life care and outcomes asssessed 261 measures described in only a 15-year time frame (Mularski et al., 2007). Yet patients' end-of-life care needs, especially when psychosocial more than medical, continue to go largely unmet (e.g., Davison, 2010; Hanson, Danis, & Garrett, 1997).

While multiple factors may contribute to this disturbing clinical picture, one common theme remains constant. When it comes to clinical communication about psychologically uncomfortable areas of care such as driving cessation, end of life and suicide, it appears effective tools, while important in *theory*, are insufficient in *practice* (see Chapters 7–9). Clinical integration with psychologists, the professionals most thoroughly trained to not only understand but effectively manage human behavior, should help.

PHYSICIAN BELIEFS

As clarified above, it is not just patients and caregivers who are guided by their beliefs. Unwavering allegiance to amyloid theories of dementia mentioned earlier represent but one piece of evidence that physicians, like nonphysicians, are similarly influenced. In a 1960 issue of *JAMA*, Newman and Nichols measured sexual activity and attitudes among older people and concluded that older people remain sexually interested and active in later life but declining health often coincides with declining sexual activity. Their take-home message for physicians was that discussion of sexual behavior should be standard in geriatric care, but all too often it is avoided. Underlying this message was a key psychological insight. Unlike other less socially stigmatized health concerns, sex is less likely to be introduced by older patients if their physician does not explicitly communicate (i.e., give permission) that doing so is acceptable. The likelihood that patients will raise the topic decreases further if they sense physicians' discomfort or worse yet, disapproval. More recent calls to address the topic (e.g., Wilson, 2003), suggest it is just as relevant and apparently difficult to heed half a century later.

Lindau and colleagues (2007) measured sexuality and health among 3005 older people aged 57–85 years old. Their data showed that prevalence of sexual activity declined with age but more than half the sample aged 65–74 was sexually active as were more than 25% of those 75–85 years old. While about half the entire sample reported at least one bothersome problem related to sexual function, only 38% of the men and 22% of the women reported ever discussing sex with their physician after turning age 50. In this context of "don't ask, don't tell" it is not surprising to learn that reported cases of both syphilis and chlamydia among adults aged 45–64 nearly tripled between 2000 and 2010 (Centers for Disease Control & Prevention). Particularly troubling and directly related is recent evidence that HIV diagnosis is more likely to come later among older patients than younger patients (e.g., Linley et al., 2012). Taylor and Gosney (2011) reviewed the literature on geriatric sexuality and concluded that clinicians' decisions about whether to discuss sex are largely informed by their own personal attitudes, value systems, and beliefs in stereotypes. Psychiatrists are no less vulnerable to such bias and when evaluating depressed patients may be less likely to elicit a sexual history from older than younger individuals (Bouman & Arcelus, 2001).

Physician belief-behavior links have been found in many other aspects of care. Harris and colleagues (2009) compared the views of primary care physicians (internists vs. family physicians) toward dementia care relative to other conditions. Among their key findings, compared to internists, family physicians more strongly believed they could improve quality of life among older patients with dementia. Not surprisingly, they also more strongly agreed that older patients should be routinely screened for dementia. Epstein and colleagues (1984) found correlations between physician attitudes about cost and placebo effects and their actual prescribing behavior. Pittet and colleagues (2004) found physician adherence to hand hygiene behavior was associated with their personal beliefs about being a role model for other colleagues, about whether they perceived hand hygiene as a behavioral norm and that nonadherence was risky, and whether they held a positive attitude toward such practice after patient contact. In a national sample, fewer primary care physicians screened for domestic violence than they did for other risks and fewer believed they knew how to screen or intervene, or that such interventions could be as successful as those for other health risks such as tobacco and HIV (Gerbert et al., 2002).

In truth, the challenge of influencing physician behavior has been documented for decades. Davis and colleagues (1995) reviewed the literature of education strategies aimed at changing physician performance and health care outcomes from 1975 to 1994. Among the 160 interventions reviewed, specific strategies included reminders, patient-mediated interventions, outreach visits, opinion leaders, and multifactorial approaches. On the whole, most strategies were ineffective at creating behavior change. Bloom's (2005) review of 26 systematic reviews yielded a similar conclusion. Many physicians, themselves, have recognized the multifactorial nature of behavior change and the fact that interventions relying primarily on information alone, such as continuing medical education credits, is unlikely to suffice (Grimshaw et al., 2001; Shearn, 2001). At the system level, attempts to mitigate the risk of physicians' own "nonadherence" to best practice guidelines (Cabana et al., 1999; Cohen, Halvorson, & Gosselink, 1994) have led to an aggressive push toward the practice of evidence-based medicine (EBM) in vogue today (Sackett, Rosenberg, Gray, Haynes, & Richardson, 1996).

Consistent with this chapter's theme, physicians' beliefs and behavior, like those of non-physicians, appear inseparable. Indeed, Street and colleagues (2003) have shown that both physician and patient beliefs about control, and the respective behaviors that follow, influence each other during medical encounters. To help physicians recognize their beliefs and positively influence their behaviors, integrated programs in schools of medicine are beginning to take shape (e.g., Bensadon & Odenheimer, 2014b; Bensadon, Teasdale, & Odenheimer, 2013).

SENSITIZING LEARNERS TO CHRONIC DISEASE IMPACT: THE OKLAHOMA EXPERIENCE

Effective integration with psychology, especially when physicians are still training (undergraduate and graduate) and developing their practice-related beliefs and behaviors, allows them to be *shown rather than told* what to do. For example, at the University of Oklahoma College of Medicine, in an effort to sensitize future physicians to the impact of incurable chronic, neurodegenerative disease on both patients and their caregivers, we exposed fourth-year medical students to two dementia support groups – one for those carrying the diagnosis, one for their caregivers – as part of a required geriatrics clerkship (see Bensadon & Odenheimer, 2014a). Each group's duration was 1.5 hours, and topics discussed included positive and negative experiences with the medical system. To assess student impact, we created and administered a brief anonymous survey to be completed immediately after the group, and asked students to submit a brief reflection essay within 48 hours.

Overall, most students were astounded. In their essays they explicitly acknowledged a large training gap that this experience filled, and some pointed out this impact was felt both in their head (i.e., cognitively) and in their gut (i.e., affectively). Interestingly, a growing body of literature has established this connection, often referred to by gastroenterologists and neuroscientists as the gut-brain axis (e.g., Mayer, 2011).

Some students cried, some called their parents to "check in," and most thanked us for the experience, stating it reminded them of why they entered medicine in the first place. One student planning a career in surgery "confessed" via email that reading support group participant bios (circulated to students in advance) depressed him so intensely that he had to stop studying for the remainder of the evening. Our findings were particularly encouraging, given the widespread stereotypes (i.e., beliefs) within medical culture that clinical years of medical school inevitably lead to empathy erosion, and that surgery is an area of low sensitivity to begin with. Some data support these ideas (e.g., Bellini & Shea, 2005; Hojat et al., 2009; Tait, Chibnall, Luebbert, & Sutter, 2005), but our intervention and other data (e.g., Mangione et al., 2002) provide an important challenge to premature fatalism.

Our support group experience led many students to reveal their own, sometimes strong, biases, such as an expectation that the group would be a "pity party." But the intervention allowed even these students to spontaneously recognize and reflect on the inaccuracy of their preconceived notions, both about dementia and therapeutic support groups. This is particularly encouraging given the major stigma associated with both. It is also to be expected, given that most students' previous exposure to this illness was limited to textbooks, neuroimaging, or inpatient settings with advance-stage patients. Additionally, their previous exposure to behavioral therapy was limited and shaped largely by that of their physician models prior to the experience. In contrast, the high-functioning, young-onset community-dwellers and their caregivers were similar in age to the medical students' parents, another reason the exposure resonated personally with many learners. Without this evocative, community-based experience, medical trainee beliefs about neurodegenerative illness are likely skewed, something the students themselves were able to recognize via a relatively brief forum for introspection.

While promising, support group exposure for practicing physicians and those in training remains virtually nonexistent. However, related attempts to destigmatize and humanize dementia are beginning to surface throughout the country, often in the guise of "mentor" or "buddy" programs matching medical trainees with volunteers living with the disease. In 2013 medical schools launching such programs included Boston University, Dartmouth, Washington University in St Louis, Kansas University, and Albany Medical College (American College of Physicians, 2014). Other experiential learning approaches that provide early introductions to aging and geriatric medicine are discussed later in this publication.

Time will tell what impact such programs have on the attitudes, beliefs, and behavior of physicians, patients, and informal caregivers, but given the large number of chronic illness support groups nationally and the growing number of patients and families attending them to cope (Davison, Pennebaker, & Dickerson, 2000), their integration in medical training is warranted.

References

Adelman, R. D., Tmanova, L. L., Delgado, D., Dion, S., & Lachs, M. S. (2014). Caregiver burden: A clinical review. *Journal of the American Medical Association, 311*(10), 1052–1060.

Ahluwalia, S. C., Levin, J. R., Lorenz, K. A., & Gordon, H. S. (2013). "There's no cure for this condition": How physicians discuss advance care planning in heart failure. *Patient Education and Counseling, 91*(2), 200–205.

Allport, G. W. (1954). *The nature of prejudice.* Reading: Addison-Wesley.

American College of Physicians (2014). Alzheimer's patients preapre, enlighten future physicians. ACP Internist website. Retrieved from: <http://www.acpinternist.org/archives/2014/05/alzheimers.htm>.

Arkes, H. R., & Blumer, C. (1985). The psychology of sunk cost. *Organizational Behavior and Human Decision Processes, 35*(1), 124–140.

Bandura, A. (1977). Self-efficacy: Toward a unifying theory of behavioral change. *Psychological Review, 84*(2), 191–215.

Bellini, L. M., & Shea, J. A. (2005). Mood change and empathy decline persist during three years of internal medicine training. *Academic Medicine, 80*(2), 164–167.

Bensadon, B.A. (2010). *Memory self-efficacy and stereotype effects in aging.* (Unpublished doctoral dissertation). Available from ProQuest Dissertations and Theses database. (Order No. 856603225). University of Florida, Gainesville, Florida.

Bensadon, B. A. (2014). Maximizing treatment adherence: Physician-patient partnerships vs. procedures. *Hypertension, 63,* e7.

Bensadon, B. A., & Odenheimer, G. L. (2013). Current management decisions in mild cognitive impairment. *Clinics in Geriatric Medicine, 29*(4), 847–871.

Bensadon, B. A., & Odenheimer, G. L. (2014a). Understanding chronic disease: Student exposure to support groups. *Medical Education, 48*(5), 526–527.

Bensadon, B. A., & Odenheimer, G. L. (2014b). Listening to our elders: A story of resilience and recovery. *Patient Education and Counseling, 95*(3), 433–434.

Bensadon, B. A., Teasdale, T. A., & Odenheimer, G. L. (2013). Attitude adjustment: Shaping medical students' perceptions of older patients with a geriatrics curriculum. *Academic Medicine, 88*(11), 1630–1634.

Berry, J. M., West, R. L., & Dennehy, D. M. (1989). Reliability and validity of the memory self-efficacy questionnaire. *Developmental Psychology, 25*(5), 701–713.

Bloom, B. S. (2005). Effects of continuing medical education on improving physician clinical care and patient health: A review of systematic reviews. *International Journal of Technology Assessment in Health Care, 21*(3), 380–385.

Bodenheimer, T., Lorig, K., Holman, H., & Grumbach, K. (2002). Patient self-management of chronic disease in primary care. *Journal of the American Medical Association, 288*(19), 2469–2475.

Bouman, W. P., & Arcelus, J. (2001). Are psychiatrists guilty of ageism when it comes to taking a sexual history? *International Journal of Geriatric Psychiatry, 16,* 27–31.

Brady, T. J., Murphy, L., O'Colmain, B. J., Beauchesne, D., Daniels, B., Greenberg, M., et al. (2013). A meta-analysis of health status, health behaviors, and health care utilization outcomes of the chronic disease self-management program. *Preventing Chronic Disease, 10,* 120112.

Brown, L. B., & Ott, B. R. (2004). Driving and dementia: A review of the literature. *Journal of Geriatric Psychiatry & Neurology, 17*(4), 232–240.

Bruckert, E., Hayem, G., Dejager, S., Yau, C., & Begaud, B. (2005). Mild to moderate muscular symptoms with high-dosage statin therapy in hyperlipidemic patients – The primo study. *Cardiovascular Drugs and Therapy, 19*(6), 403–414.

Burnier, M., Wuerzner, G., Struijker-Boudier, H., & Urquhart, J. (2013). Measuring, analyzing, and managing drug adherence in resistant hypertension. *Hypertension, 62,* 218–225.

Butler, R. N. (1969). Ageism: Another form of bigotry. *Gerontologist, 9,* 243–246.

Butler, R. N. (1975). *Why Survive? Being Old in America*. New York: Harper & Row.

Butterfield, S. (2014, May). Treat the epidemic of medical nonadherence. ACP Internist website. Retrieved from: <http://www.acpinternist.org/archives/2014/05/nonadherence.htm>.

Cabana, M. D., Rand, C. S., Powe, N. R., Wu, A. W., Wilson, M. H., Abboud, P. A. C., et al. (1999). Why don't physicians follow clinical practice guidelines? A framework for improvement. *Journal of the American Medical Association, 282*(15), 1458–1465.

Cain, D. M., & Detsky, A. S. (2008). Everyone's a little bit biased (even physicians). *Journal of the American Medical Association, 299*(24), 2893–2895.

Carr, D. B., & Ott, B. R. (2010). The older adult driver with cognitive impairment "It's a very frustrating life.". *Journal of the American Medical Association, 303*(16), 1632–1641.

Chien, L. Y., Chu, H., Guo, J. L., Liao, Y. M., Chang, L. I., Chen, C. H., et al. (2011). Caregiver support groups in patients with dementia: a meta-analysis. *International Journal of Geriatric Psychiatry, 26*(10), 1089–1098.

Cohen, S. J., Halvorson, H. W., & Gosselink, C. A. (1994). Changing physician behavior to improve disease prevention. *Preventive Medicine, 23*(3), 284–291.

Dark-Freudeman, A., West, R. L., & Viverito, K. M. (2006). Future selves and aging: Older adults' memory fears. *Educational Gerontology, 32*(2), 85–109.

Davis, D. A., Thomson, M. A., Oxman, A. D., & Haynes, R. B. (1995). Changing physician performance: A systematic review of the effect of continuing medical education strategies. *Journal of the American Medical Association, 274*(9), 700–705.

Davison, K. P., Pennebaker, J. W., & Dickerson, S. S. (2000). Who talks? The social psychology of illness support groups. *American Psychologist, 55*(2), 205–217.

Davison, S. N. (2010). End-of-life care preferences and needs: Perceptions of patients with chronic kidney disease. *Clinical Journal of the American Society of Nephrology, 5*(2), 195–204.

DeSalvo, K. B., Bloser, N., Reynolds, K., He, J., & Muntner, P. (2006). Mortality prediction with a single general self-rated health question: A meta-analysis. *Journal of General Internal Medicine, 21*(3), 267–275.

DeSalvo, K. B., & Muntner, P. (2011). Discordance between physician and patient self-rated health and all-cause mortality. *The Ochsner Journal, 3*, 232–240.

Dunkin, J. J., & Anderson-Hanley, C. (1998). Dementia caregiver burden: A review of the literature and guidelines for assessment and intervention. *Neurology, 51*(1), S53–S60.

Epstein, A. M., Read, J. L., & Winickoff, R. (1984). Physician beliefs, attitudes, and prescribing behavior for anti-inflammatory drugs. *The American Journal of Medicine, 77*(2), 313–318.

Evans, M. A., & Golomb, B. A. (2009). Statin-associated adverse cognitive effects: Survey results from 171 patients. *Pharmacotherapy: The Journal of Human Pharmacology & Drug Therapy, 29*(7), 800–811.

Folstein, M. F., Folstein, S. E., & McHugh, P. R. (1975). "Mini-mental state": A practical method for grading the cognitive state of patients for the clinician. *Journal of Psychiatric Research, 12*(3), 189–198.

Friedman, M., & Rosenman, R. H. (1959). Association of specific overt behavior pattern with blood and cardiovascular findings: Blood cholesterol level, blood clotting time, incidence of arcus senilis, and clinical coronary artery disease. *Journal of the American Medical Association, 169*(12), 1286–1296.

Friedman, M., & Rosenman, R. H. (1974). *Type A Behavior and Your Heart*. New York: Knopf.

Friedrich, M. J. (2012). New research on Alzheimer treatments ventures beyond plaques and tangles. *Journal of the American Medical Association, 308*(24), 2553–2555.

Friedrich, M. J. (2014). Researchers test strategies to prevent Alzheimer disease. *Journal of the American Medical Association, 311*(16), 1596–1598.

Gauthier, S., & Touchon, J. (2005). Mild cognitive impairment is not a clinical entity and should not be treated. *Archives of Neurology, 62*(7), 1164–1166.

Gauthier, S., Reisberg, B., Zaudig, M., Petersen, R. C., Ritchie, K., & Broich, K., et al. (2006). Mild cognitive impairment. *The Lancet, 367*(9518), 1262–1270.

George, D. R., & Whitehouse, P. J. (2014). Chasing the "White Whale" of Alzheimer's. *Journal of the American Geriatrics Society, 62*(3), 588–589.

Gerbert, B., Gansky, S. A., Tang, J. W., McPhee, S. J., Carlton, R., Herzig, K., et al. (2002). Domestic violence compared to other health risks: a survey of physicians' beliefs and behaviors. *American Journal of Preventive Medicine, 23*(2), 82–90.

Golomb, B. A., McGraw, J. J., Evans, M. A., & Dimsdale, J. E. (2007). Physician response to patient reports of adverse drug effects. *Drug Safety, 30*(8), 669–675.

Greenaway, M. C., Duncan, N. L., & Smith, G. E. (2013). The memory support system for mild cognitive impairment: Randomized trial of a cognitive rehabilitation intervention. *International Journal of Geriatric Psychiatry, 28*(4), 402–409.

Grimshaw, J. M., Shirran, L., Thomas, R., Mowatt, G., Fraser, C., Bero, L., et al. (2001). Changing provider behavior: An overview of systematic reviews of interventions. *Medical Care, 39,* II2–II45.

Hanson, L. C., Danis, M., & Garrett, J. (1997). What is wrong with end-of-life care? Opinions of bereaved family members. *Journal of the American Geriatrics Society, 45*(11), 1339–1344.

Harris, D. P., Chodosh, J., Vassar, S. D., Vickrey, B. G., & Shapiro, M. F. (2009). Primary care providers' views of challenges and rewards of dementia care relative to other conditions. *Journal of the American Geriatrics Society, 57*(12), 2209–2216.

Hess, T. M., Auman, C., Colcombe, S. J., & Rahhal, T. A. (2003). The impact of stereotype threat on age differences in memory performance. *Journals of Gerontology: Psychological Sciences, 58B*(1), P3–P11.

Hess, T. M., & Hinson, J. T. (2006). Age-related variation in the influences of aging stereotypes on memory in adulthood. *Psychology and Aging, 21*(3), 621–625.

Hess, T. M., Hinson, J. T., & Hodges, E. A. (2009). Moderators of and mechanisms underlying stereotype threat effects on older adults' memory performance. *Experimental Aging Research, 35*(2), 153–177.

Hess, T. M., Hinson, J. T., & Statham, J. A. (2004). Explicit and implicit stereotype activation effects on memory: Do age and awareness moderate the impact of priming? *Psychology and Aging, 19*(3), 495–505.

Hofmann, J. C., Wenger, N. S., Davis, R. B., Teno, J., Connors, A. F., Desbiens, N., et al. (1997). Patient preferences for communication with physicians about end-of-life decisions. *Annals of Internal Medicine, 127*(1), 1–12.

Hojat, M., Vergare, M. J., Maxwell, K., Brainard, G., Herrine, S. K., Isenberg, G. A., et al. (2009). The devil is in the third year: A longitudinal study of erosion of empathy in medical school. *Academic Medicine, 84*(9), 1182–1191.

Hundt, N. E., Bensadon, B. A., Stanley, M. A., Petersen, N. J., Kunik, M. E., Kauth, M. R., et al. (2013). Coping mediates the relationship between disease severity and illness intrusiveness among chronically ill patients. *Journal of Health Psychology* Epub 2013 December 1.

Idler, E., & Benyamini, Y. (1997). Self-rated health and mortality: A review of twenty-seven community studies. *Journal of Health and Social Behavior, 38,* 21–37.

Jang, R. W., Man-Son-Hing, M., Molnar, F. J., Hogan, D. B., Marshall, S. C., Auger, J., et al. (2007). Family physicians' attitudes and practices regarding assessments of medical fitness to drive in older persons. *Journal of General Internal Medicine, 22*(4), 531–543.

Knight, K. M., McGowan, L., Dickens, C., & Bundy, C. (2006). A systematic review of motivational interviewing in physical health care settings. *British Journal of Health Psychology, 11*(2), 319–332.

Kotter-Gruhn, D., & Hess, T. M. (2012). The impact of age stereotypes on self-perceptions of aging across the adult lifespan. *Journals of Gerontology B: Psychological Sciences & Social Sciences, 67*(5), 563–571.

Kurz, A., Pohl, C., Ramsenthaler, M., & Sorg, C. (2009). Cognitive rehabilitation in patients with mild cognitive impairment. *International Journal of Geriatric Psychiatry, 24*(2), 163–168.

Lau, F., Cloutier-Fisher, D., Kuziemsky, C., Black, F., Downing, M., Borycki, E., et al. (2007). A systematic review of prognostic tools for estimating survival time in palliative care. *Journal of Palliative Care, 23*(2), 93–112.

Lee, M. A., Brummel-Smith, K., Meyer, J., Drew, N., & London, M. R. (2000). Physician orders for life-sustaining treatment (POLST): Outcomes in a PACE program. Program of All-Inclusive Care for the Elderly. *Journal of the American Geriatrics Society, 48*(10), 1219–1225.

Lenehan, M. E., Klekociuk, S. Z., & Summers, M. J. (2012). Absence of a relationship between subjective memory complaint and objective memory impairment in mild cognitive impairment (MCI): Is it time to abandon subjective memory complaint as an MCI diagnostic criterion? *International Psychogeriatrics, 24*(9), 1505–1514.

Levy, B. (1996). Improving memory in old age through implicit self-stereotyping. *Journal of Personality and Social Psychology, 71*(6), 1092–1107.

Levy, B. (2000). Handwriting as a reflection of aging self-stereotypes. *Journal of Geriatric Psychiatry*.

Levy, B. R. (2003). Mind matters: Cognitive and physical effects of aging self-stereotypes. *Journals of Gerontology: Psychological Sciences, 58B*(4), P203–P211.

Levy, B. (2009). Stereotype embodiment: A psychosocial approach to aging. *Current Directions in Psychological Science, 18*(6), 332–336.

Levy, B.R., & Banaji, M.R. (2002). Implicit ageism. In T.D. Nelson (Ed.): Ageism: Stereotyping and Prejudice Against Older Persons, 49–75.

Levy, B. R., Hausdorff, J. M., Hencke, R., & Wei, J. Y. (2000). Reducing cardiovascular stress with positive self-stereotypes of aging. *The Journals of Gerontology Series B: Psychological Sciences and Social Sciences, 55*(4), P205–P213.

Levy, B. R., Slade, M. D., Kunkel, S. R., & Kasl, S. V. (2002). Longevity increased by positive self-perceptions of aging. *Journal of Personality and Social Psychology, 83*(2), 261–270.

Levy, B., & Langer, E. (1994). Aging free from negative stereotypes: Successful memory in China among the American deaf. *Journal of Personality and Social Psychology, 66*(6), 989–997.

Levy, B. R., Zonderman, A. B., Slade, M. D., & Ferrucci, L. (2009). Age stereotypes held earlier in life predict cardiovascular events in later life. *Psychological Science, 20*(3), 296–298.

Levy, B. R., Zonderman, A. B., Slade, M. D., & Ferrucci, L. (2012). Memory shaped by age stereotypes over time. *The Journals of Gerontology Series B: Psychological Sciences and Social Sciences, 67*(4), 432–436.

Levy, B. R., Slade, M. D., & Kasl, S. V. (2002). Longitudinal benefit of positive self-perceptions of aging on functional health. *The Journals of Gerontology Series B: Psychological Sciences and Social Sciences, 57*(5), P409–P417.

Levy, B. R., Slade, M. D., Chung, P. H., & Gill, T. M. (2014). Resiliency over time of elders' age stereotypes after encountering stressful events. *Journals of Gerontology B: Psychological Sciences & Social Sciences, 61B,* P82–P87.

Levy, B. R., Slade, M. D., Murphy, T. E., & Gill, T. M. (2012). Association between positive age stereotypes and recovery from disability in older persons. *Journal of the American Medical Association, 308*(19), 1972–1973.

Lindau, S. T., Schumm, L. P., Laumann, E. O., Levinson, W., O'Muircheartaigh, C. A., & Waite, L. J. (2007). A study of sexuality and health among older adults in the United States. *New England Journal of Medicine, 357*(8), 762–774.

Linley, L., Prejean, J., An, Q., Chen, M., & Hall, H. I. (2012). Racial/ethnic disparities in HIV diagnoses among persons aged 50 years and older in 37 US states, 2005–2008. *American Journal of Public Health, 102*(8), 1527–1534.

Lorig, K. R., Ritter, P., Stewart, A. L., Sobel, D. S., Brown, B. W., Jr., Bandura, A., et al. (2001). Chronic disease self-management program 2-year health status and health care utilization outcomes. *Medical Care, 39*(11), 1217–1223.

Madson, M. B., Loignon, A. C., & Lane, C. (2009). Training in motivational interviewing: A systematic review. *Journal of Substance Abuse Treatment, 36*(1), 101–109.

Mangione, S., Kane, G. C., Caruso, J. W., Gonnella, J. S., Nasca, T. J., & Hojat, M. (2002). Assessment of empathy in different years of internal medicine training. *Medical Teacher*, 24(4), 370–373.

Mann, J. J., Apter, A., Bertolote, J., Beautrais, A., Currier, D., Haas, A., et al. (2005). Suicide prevention strategies: A systematic review. *Journal of the American Medical Association*, 294(16), 2064–2074.

Martin, A. J., Marottoli, R., & O'Neill, D. (2013). Driving assessment for maintaining mobility and safety in drivers with dementia. *Cochrane Database Systematic Review*, 8.

Mayer, E. A. (2011). Gut feelings: the emerging biology of gut-brain communication. *Nature Reviews Neuroscience*, 12, 453–466.

McGuinness, B., O'Hare, J., Craig, D., Bullock, R., Malouf, R., & Passmore, P. (2013). Cochrane review on 'statins for the treatment of dementia'. *International Journal of Geriatric Psychiatry*, 28(2), 119–126.

Miller, W. R. (1982). Motivational interviewing with problem drinkers. *Behavioural Psychotherapy*, 11(2), 147–172.

Mossey, J. M., & Shapiro, E. (1982). Self-rated health: A predictor of mortality among the elderly. *American Journal of Public Health*, 72(8), 800–808.

Mularski, R. A., Dy, S. M., Shugarman, L. R., Wilkinson, A. M., Lynn, J., Shekelle, P. G., et al. (2007). A systematic review of measures of end-of-life care and its outcomes. *Health Services Research*, 42(5), 1848–1870.

Newman, G., & Nichols, C. R. (1960). Sexual activities and attitudes in older persons. *Journal of the American Medical Association*, 173(1), 33–35.

O'Leary, A. (1985). Self-efficacy and health. *Behaviour Research and Therapy*, 23(4), 437–451.

Perri, R., Carlesimo, G. A., Serra, L., & Caltagirone, C. (2009). When the amnestic mild cognitive impairment disappears. *Cognitive Behavioral Neurology*, 22(2), 109–116.

Perri, R., Serra, L., Carlesimo, G. A., & Caltagirone, C. (2007). Preclinical dementia: An Italian multicenter study on amnestic mild cognitive impairment. *Dementia and Geriatric Cognitive Disorders*, 23, 289–300.

Petersen, R. C., Roberts, R. O., Knopman, D. S., Boeve, B. F., Geda, Y. E., Ivnik, R. J., et al. (2009). Mild cognitive impairment: Ten years later. *Archives of Neurology*, 66(12), 1447–1455.

Petersen, R. C., Smith, G. E., Ivnik, R. J., Tangalos, E. G., & Kokmen, E. (1994). Memory function in very early Alzheimer's. *Neurology*, 44(5), 867–872.

Petersen, R. C., Smith, G. E., Waring, S. C., Ivnik, R. J., Tangalos, E. G., & Kokmen, E. (1999). Mild cognitive impairment: clinical characterization and outcome. *Archives of Neurology*, 56(3), 303–308.

Pittet, D., Simon, A., Hugonnet, S., Pessoa-Silva, C., Sauvan, V., & Perneger, T. V. (2004). Hand hygiene among physicians: Performance, beliefs, and perceptions. *Annals of Internal Medicine*, 141, 1–8.

Range, L. M., & Knott, E. C. (1997). Twenty suicide assessment instruments: Evaluation and recommendations. *Death Studies*, 21(1), 25–58.

Raschetti, R., Albanese, E., Vanacore, N., & Maggini, M. (2007). Cholinesterase inhibitors in mild cognitive impairment: A systematic review of randomised trials. *PLoS Medicine*, 4(11), e338.

Regan, B., & Varanelli, L. (2013). Adjustment, depression, and anxiety in mild cognitive impairment and early dementia: A systematic review of psychological intervention studies. *International Psychogeriatrics*, 25(12), 1963–1984.

Reuben, D., Levin, J., Frank, J., Hirsch, S., McCreath, H., Roth, C., et al. (2009). Closing the dementia care gap: Can referral to Alzheimer's Association chapters help? *Alzheimer's & Dementia: The Journal of the Alzheimer's Association*, 5(6), 498–502.

Reuben, D. B., Roth, C. P., Frank, J. C., Hirsch, S. H., Katz, D., & McCreath, H., et al. (2010). Assessing care of vulnerable elders—Alzheimer's disease: A pilot study of a practice redesign intervention to improve the quality of dementia care. *Journal of the American Geriatrics Society*, 58(2), 324–329.

Roberts, R. O., Knopman, D. S., Mielke, M. M., Cha, R. H., Pankratz, V. S., Christianson, T. J., et al. (2014). Higher risk of progression to dementia in mild cognitive impairment cases who revert to normal. *Neurology, 82*(4), 31–325.

Sackett, D. L., Rosenberg, W., Gray, J. A., Haynes, R. B., & Richardson, W. S. (1996). Evidence based medicine: What it is and what it isn't. *British Medical Journal, 312*(7023), 71–72.

Shearn, D. (2001). Changing physician behavior: What does it take? *Western Journal of Medicine, 175*(3), 167.

Smedslund, G., Berg, R. C., Hammerstrøm, K. T., Steiro, A., Leiknes, K. A., Dahl, H. M., et al. (2011). Motivational interviewing for substance abuse. *Cochrane Database Systematic Reviews*(5), CD008063.

Smith, G. E., Petersen, R. C., Parisi, J. E., Ivnik, R. J., Kokmen, E., Tangalos, E. G., et al. (1996). Definition, course, and outcome of mild cognitive impairment. *Aging Neuropsychology & Cognition, 3,* 131–147.

Steele, C. M., & Aronson, J. (1995). Stereotype threat and the intellectual test performance of African Americans. *Journal of Personality and Social Psychology, 69*(5), 797–811.

Steele, C. M. (1997). A threat in the air: How stereotypes shape intellectual identity and performance. *American Psychologist, 52*(6), 613–629.

Street, R. L., Krupat, E., Bell, R. A., Kravitz, R. L., & Haidet, P. (2003). Beliefs about control in the physician-patient relationship. *Journal of General Internal Medicine, 18*(8), 609–616.

Tait, R. C., Chibnall, J. T., Luebbert, A., & Sutter, C. (2005). Effect of treatment success and empathy on surgeon attributions for back surgery outcomes. *Journal of Behavioral Medicine, 28*(4), 301–312.

Taylor, A., & Gosney, M. A. (2011). Sexuality in older age: Essential considerations for health care professionals. *Age and Ageing, 40*(5), 538–543.

Thompson, C. A., Spilsbury, K., Hall, J., Birks, Y., Barnes, C., & Adamson, J. (2007). Systematic review of information and support interventions for caregivers of people with dementia. *BMC Geriatrics, 7*(1), 18.

Tulsky, J. A., Fischer, G. S., Rose, M. R., & Arnold, R. M. (1998). Opening the black box: How do physicians communicate about advance directives? *Annals of Internal Medicine, 129*(6), 441–449.

Tversky, A., & Kahneman, D. (1974). Judgment under uncertainty: Heuristics and biases. *Science, 185*(4157), 1124–1131.

Weinstein, A. M., Barton, C., Ross, L., Kramer, J. H., & Yaffe, K. (2009). Treatment practices of mild cognitive impairment in California Alzheimer's disease centers. *Journal of the American Geriatrics Society, 57*(4), 686–690.

West, R. L., Bagwell, D. K., & Dark-Freudeman, A. (2005). Memory and goal setting: The response of older and younger adults to positive and objective feedback. *Psychology & Aging, 20*(2), 195–201.

West, R. L., Bagwell, D. K., & Dark-Freudeman, A. (2008). Self-efficacy and memory aging: The impact of a memory intervention based on self-efficacy. *Aging, Neuropsychology, and Cognition, 15*(3), 302–329.

West, R. L., Crook, T. H., & Barron, K. L. (1992). Everyday memory performance across the life span: Effects of age and noncognitive individual differences. *Psychology and Aging, 7*(1), 72–82.

West, R. L., Dark-Freudeman, A., & Bagwell, D. K. (2009). Goals-feedback conditions and memory: Mechanisms for memory gains in older and younger adults. *Memory, 17*(2), 233–244.

West, R. L., Dennehy-Basile, D., & Norris, M. P. (1996). Memory self-evaluation: The effects of age and experience. *Aging, Neuropsychology, and Cognition, 3*(1), 67–83.

West, R. L., Thorn, R. M., & Bagwell, D. K. (2003). Memory performance and beliefs as a function of goal setting and aging. *Psychology and Aging, 18*(1), 111–125.

West, R. L., Welch, D. C., & Knabb, P. D. (2002). Gender and aging: Spatial self-efficacy and location recall. *Basic and Applied Social Psychology, 24*(1), 71–80.

West, R. L., Welch, D. C., & Thorn, R. M. (2001). Effects of goal-setting and feedback on memory performance and beliefs among older and younger adults. *Psychology and Aging, 16,* 240–250.

West, R. L., & Yassuda, M. S. (2004). Aging and memory control beliefs: Performance in relation to goal setting and memory self-evaluation. *Journals of Gerontology: Psychological Sciences, 59B*(2), 56–65.

Wilson, M. M. (2003). Sexually transmitted diseases. *Clinics in Geriatric Medicine, 19*(3), 637–655.

Zarit, S. H., Reever, K. E., & Bach-Peterson, J. (1980). Relatives of the impaired elderly: Correlates of feelings of burden. *The Gerontologist, 20*(6), 649–655.

Zarit, S. H., Todd, P. A., & Zarit, J. M. (1986). Subjective burden of husbands and wives as caregivers: A longitudinal study. *The Gerontologist, 26*(3), 260–266.

Zullig, L. L., Peterson, E. D., & Bosworth, H. B. (2013). Ingredients of successful interventions to improve medication adherence. *Journal of the American Medical Association, 310*(24), 2611–2612.

4

Communication

Tricia A. Miller, and M. Robin DiMatteo

University of California Riverside, Riverside, California, USA

INTRODUCTION

By the year 2030, approximately 71.5 million Americans will be age 65 or older, representing nearly 20% of the total U.S. population (U.S. Census Bureau, 2004). As a result, demands on the U.S. health care system will increase; shortages of health care professionals providing effective geriatric care are predicted; and training in geriatrics for health professionals at all levels will likely remain limited (Kovner, Mezey, & Harrington, 2002; Schonfeld, Stevens, Lampman, & Lyons, 2012).

In the U.S., older patients visit their primary care physicians on average 3.9 times per year and their specialist 4.3 times per year (Starfield, Lemke, Herbert, Pavlovich, & Anderson, 2005). Such frequent medical visits with multiple providers offer opportunities for the medical team to provide psychosocial care in addition to care that is purely biomedical. Effective communication with the medical team can serve as an important source of connection and encouragement for many older patients who face illness-related challenges (and life) either alone or with minimal support (Williams, Haskard, & DiMatteo, 2007). Clinical psychologists on the medical team can take the lead in meeting these patients' needs (Williams et al., 2007), using several communication strategies, described later, that are valuable to both patient care and training of other health care team members.

The health and well-being of geriatric patients can be affected by the many different challenges of aging, including changes in health status, income levels, and insurance coverage (Adelman, Greene, & Ory, 2000; Williams et al., 2007). What remains constant, however, is the clear value of effective physician–patient communication, shown to support enhanced adaptation at multiple levels (Price, Bereknyei, Kuby, Levinson, & Braddock, 2012). Health care professionals are called upon to exchange

B. Bensadon (Ed): Psychology and Geriatrics.
DOI: http://dx.doi.org/10.1016/B978-0-12-420123-1.00004-6

69

both biomedical and psychosocial information with their older patients. Ideally, the latter includes provision of affective and emotional care, though evidence suggests this is significantly less likely to occur with geriatric patients (Greene, Hoffman, Charon, & Adelman, 1987). In each of these realms, effective communication is inseparable from a trusting therapeutic relationship and the art and science of healing (Williams et al., 2007).

Decades of empirical research have linked effective physician–patient communication with positive patient outcomes, and now, importantly, emerging research evidence demonstrates the central role of psychological insight in maximizing clinical effectiveness. This chapter will identify communication challenges especially common in geriatrics and examine the fundamental role that clinical psychologists can play in improving communication in clinical encounters. The effectiveness of communication training will be evaluated, and recommendations for optimizing geriatric management and health outcomes will be provided.

High-quality communication between clinicians and their older patients is vital to ensuring patient comprehension of medical information and subsequent adherence to treatment (Giampieri, 2012; Robinson & Reiter, 2007). However, older patients often struggle to discuss with physicians nearly half of the serious medical and psychosocial challenges they experience while living with illness (Rost & Frankel, 1993). But why?

Much of the medical visit often centers on the patient's disease state(s), leaving little time for psychosocial discussion or health behavior counseling. For many older patients, the medical visit can be emotionally overwhelming, and the pressures of time limitations can lead to confusion and forgetfulness (Rost & Frankel, 1993). In other instances, visits are simply intimidating. For example, Hudak and colleagues (2008) examined older patients' unexpressed concerns about orthopaedic surgery during 886 medical encounters. Patients raised 53% of their actual concerns, and were selective about what they disclosed. They did not raise *emotion*-based concerns about the surgeons or their own ability to meet the demands of the surgery, but did raise *fact*-based concerns about procedure timing and care facility.

Medical psychologist Edward Callahan and colleagues (2000) suggest a patient's chronological age also plays an important role in communication and can influence physicians' behaviors during the medical encounter. Compared to younger patients, for example, older patients are less likely to receive instructions and guidance about the procedures of a physical examination (Callahan et al., 2000). Yet in contrast, physicians often devote more time to medical history-taking and questions regarding prior medication adherence during visits with older patients than with younger patients. As noted previously, because older patients often present with multimorbidity, adequately addressing these medical concerns may leave little time for patients' psychosocial and emotional needs (Callahan et al.,

2000). Some research suggests physicians make extra efforts to be non-verbally responsive, egalitarian, and supportive (using back-channels of communication such as "hmm" and "uh-huh") with their older patients (Montague, Chen, Xu, Chewning, & Barrett, 2013). Yet good intentions alone are insufficient and health care communication quality as a whole remains poor.

COMMUNICATION TRAINING

As discussed throughout this publication, even with the integration of clinical psychologists in standard care, physicians' clinical acumen must expand beyond managing patients' physical concerns to include their emotional needs as well. Care delivery must be clear and commensurate with patients' expectations once they are identified. This is trainable. (e.g., Riess, Kelley, Bailey, Dunn, & Phillips, 2012; Smith et al., 2007). But because most people (physicians and others) believe they are already effective communicators, training in communication is hard to implement. Evidence suggests, however, it is well worth the effort. And while training format, trainer characteristics, and their interface with learners all can influence training success and long-term impact, when implemented, training physicians in communication skills has resulted in substantial and significant improvements in patient adherence, satisfaction with care, and improved health status (Haskard et al., 2008). Haskard-Zolnierek and DiMatteo (2009) conducted a meta-analysis of 59 years of research (127 studies) targeting physician communication, related training, and impact on patient adherence to treatment regimens. Notably, data revealed the odds of patient adherence nearly doubled when clinicians received communication training compared to when they did not.

In spite of the evidence, such training continues to fall outside the areas of major emphasis in medical education and care. The ubiquitous absence of clinical psychologists, both on health care teams and in medical training, is likely relevant to this problem. Other barriers to optimal clinical communication in geriatrics include cognitive, functional, and psychological challenges, as well as the frequent presence of a third party during the medical encounter.

COGNITION

Certainly, cognitive dysfunction can increase with age and influence health care communication in significant ways (Adelman et al., 2000). Progressive declines in memory or other cognitive domains can impair psychological, social, and occupational functioning. Alzheimer's disease and related disorders (ADRD) occur in one of every nine individuals aged 65 and older (Alzheimer's Association, 2014; Antoine & Pasquier, 2013). Dementia is the primary cause of disability among older adults, and research has demonstrated several important behavioral correlates, including depression and smoking (Sosa-Ortiz, Acosta-Castillo & Prince, 2012).

As mentioned elsewhere in this publication, it is particularly challenging for clinicians to obtain accurate objective assessments of patients with dementia. Primary care physicians often *prematurely* associate a patient's diagnosis of dementia with total cognitive impairment in all dimensions of intellect, emotion, and behavior. Erroneous assumptions are then made that patients are incapable of participating in their own care – a term known as *dementiaism* (Adelman et al., 2000). In part this is due to the insidious onset of many dementias, which poses a major challenge to timely diagnosis. There are often delays (1 to 5 years from the first sign of symptoms) in diagnoses until symptoms are prevalent and severely disabling (Salloway & Correia, 2009). Diagnostic complexity is compounded by the fact that many patients, especially early in their disease process, can often hide and compensate for their disease-related symptoms, which may fall under physicians' radar. Dutch psychologist Deliane Van Vliet and colleagues (2013) describe failures to recognize early dementia symptoms, lack of confidence in diagnosing dementia, and patients' lack of social support as barriers to early detection in primary care settings. This failure to recognize dementia underscores the fundamental need for a team approach in which clinical geropsychologists assess, diagnose, and provide management support to cognitively impaired older patients and their caregivers.

Elderly patients often experience communication problems as a result of primary aging. These include sensory impairment (e.g., hearing and vision loss), functional and mobility limitations, and communication deficits such as word-finding difficulty (Toner, Shadden, & Gluth, 2011). Evidence suggests clinicians inaccurately assess older patients' communication ability, often underestimating it (Toner et al., 2011; Williams, Herman, Gajewski, & Wilson, 2009). This often leads to addressing older patients with exaggerated intonation patterns, higher pitch and volume, and simpler vocabulary and grammar. Clinicians also speak more slowly than they do to younger patients. Though at times this adjustment may be clinically indicated, indiscriminate use of this approach is known as *elderspeak* (Thomas, 2010), the equivalent of babytalk but applied to older people. This can be demeaning and undermining of the patient–physician relationship.

Oversimplified communication style with geriatric patients, such as *"Are we ready for our bath?"* or *"You want to get up now, don't you?"* is not only insulting but implies that elders are incapable of independent choice (Kemper & Harden, 1999; Williams et al., 2009). Worse yet, in some ways elderspeak becomes a self-fulfilling prophecy, creating the very problems it is mistakenly implemented to assist. A qualitative review by Thomas (2010) has shown that elderspeak can cause patients to actually lose confidence in their own communication ability, and it can decrease comprehension and interpretation of statements because unimportant words are often emphasized with inappropriate rises in pitch and intonation. Additionally, when health professionals speak extremely slowly they can reduce the elderly patient's ability to focus and remember important information (Thomas, 2010). Again, often well-intentioned desire to help may inadvertently prevent opportunities for older patients to demonstrate their true functional or cognitive capacity, and may even be iatrogenic in accelerating their trajectory of decline.

Older patients may notice these speech patterns, or the fact that clinicians tend to speak *about* rather than directly *to* them, but keep related complaints to themselves. Though challenging to measure empirically, anecdotal concerns about becoming a burden are common in the aged, and some physicians, themselves, have poignantly illustrated insight into the unexpressed shame, anger, and desperation internalized by many older patients (e.g., Delaplain, 2011).

MOOD

Risk of depression and other psychological morbidity can increase with age. The prevalence of depressive symptoms can be as high as 40% of patients aged 65 and older (Chen & Landefeld, 2007). Depression has been associated with increased medical comorbidity and higher rates of relapse (Mitchell & Subramaniam, 2005). Serious chronic disease challenges in older age can increase the likelihood of depression (Mitchell & Subramaniam, 2005; Williams et al., 2007), and major depression is common among the elderly who attempt suicide (Lapierre et al., 2011; Szanto, Prigerson, & Reynolds III, 2001). A 2013 review of screening for and treatment of suicide risk relevant to primary care found, among suicide completers, 50–70% were seen in primary care within the prior month. Clinical psychologist presence could enhance detection of those at greatest risk and lead to intervention such as psychotherapy, which, the review concluded, may reduce suicide attempts (O'Connor, Gaynes, Burda, Soh, & Whitlock, 2013).

The most common risk factors for geriatric suicide include serious medical conditions or illness, stressful life events (e.g., loss of a spouse), and social isolation (Lapierre et al., 2011). While the medical factors may be familiar territory for physicians, the psychological and emotional ones may not be, and patients, especially if depressed and/or suicidal, may recognize that. This can influence what and how much related information they choose to disclose.

As demonstrated elsewhere in this publication, lack of familiarity, training, and related discomfort may explain, in part, why suicide assessments in the primary care setting continue to occur infrequently and insufficiently (Crawford et al., 2011). General practitioners may worry that such assessment or screening may induce or "plant" suicidal thoughts and behaviors or will be too time consuming. In fact physicians, themselves, have reported they do not have the training or skill to conduct such assessments adequately (Crawford et al., 2011). Conversely, clinical psychologists are trained to routinely assess, treat, and manage suicidal patients (Fowler, 2012). Indeed, from the start of their clinical training, this assessment is not merely an option but a requirement, at every intake (i.e., initial) encounter.

This highlights again the clear need and potential value of integration. While some may advocate for physician–psychologist collaboration to recognize and manage psychosocial components of suicide risk, research attempting to identify genetic biomarkers for suicidal behavior has already begun (e.g., Guintivano et al., 2014).

FUNCTION AND STIGMA

Functional and mobility deficits can further inhibit communication during the medical visit. Many older patients face limitations in activities of daily living (ADL) such as bathing, toileting, or even ambulating independently. Moving from waiting room chair to examination table can be taxing, both emotionally and physically. Without support, these patients may see the medical visit as an ordeal that is more trouble than it's worth. Even when older patients do decide to attend their appointments, their complex medical challenges may be anxiety provoking. What's more, they may feel rushed or stressed by the need to express all of their concerns in a limited time frame, especially if they sense clinicians are not listening or interested. Even those older patients who are more accepting of an authoritative communication style (Haug, 1979) may still prefer physicians who share laughter, provide supportive interpersonal warmth, and an opportunity to raise issues and questions on their (patients') own "agenda" (Greene, Adelman, Friedman, & Charon, 1994).

It is not uncommon to hear older patients express concern about "bothering" a busy physician. Some data suggest this may stem from patient uncertainty about their own perceived "worth" as patients (e.g., Clarke, Bennett, & Korotchenko, 2014). Clinical communication informed by societal bias (i.e., ageism) does not help. Some patients may experience shame in discussing socially stigmatized symptoms such as incontinence, cognitive impairment, or sexual dysfunction (Min et al., 2011). If patient ambivalence and embarrassment are undetected and unaddressed, delicate issues may not be raised. Worse yet, if clinicians hold similar bias themselves, these delicate matters are even less likely to be voiced. For these reasons psychologists can play a central role in sensitively recognizing, managing, and minimizing patients' discomfort by normalizing patient emotions and validating their concerns. Ideally, integration can help both clinicians and patients recognize and manage related anxiety and focus on treatment adherence (DiMatteo, 2004).

PRESENCE OF A THIRD PERSON

One important distinction in geriatrics is that older patients are often accompanied by a third person (e.g., spouse, adult child, other family member, friend or professional caregiver). Such individuals can serve as a means of support and are often necessary for elderly patients who are both physically and cognitively vulnerable (Adelman et al., 2000; Greene & Adelman, 2003). However, the presence of a third person can also inhibit and further complicate the development and maintenance of a trusting relationship between patient and physician (Greene & Adelman, 2013). When these encounters are not managed effectively, older patients ask fewer questions, are less expressive and responsive in their questioning, and participate less in shared decision-making (Greene & Adelman, 2003). Thus, it is important that physicians recognize how much influence or involvement third-party caregivers play in their patients' care. In doing so, they can involve caregivers more effectively and acknowledge not only the patients' needs and concerns but also validate those of the caregiver (Bevans & Sternberg, 2012). Indirectly, via consultation and communication with team members, psychologists can recognize potential elder exploitation (e.g., financial), identify elder abuse, reconcile conflicting treatment preferences, and address end-of-life concerns.

CAREGIVER BURNOUT

Informal caregivers often receive inadequate support from health care providers and report feeling abandoned and unrecognized by the health care system (Lilly, Robinson, Holtzman, & Bottorff, 2012). This can result in caregiver burnout (Bevans & Sternberg, 2012) and psychological, behavioral, and physiologic effects associated with impaired immune functioning, coronary heart disease, and even early death (Bevans & Sternberg, 2012; Gouin, Hantsoo, & Kiecolt-Glaser, 2008; Lee, Colditz, Berkman, & Kawachi, 2003; Schulz & Beach, 1999).

Through geropsychology consultation, brief screening (measuring emotional and physical distress), and direct care, psychologists can help mitigate caregivers' stress associated with patient care and recommend behavioral interventions to attenuate their negative experiences. Through effective communication, psychologists can, often more comfortably and effectively than physicians, provide support and guidance about emotionally sensitive subjects to help equip caregivers for challenges of end-of-life care, maintenance of family and marital relationships, and the importance of caregivers' own self-care, which guilt and other emotions often inhibit (Bevans & Sternberg, 2012).

BREAKING BAD NEWS

In 1969 psychologist Ezra Saul led a study of first-year medical students at Tufts University. The goal was to identify which physician roles were viewed with greatest anticipatory anxiety. Potentially stressful hypothetical clinical scenarios were shown and students rated physical symptoms consistent with anxiety (e.g., dry mouth, increased heart rate, perspiration) on a 5-point Likert scale. The two most anxiety-inducing situations were discussion of fatal illness, and telling a relative that a patient (i.e., family member) died. While nearly 50 years have passed, little has changed. This can be said for both psychological discomfort and related training that might alleviate or reduce it.

Orlander and colleagues (2002) found, among 129 internal medicine residents surveyed, only 5% recalled their first experience giving bad news actually included the presence of an attending physician. Nearly 75% of the sample first delivered such news as medical students or first-year residents. In more than half the cases (61%), they knew the patient for a matter of days or hours. Interestingly, almost half those sent the study survey did not return it.

At the same time, situations requiring bad news delivery can be common. A global sample of 167 oncologists reported giving bad news on average 35 times per month – that is, more than once a day (Baile, Lenzi, Parker, Buckman, & Cohen, 2002). And evidence suggests conversation about related topics such as advance directives are suboptimal in terms of both quality and frequency. Tulsky, Fischer, Rose, and Arnold (1998) examined audiotaped discussion from 56 internists and 56 of their established patients, age 65 and older. Related discussion averaged 5.6 minutes and physicians spoke for two-thirds of the time. While physicians discussed dire scenarios and surrogate decision-making in almost all cases, less than half asked patients about their preferences in reversible situations. Even when patients, themselves, attempt to raise such discussion, physicians have been found to avoid them by either "terminating the conversation, hedging their responses, denying the patient's expressed emotion, or inadequately acknowledging the sentiment underlying the patient's statement" (Ahluwalia, Levin, Lorenz, & Gordon, 2012).

Most articles in medical journals view delivering bad news as one moment in time (i.e., disclosure). However, social scientists have demonstrated evidence that patients consider the larger process, especially in the case of cancers, that culminates in this diagnostic event (Schaepe, 2011). Similarly, the prevailing wisdom in medical training is that such skills come with time and practice. But decades of data do not support this and some studies actually suggest a decline in communication ability even within the 4 years of medical school (Hook & Pfeiffer, 2007; Pfeiffer, Madray, Ardolino, & Willms, 1998). This disconnect between patients' and clinicians' experiences is rarely addressed in formal training. Based on their literature review of how such training occurs, when it does indeed occur, Rosenbaum and colleagues (2004) identified six key ingredients that can maximize effectiveness and result in lasting improvement:

- Multiple sessions
- Opportunities for actual demonstration
- Reflection
- Discussion
- Practice
- Feedback

Receiving bad news is never pleasant but patients do have preferences about what is more or less desirable, and these have been measured. Ptacek and Ptacek (2001) surveyed 120 people with cancer – mostly of the breast, prostate, or lung – about their satisfaction level with how they received bad news. Those reporting higher stress reported lower satisfaction and those with higher satisfaction reported better adjustment to the diagnosis. Importantly, satisfaction was not achieved randomly. Rather, the odds of being satisfied were higher when news was received in a comfortable location, the exchange was free of interruptions, physicians sat close to patients, attempted to empathize with their feelings, and provided a warning that bad news was coming. Other studies have revealed similar preferences that physicians sit rather than stand (Bruera et al., 2007), and reduce their speech rate and voice pitch (McHenry, Parker, Baile, & Lenzi, 2011).

While some age-based trends in patient preferences exist, there is no *one size fits all* model (Benbassat, Pilpel, & Tidhar, 1998). Rather, the needed skill is to recognize and tailor communication delivery appropriately. This flexibility is core to clinical geropsychologists' training and experience, and their integration may create opportunities to discuss fears and concerns that patients and family are not comfortable bringing to the physician; indeed psychologists may recognize patient and caregiver distress that physicians fail to see, or feel ill-equipped to manage.

TIME

Many of the communication skills described may seem fundamental, yet empirical evidence shows they are far from rudimentary, not applied systematically, and may be taken for granted. In fact, simply allowing patients to speak uninterrupted often distresses physicians. On average, physicians interrupt patients within 18 seconds (Martin, Haskard-Zolnierek, & DiMatteo, 2010). This is understandable since physicians are increasingly pressed for time (Levinson & Pizzo, 2011) and often worry that patients will use up this scarce commodity if allowed to speak freely. But as psychologists are well aware, fear is shaped by perception, and remains a powerful predictor of behavior, regardless of objective or actual threat.

When allowed to speak without interruption, patients take about 30 seconds in primary care settings and 90 seconds in specialty care settings (Rabinowitz, Luzzatti, Tamir, & Reis, 2004). Olsburgh and Jelley (1989) found that across 100 patients seen, when uninterrupted, only one spoke for more than 2 minutes and 87% spoke for less than a minute. The mean length of speech was 35 seconds. Similarly, Langewitz and colleagues (2002) recorded a mean speaking time of 92 seconds among 330 patients seen by 14 different physicians; 78% had completed their initial statement in 2 minutes and only 7 patients spoke for more than 5 minutes. Tragically, in practice, physician behavior is guided by subjective worry more than objective data. Geriatric patients are especially at risk. "Jokes" are made by clinicians who intentionally redirect older patients to avoid "opening a can of worms" that they fear would lead to "excessive" conversation. Marvel, Epstein, Flowers, and Beckman (1999) measured this trend of redirection in a sample of physicians, one-third of whom had Fellowship training in communication and family counseling. Only 28% of the patient sample was allowed by physicians to complete their initial statements. Patients were redirected after a mean of 23.1 seconds. Those who were allowed to complete their statement did so in only 6 more seconds than those who were redirected. Interestingly, physicians with communications training were twice as likely to allow patients to complete their initial statements (44% vs. 22%). Even adjusting one word during a clinical visit can have an impact. Heritage, Robinson, Elliott, Beckett, and Wilkes (2007) compared the impact of two questions – is there *any*thing else you want to address in the visit today vs. is there *some*thing else you want to address in the visit today? – on patients' unmet concerns. The latter eliminated 78% of unmet concerns. Again, while health care providers have timetables, patients have (often unmet) needs. Physician–psychologist integration can address both.

Physicians themselves have recognized some of these current system and training gaps. Ekdahl, Hellstrom, Andersson, and Friedrichsen (2012) interviewed 30 physicians and found self-identified lack of competence in geriatric care, concerns about the need for time-consuming care and communication with multiple caregivers, and challenges of older patients' set routines, were all identified as impediments to optimal shared decision-making.

TRAINING TARGETS

Information Exchange

Effective information exchange (e.g., explanations of diagnoses, acknowledgment of emotions, treatment instructions) between physician and patient is central to quality medical visits. Not just what but the *way* information is provided can influence patients' satisfaction with care, their adherence to medical treatment, and ultimately their treatment outcomes (DiMatteo, 2004; DiMatteo, Giordani, Lepper, & Croghan, 2002). As discussed previously, research suggests that older patients receive less information from their physicians during encounters than do younger patients, perhaps in some cases because limited visit time is consumed with complex diagnosis and treatment activities, and/or because physicians hold stereotyped expectations that older patients will not understand their explanations (Greene et al., 1994).

It follows that older patients are typically less satisfied with the information they receive, in part because physicians have difficulty gauging the appropriate amount of information to provide. While it is important to inform older patients about their responsibilities in actively managing their health, physicians must transfer the right balance of information about what patients need to know and do, without overwhelming them with information that will not be comprehended or remembered. Otherwise, patients feel distressed or confused (Beach, Roter, Wang, Duggan, & Cooper, 2006). Providing just the right amount of information is not easy for physicians, and here too, psychologists who are trained in learning and memory can help by providing health literacy-related information directly and/or by teaching medical professionals to do so (Nash, McKay, Vogel, & Masters, 2012; Quill & Holloway, 2012).

Equipping patients to be active participants in their own care is an important aspect of information exchange in the physician–patient relationship. Research comparing participatory versus paternalistic physician communication styles has found that older patients are typically offered less involvement in their own care compared with patients who are younger than 30 years of age (Kaplan, Greenfield, Gandek, Rogers, & Ware, 1996). Other factors, such as patients' ethnicity and type of insurance, can also influence the level of information, explanation, and referrals that physicians offer to geriatric patients (Stepanikova & Cook, 2004).

A patient-centered approach to medical care aspires to provide collaboration and cooperation among physicians and their patients. Important aspects of patient-centered communication include psychosocial talk, information giving, and expressions of partnership and therapeutic alliance through shared decision-making (Street, Krupat, Bell, Kravitz, & Haidet, 2003; Williams et al., 2007).

Teach-Back Method

The *teach-back* method allows health care professionals to enhance communication and patients' comprehension of medical directives. Such a technique has significant value in the care of all patient populations and especially in geriatrics. Patients are asked to repeat and explain in their own words (i.e., teach back) any treatment information that was discussed in the medical interaction (Kripalani, Bengtzen, Henderson, & Jacobson, 2008). This approach allows all involved clinicians to confirm the degree to which the patient knows what is necessary to adhere to treatment, and how he or she intends to do it. This technique also allows clinicians to check for any lapses in recall and understanding, and reinforces open dialogue with patients about their role and commitment to the treatment plan (White, Garbez, Carroll, Brinker, & Howie-Esquivel, 2013).

Psychosocial Talk

As noted earlier, communication in which physicians seek to address verbally (or nonverbally) both the biomedical and psychosocial needs of their geriatric patients is essential for successful health outcomes (Pawlikowska, Zhang, Griffiths, Van Dalen, & van der Vleuten, 2012). In the context of a patient-centered approach to care, physicians must elicit and acknowledge their patients' concerns and reasons for their visit by means of *psychosocial talk*. If done effectively, this communication style formally grants patients permission to tell their personal story of living with illness, thus validating the importance and clinical relevance of patient perspectives (i.e., how the illness or disease affects the patient's quality of life, daily functioning, social and professional relationships, and the patient's own feelings and emotions). Psychosocial talk allows patients to explore what their illness means to them, and to integrate and interpret their experience (Rotar, 2000). A physician's awareness of psychosocial factors that may challenge a patient's ability to cope with disease is critical to establishing authentic dialogue within the therapeutic relationship (Cousin, Schmid Mast, Rotar, & Hall, 2012). Yet, as addressed in the training section of this publication, physicians are traditionally trained to manage patients' biomedical needs, while receiving little to no training in identifying or meeting patients' psychosocial needs (Cousin, Schmid

Mast, Roter, & Hall, 2012). As a consequence, some physicians feel that caring for their patient's psychological challenges falls well beyond the scope of the services they can provide. When that is the case, consultation with a clinical psychologist is in order. Such a consultation is not only helpful to the patient, but also assists the physician in managing his or her time and services efficiently.

The traditional model separating psychosocial and biomedical aspects of care may be changing, however. Interpersonal communication skills have been identified as a core competency of medical residency training (Accreditation Council for Graduate Medical Education, ACGME) and are formally assessed during the United States Medical Licensing Examination (Duffy et al., 2004). Multicultural sensitivity, termed cultural competence when applied to medical communication, has also become a formal priority (Anderson, Scrimshaw, Fullilove, Fielding, & Normand, 2003). And of course the Medical College Admission Test (MCAT) has expanded to include psychological and behavioral science content for the first time in its history. Though their long-term implications are unknown, these changes underscore the concept that physicians' interviewing skills and attention to psychosocial aspects of care are important and trainable. Integrated clinical psychologists can apply related best practice behavioral health guidelines to ensure that patients' psychosocial needs are adequately addressed (Kearney, Post, Pomerantz, & Zeiss, 2014).

Shared Decision-Making

Over the past several decades there has been increasing support for patients' participation in the medical decision-making process. In contrast to a paternalistic approach to care, where physicians make all treatment decisions and dictate to the patient what must be done to comply, health care providers have begun to move towards a model of care known as shared decision-making (Elwyn et al., 2012). Shared decision-making (SDM) is a process by which physicians and patients work together in mutual partnership towards a treatment plan that is most conducive to the specific needs of the patient. This model also enables patients to feel that their physician values their personal preferences and goals for treatment (Elwyn et al., 2012; Frosch & Kaplan, 1999). Active communication, within SDM, can help increase patients' knowledge of their disease and enable them to better convey important health information to their physicians (Greene & Hibbard, 2012).

Studies have shown that rates of medication adherence increase when physicians and patients work together in deciding which among various medications to take, devising specific medication schedules, and discussing potential side effects (Jahng, Martin, Golin, & DiMatteo, 2005). As shown by the hazardous correlates of polypharmacy, such a collaborative approach is particularly important for older patient safety, as geriatric patients often struggle to both remember and manage multiple and complex medication regimens (Ownby, Hertzog, Crocco, & Duara, 2006).

Not all patients want to participate in medical decisions to the same degree, however. Some patients prefer to discuss treatments with their physicians but then rely entirely on their physicians to make decisions on their behalf (Levinson, Kao, Kuby, & Thisted, 2004). Others want all decisions to be joint decisions. Physicians should offer patients the opportunity to participate by sharing information and responsibilities and actively communicating with patients at every step of the decision-making process (Levinson et al., 2004). Psychologists can be particularly helpful with SDM using "active listening" or "attentive listening" to receive, construct meaning from, and respond to patients' verbal and nonverbal messages regarding their needs and preferences. Active listening skills have been associated with reductions in patient stress, increases in joint decision-making, and increases in patient confidence in treatment and therapy (Jagosh, Boudreau, Steinert, MacDonald, & Ingram, 2011).

Empathy

A physician's ability to empathize with patients is fundamental to developing and sustaining the therapeutic relationship (Roter & Hall, 1989). Unlike sympathizing, which connotates a *sharing* of emotion (Nightingale, Yarnold, & Greenberg, 1991; Wispe, 1968), empathizing requires accurate *understanding* of patients' experiences and emotional states. As described below, physicians must convey this understanding through words of comfort, body gestures, and positive nonverbal feedback (Hojat, Spandorfer, Louis, & Gonnella, 2011; Williams et al., 2007). In spite of continued debate about a precise definition, several validated instruments target empathy measurement. Some of the most widely used include the Jefferson Scale of Physician Empathy (JSPE), the Questionnaire Measure of Emotional Empathy, and the Empathy Construct Scale (Hemmerdinger, Stoddart, & Lilford, 2007; Hojat et al., 2001; La Monica, 1981).

Sleath, Rubin, and Arrey-Wastavino (2000) found that empathy can reduce patients' experiences of alienation from others and can be expressed through both verbal and nonverbal communication (Riess & Kraft-Todd, 2014). For example, verbal expressions of empathy include words of support or expressions of understanding, where patients are invited to tell their story of living and coping with illness (Williams et al., 2007). Physicians' empathic tones of voice are associated with better patient outcomes and fewer malpractice claims (Ambady et al., 2002). Narrative medicine is a popular clinical model described by physicians (e.g., Charon, 2001) to emphasize "the ability to acknowledge, absorb, interpret, and act on the stories and plights of others" (p. 1897), and while it may seem controversial given the current shift toward evidence-based medicine, the two are compatible (Charon & Wyer, 2008).

Clinical relevance and impact of congruence (i.e., match) between patients sharing and physicians understanding their "story" was elucidated by humanistic psychologist Carl Rogers nearly 75 years ago (e.g., Rogers, 1942, 1949, 1957). In fact overlap is quite clear and frequent when examining the Rogerian method of *client-centered* therapy then and the tenets of *patient-centered* medicine promoted today; but only when clinicians from both medicine and psychology disciplines can communicate with each other.

FINAL RECOMMENDATIONS

Current research on the physician–patient relationship suggests some important clinical recommendations to apply when caring for older patients. First, health care professionals must seek to elicit and actively document geriatric patients' therapeutic goals. Goal Attainment Scaling (GAS) aids efforts to understand individual patients' personal conceptualization of a good quality of life. This includes setting goals related to functional status, social, and role function (Reuben & Tinetti, 2012; Rockwood et al., 2003; Williams et al., 2007). As addressed earlier in this publication, this goal-oriented model has several advantages, including the ability to focus physician–patient discussions on patients' individual concerns and desired health outcomes. This customized approach makes decision-making easier for patients; prompts patients to articulate and prioritize their health needs (i.e., patient comorbidity); and facilitates a therapeutic relationship based on shared decision-making (Reuben & Tinetti, 2012).

Second, clinicians must provide patients frequent opportunities to share their medical narrative and current experience of living with illness (including treatment challenges and concerns), and encourage patients to be active participants in their own care (Ashton et al., 2003). When done effectively, this process may reveal important health information that might otherwise be unavailable. Physicians must actively listen and express accurate empathy (both verbally and nonverbally) that conveys to patients they are understood *as people* and not viewed merely as their disease or medical condition (Adelman et al., 2000).

Third, physicians should seek to evaluate the effectiveness of their own communication style. Often, physicians are primarily open to and trusting of guidance from other physicians (Kane & West, 2005). As shown throughout this chapter, this is unlikely to help in evaluating communication style. This cultural trend aside, physicians who practice within accountable care organizations (ACOs) might be motivated financially to improve their communication skills. Assessments of patient satisfaction, such as the Medicare Health Plan Quality and Performance Ratings, include ratings of providers' responsiveness and can affect practice reimbursements. Survey questions ask Medicare patients about their experience of being listened to, respected, receiving necessary explanations, and having appropriate time offered to them in their care (Agency for Health care Research Quality, 2014). These perceptions are often directly shaped by clinical communication style. Again, while this behavioral awareness is core to clinical psychology training and practice, it is comparatively new to clinical medicine. Ultimately, reimbursement changes may incentivize better collaboration and integration in an effort to improve patient satisfaction via more effective patient-centered communication.

Post-visit questionnaires administered by medical staff can uncover information about the patient's life, including socially stigmatized disease-specific details that may not have been mentioned to the physician. Physicians might also consider audio-recording selected medical visits (with permission of the patient) and reviewing them alone or with a clinical psychologist to assess the strengths and weaknesses of their own communication style and develop workable strategies for improvement (Williams et al., 2007).

Psychologists Van Ryn, Burgess, Malat, and Griffin (2006) suggest that physicians consider training programs targeting culturally competent communication. A patient's culture can determine trust, beliefs regarding mental health, chronic disease, and the role of lifestyle as well as other behaviors related to health and illness. It can also determine whether or not patients seek health care at all (González, Vega, & Tarraf, 2010). Though increasingly viewed as vital to quality medical care, literature review reveals formal training is far from standard (Green et al., 2007). Clinical psychologists can collaborate with physicians to model diversity awareness and identify strategies to optimally meet the behavioral needs of patients from diverse backgrounds. Academic approaches may utilize culturally diverse standardized patients (e.g., Bensadon & Servoss, 2014). Clinically, these opportunities might include community-based health promotion screening activities, comprehensive preventive medicine education programs, and chronic illness management programs.

FUTURE

The Patient Protection and Affordable Care Act of 2010 includes the "medical home" model of care delivery. Initially introduced in 1967 by the American Academy of Pediatrics, the patient-centered medical home (PCMH) is an interdisciplinary care approach guided directly by values and preferences of patients and their families. Given their training in active listening and understanding of both verbal and nonverbal communication behavior, clinical psychologists can ensure patient-centered orientation and sustained focus on the patient's own perceptions of illness and health. This includes satisfaction with care, disease-specific education, behavioral strategies for effective self-management, treatment adherence, and management of depression and anxiety, among other goals (McDaniel & Fogarty, 2009).

Behavioral emphasis is core to effective management of most chronic diseases, particularly the multimorbidity common in older age. Health psychologists have adapted readily to the PCMH model, targeting "patient goals" and holistic care of the person, rather than focusing solely on disease-specific interventions (Kearney et al., 2014). Perhaps nowhere are effective communication and care of the "whole person" more important than in geriatrics.

In addition, psychologists can enhance collaboration and mutual understanding between members of the health care team, patients, patients' family members and other support systems, throughout the diagnosis and treatment process (McDaniel & Fogarty, 2009). In some health care delivery systems, such as the Veterans Health Administration (VHA), the role of clinical psychologists in biopsychosocial patient care is already standard (Kearney et al., 2014). In 2007, for example, the VHA initiated collaborative care management via primary care mental health implementation. In fact, the VHA has mandated the presence of clinical psychologists on integrated health care teams throughout their hospitals (Zeiss & Karlin, 2008), including Patient Aligned Care Teams (PACT), the VHA version of the PCMH (Kearney, Post, Zeiss, Goldstein, & Dundon, 2011). This is even more notable in primary care, where psychologist offices are intentionally co-located (i.e., same hallway) with primary care physicians and nurse practitioners to facilitate warm handoffs, nonfragmented communication, and patient follow-up, all while minimizing possible stigma due to separation of "mental" health.

Quality of health care communication is essential to maximizing a therapeutic relationship with older patients. Mutual collaboration fosters greater patient satisfaction, reduces the risks of nonadherence, improves patient health outcomes, and allows patients to build trusting relationships with their clinicians. Physicians, like psychologists, who effectively express empathy, engage in active listening, and offer practical, comprehensible assistance via transparent, egalitarian communication, can optimize their clinical impact. Through shared decision-making and a collaborative partnership, physicians can assess and manage their older patients' biomedical and psychosocial needs (Williams et al., 2007). Decades of research have shown this to be a difficult task to accomplish. A concomitant challenge has been integration of clinical psychologists. Integration can help assure implementation of effective communication strategies into everyday practice. Standard roles in both training and care provision will maximize the likelihood of improvement. As life expectancy increases, so will the need for these skills.

References

Adelman, R. D., Greene, M. G., & Ory, M. G. (2000). Communication between older patients and their physicians. *Clinics in Geriatric Medicine, 16*(1), 1–24.

Agency for Health care Research Quality (2014). *The CAHPS program.* Retrieved from: <https://cahps.ahrq.gov/about-cahps/cahps-program/index.html>.

Ahluwalia, S. C., Levin, J. R., Lorenz, K. A., & Gordon, H. S. (2012). Missed opportunities for advance care planning communication during outpatient clinic visits. *Journal of General Internal Medicine, 27*(4), 445–451.

Alzheimer's Association, (2014). Retrieved from: <www.alz.org/>August 20, 2014.

Ambady, N., Laplante, D., Nguyen, T., Rosenthal, R., Chaumeton, N., & Levinson, W. (2002). *Surgery, 132*(1), 5–9.

Anderson, L. M., Scrimshaw, S. C., Fullilove, M. T., Fielding, J. E., Normand, J., & Task Force on Community Health Services, (2003). Culturally competent health care systems: A systematic review. *American Journal of Preventive Medicine, 24*(3), 68–79.

Antoine, P., & Pasquier, F. (2013). Emotional and psychological implications of early AD diagnosis. *Medical Clinics of North America, 97*(3), 459–475.

Ashton, C. M., Haidet, P., Paterniti, D. A., Collins, T. C., Gordon, H. S., O'Malley, K., et al. (2003). Racial and ethnic disparities in the use of health services. *Journal of General Internal Medicine, 18*(2), 146–152.

Baile, W. F., Lenzi, R., Parker, P. A., Buckman, R., & Cohen, L. (2002). Oncologists' attitudes toward and practices in giving bad news: An exploratory study. *Journal of Clinical Oncology, 20*(8), 2189–2196.

Beach, M. C., Roter, D. L., Wang, N., Duggan, P. S., & Cooper, L. A. (2006). Are physicians' attitudes of respect accurately perceived by patients and associated with more positive communication behaviors? *Patient Education and Counseling, 62*(3), 347–354.

Benbassat, J., Pilpel, D., & Tidhar, M. (1998). Patients' preferences for participation in clinical decision making: A review of published surveys. *Behavioral Medicine, 24*(2), 81–88.

Bensadon, B.A., & Servoss, J.C. (2014). *Simulation-based training in cultural competence: The ccOSCE.* Poster presented at the Minority Health & Health Disparities Grantees' Conference: Transdisciplinary Collaborations: Evolving Dimensions of US and Global Health Equity. National Harbor, MD.

Bevans, M., & Sternberg, E. M. (2012). Caregiving burden, stress, and health effects among family caregivers of adult cancer patient. *Journal of the American Medical Association, 307*(4), 398–403.

Bruera, E., Palmer, J. L., Pace, E., Zhang, K., Willey, J., Strasser, F., et al. (2007). A randomized, controlled trial of physician postures when breaking bad news to cancer patients. *Palliative Medicine, 21*(6), 501–505.

Callahan, E. J., Bertakis, K. D., Azari, R., Robbins, J. A., Helms, L. J., & Chang, D. W. (2000). The influence of patient age on primary care resident physician–patient interaction. *Journal of American Geriatrics Society, 48*(1), 30–35.

Charon, R. (2001). Narrative medicine: A model for empathy, reflection, profession, and trust. *Journal of the American Medical Association, 286*(15), 1897–1902.

Charon, R., & Wyer, P. (2008). Narrative evidence based medicine. *The Lancet, 371*(9609), 296–297.

Chen, H., & Landefeld, S. C. (2007). The hidden poor: Care of the elderly. In W. M. King (Ed.), *Medical management of vulnerable and underserved patients* (pp. 199–209). New York, NY: McGraw-Hill.

Clarke, L. H., Bennett, E. V., & Korotchenko, A. (2014). Negotiating vulnerabilities: How older adults with multiple chronic conditions interact with physicians. *Canadian Journal on Aging, 33*(1), 26–37.

Cousin, G., Schmid Mast, M., Roter, D. L., & Hall, J. A. (2012). Concordance between physician communication style and patient attitudes predicts patient satisfaction. *Patient Education and Counseling, 87*(2), 193–197.

Crawford, M. J., Thana, L., Methuen, C., Ghosh, P., Stanely, S. V., Ross, J., et al. (2011). Impact of screening for risk of suicide: Randomised controlled trial. *The British Journal of Psychiatry, 198,* 379–384.

Delaplain, T. (2011). Failing. *Journal of General Internal Medicine, 26*(7), 819.

DiMatteo, M. R. (2004). Variations in patients' adherence to medication recommendations: A quantitative review of 50 years of research. *Medical Care, 42*(3), 200–209.

DiMatteo, M. R., Giordani, P. J., Lepper, H. S., & Croghan, T. W. (2002). Patient adherence and medical treatment outcomes: A meta-analysis. *Medical Care, 40,* 794–811.

Duffy, F. D., Gordon, G. H., Whelan, G., Cole-Kelly, K., Frankel, R., & Buffone, N. (2004). Assessing competence in communication and interpersonal skills: The Kalamazoo II Report. *Academic Medicine, 79*(6), 495–507.

Ekdahl, A. W., Hellstrom, I., Andersson, L., & Friedrichsen, M. (2012). Too complex and time-consuming to fit in! Physicians' experiences of elderly patients and their participation in medical decision making: A grounded theory study. *British Medical Journal, 2,* 1–7.

Elwyn, G., Frosch, D., Thomson, R., Joseph-Williams, N., Lloyd, A., Kinnersley, P., et al. (2012). Shared decision making: A model for clinical practice. *Journal of General Internal Medicine, 27*(10), 1361–1367.

Fowler, J. C. (2012). Suicide risk assessment in clinical practice: Pragmatic guidelines for imperfect assessments. *Psychotherapy, 49*(1), 81–90.

Frosch, D. L., & Kaplan, R. M. (1999). Shared decision making in clinical medicine: Past research and future directions. *American Journal of Preventive Medicine, 7*(4), 285–293.

Giampieri, M. (2012). Communication and informed consent in elderly people. *Minerva Anestesiologica, 78*(2), 236–242.

González, M. H., Vega, A. W., & Tarraf, W. (2010). Health care quality perceptions among foreign-born Latinos and the importance of speaking the same language. *The Journal of the American Board of Family Medicine, 23,* 745–752.

Gouin, J. P., Hantsoo, L., & Kiecolt-Glaser, J. K. (2008). Immune dysregulation and chronic stress among older adults: A review. *Neuroimmunomodulation, 15*(4–6), 251–259.

Green, A. R., Miller, E., Krupat, E., White, A., Taylor, W. C., Hirsh, D. A., et al. (2007). Designing and implementing a cultural competence OSCE: Lessons learned from interviews with medical students. *Ethnicity & Disease, 17*(2), 344–350.

Greene, J., & Hibbard, J. H. (2012). Why does patient activation matter? An examination of the relationship between patient activation and health-related outcomes. *Journal of General Internal Medicine, 27*(5), 520–526.

Greene, M. G., & Adelman, R. D. (2003). Physician–older patient communication about cancer. *Patient Education and Counseling, 50,* 55–60.

Greene, M. G., & Adelman, R. D. (2013). Beyond the dyad: Communication in triadic (and more) medical encounters. In L. R. Martin & M. R. DiMatteo (Eds.), *The oxford handbook of health communication, behavior change, and treatment adherence.* New York, NY: Oxford University Press.

Greene, M. G., Adelman, R. D., Friedmann, E., & Charon, R. (1994). Older patient satisfaction with communication during an initial medical encounter. *Social Science & Medicine, 38*(9), 1279–1288.

Greene, M. G., Hoffman, S., Charon, R., & Adelman, R. (1987). Psychosocial concerns in the medical encounter: A comparison of the interactions of doctors with their old and young patients. *The Gerontologist, 27*(2), 164–168.

Guintivano, J., Brown, T., Newcomer, A., Jones, M., Cox, O., Maher, B. S., et al. (2014). Identification and replication of a combined epigenetic and genetic biomarker predicting suicide and suicidal behaviors. *American Journal of Psychiatry, 2014.*

Haskard, K. B., Williams, S. L., DiMatteo, M. R., Rosenthal, R., White, M. K., & Goldstein, M. G. (2008). Physician and patient communication training in primary care: Effects on participation and satisfaction. *Health Psychology, 27*(5), 513–522.

Haskard-Zolnierek, K. B., & DiMatteo, M. R. (2009). Physician communication and patient adherence to treatment: A meta-analysis. *Medical Care, 47*, 826–834.

Haug, M. (1979). Doctor–patient relationships and the older patient. *Journal of Gerontology, 34*(6), 852–860.

Hemmerdinger, J. M., Stoddart, S. D., & Lilford, R. J. (2007). A systematic review of tests of empathy in medicine. *BMC Medical Education, 7*(24), 1–8.

Heritage, J., Robinson, J. D., Elliott, M. N., Beckett, M., & Wilkes, M. (2007). Reducing patients' unmet concerns in primary care: The difference one word can make. *Journal of General Internal Medicine, 22*(10), 1429–1433.

Hojat, M., Mangione, S., Nasca, T. J., Cohen, M. J., Gonnella, J. S., Erdmann, J. B., et al. (2001). The Jefferson Scale of Physician Empathy: Development and preliminary psychometric data. *Educational and Psychological Measurement, 61*(2), 349–365.

Hojat, M., Spandorfer, J., Louis, D. Z., & Gonnella, J. S. (2011). Empathic and sympathetic orientations toward patient care: Conceptualization, measurement, and psychometrics. *Academic Medicine, 86*(8), 989–995.

Hook, K. M., & Pfeiffer, C. A. (2007). Impact of a new curriculum on medical students' interpersonal and interviewing skills. *Medical Education, 41*(2), 154–159.

Hudak, P. L., Armstrong, K., Braddock, C., III, Frankel, R. M., & Levinson, W. (2008). Older patients' unexpressed concerns about orthopaedic surgery. *The Journal of Bone & Joint Surgery, 90*(7), 1427–1435.

Jagosh, J., Boudreau, J. D., Steinert, Y., MacDonald, M. E., & Ingram, L. (2011). The importance of physician listening from the patients' perspective: Enhancing, diagnosis, healing, and the doctor–patient relationship. *Patient Education and Counseling, 85,* 369–374.

Jahng, K. H., Martin, L. R., Golin, C. E., & DiMatteo, M. R. (2005). Preferences for medical collaboration: Patient-physician congruence and patient outcomes. *Patient Education and Counseling, 57*(3), 308–314.

Kane, R. L., & West, J. C. (2005). *It shouldn't be this way: The failure of long-term care.* Nashville, TN: Vanderbilt University Press.

Kaplan, S. H., Greenfield, S., Gandek, B., Rogers, W. H., & Ware, J. E., Jr (1996). Characteristics of physicians with participatory decision-making styles. *Annals of Internal Medicine, 124*(5), 497–504.

Kearney, L. K., Post, E. P., Pomerantz, A. S., & Zeiss, A. (2014). Applying the interprofessional patient aligned care team in the department of Veterans Affairs. *American Psychologist, 69*(4), 399–408. Ethics and Human Research, 30(20), 13–19.

Kearney, L. K., Post, E. P., Zeiss, A., Goldstein, M. G., & Dundon, M. (2011). The role of mental and behavioral health in the application of the patient-centered medical home in the Department of Veterans Affairs. *Translational Behavioral Medicine, 1*(4), 624–628.

Kemper, S., & Harden, T. (1999). Experimentally disentangling what's beneficial about elderspeak from what's not. *Psychology and Aging, 14,* 656–670.

Kovner, C. T., Mezey, M., & Harrington, C. (2002). Who cares for older adults? Workforce implications of an aging society. *Health Affairs, 21*(5), 78–89.

Kripalani, S., Bengtzen, R., Henderson, L.E., & Jacobson, T.A. (2008). Clinical research in low-literacy populations: Using teach-back to assess comprehension of informed consent and privacy information.

La Monica, E. L. L. (1981). Construct validity of an empathy instrument. *Research in Nursing and Health, 4*(4), 389–400.

Langewitz, W., Denz, M., Keller, A., Kiss, A., Rütimann, S., & Wössmer, B. (2002). Spontaneous talking time at start of consultation in outpatient clinic: Cohort study. *BMJ, 325*(7366), 682–683.

Lapierre, S., Erlangsen, A., Waern, M., Leo, D. D., Oyama, H., & Scocco, P. (2011). The International Research Group for Suicide among the Elderly. *Crisis, 32*(3), 88–98.

Lee, S., Colditz, G. A., Berkman, L. F., & Kawachi, I. (2003). Caregiving and risk of coronary heart disease in US women: A prospective study. *American Journal of Preventive Medicine, 24*(2), 113–119.

Levinson, W., Kao, A., Kuby, A., & Thisted, R. A. (2004). Not all patients want to participate in decision making: A nation study of public preferences. *Journal of General Internal Medicine, 20*, 531–535.

Levinson, W., & Pizzo, P. A. (2011). Patient-physician communication: It's about time. *Journal of the American Medical Association, 305*(17), 1802–1803.

Lilly, M. B., Robinson, C. A., Holtzman, S., & Bottorff, J. L. (2012). Can we move beyond burden and burnout to support the health and wellness of family caregivers to persons with dementia? Evidence from British Columbia, Canada. *Health & Social Care in the Community, 20*(1), 103–112.

Martin, L. R., Haskard-Zolnierek, K. B., & DiMatteo, M. R. (2010). *Health behavior change and treatment adherence: Evidence-based guidelines for improving health care*. New York, NY: Oxford University Press.

Marvel, M. K., Epstein, R. M., Flowers, K., & Beckman, H. B. (1999). Soliciting the patient's agenda: Have we improved? *Journal of the American Medical Association, 281*(3), 283–287.

McDaniel, S. H., & Fogarty, C. T. (2009). What primary care psychology has to offer the patient-centered medical home. *Professional Psychology: Research and Practice, 40*(5), 483–492.

McHenry, M., Parker, P. A., Baile, W. F., & Lenzi, R. (2011). Voice analysis during bad news discussion in oncology: Reduced pitch, decreased speaking rate, and nonverbal communication of empathy. *Support Care Cancer, 20*(5), 1073–1078.

Min, L. C., Reuben, D. B., Keeler, E., Ganz, D. A., Fung, C. H., Shekelle, P., et al. (2011). Is patient-perceived severity of a geriatric condition related to better quality of care? *Medical Care, 49*(1), 101–107.

Mitchell, A. J., & Subramaniam, H. (2005). Prognosis of depression in old age compared to middle age: A systematic review of comparative studies. *American Journal of Psychiatry, 162*(9), 1588–1601.

Montague, E., Chen, P., Xu, J., Chewning, B., & Barrett, B. (2013). Nonverbal interpersonal interactions in clinical encounters and patient perceptions of empathy. *Journal of Participatory Medicine, 5*.

Nash, J. M., McKay, K. M., Vogel, M. E., & Masters, K. S. (2012). Functional roles and foundational characteristics of psychologists in integrated primary care. *Journal of Clinical Psychology in Medical Settings, 19*, 93–104.

Nightingale, S. D., Yarnold, P. R., & Greenberg, M. S. (1991). Sympathy, empathy, and physician resource utilization. *Journal of General Internal Medicine, 6*(5), 420–423.

Olsburgh, B., & Jelley, D. M. (1989). Time to let the patient speak. *British Medical Journal, 298*(6671), 458.

Orlander, J. D., Graeme Fincke, B., Hermanns, D., & Johnson, G. A. (2002). Medical residents' first clearly remembered experiences of giving bad news. *Journal of General Internal Medicine, 17*(11), 825–840.

Ownby, R. L., Hertzog, C., Crocco, E., & Duara, R. (2006). Factors related to medication adherence in memory disorder in clinic. *Aging and Mental Health, 10*(4), 378–385.

O'Connor, E., Gaynes, B. N., Burda, B. U., Soh, C., & Whitlock, E. P. (2013). Screening for and treatment of suicide risk relevant to primary care: A systematic review for the US Preventive Services Task Force. *Annals of Internal Medicine, 158*(10), 741–754.

Pawlikowska, T., Zhang, W., Griffiths, F., Van Dalen, J., & van der Vleuten, C. (2012). Verbal and nonverbal behavior of doctors and patients in primary care consultations – How this relates to patient enablement. *Patient Education and Counseling, 86*, 70–76.

Pfeiffer, C., Madray, H., Ardolino, A., & Willms, J. (1998). The rise and fall of students' skill in obtaining a medical history. *Medical Education, 32*(3), 283–288.

Price, E. L., Bereknyei, S., Kuby, A., Levinson, W., & Braddock, C. H. (2012). New elements for informed decision making: A qualitative study of older adults' views. *Patient Education and Counseling, 86,* 335–341.

Ptacek, J. T., & Ptacek, J. J. (2001). Patients' perceptions of receiving bad news about cancer. *Journal of Clinical Oncology, 19*(21), 4160–4164.

Quill, T. E., & Holloway, R. G. (2012). Evidence, preferences, recommendations – Finding the right balance in patient care. *The New England Journal of Medicine, 366,* 1653–1655.

Rabinowitz, I., Luzzatti, R., Tamir, A., & Reis, S. (2004). Length of patient's monologue, rate of completion, and relation to other components of the clinical encounter: Observational intervention study in primary care. *British Medical Journal, 328,* 501–502.

Reuben, D. B., & Tinetti, M. E. (2012). Goal-oriented patient care: An alternative health outcomes paradigm. *New England Journal of Medicine, 366*(9), 777–779.

Riess, H., Kelley, J. M., Bailey, R. W., Dunn, E. J., & Phillips, M. (2012). Empathy training for resident physicians: A randomized controlled trial of a neuroscience-informed curriculum. (2012). *Journal of General Internal Medicine, 10,* 1280–1286.

Riess, H., & Kraft-Todd, G. (2014). E.M.P.A.T.H.Y.: A tool to enhance nonverbal communication between clinicians and their patients. *Academic Medicine, 89*(8), 1108–1112.

Robinson, P. J., & Reiter, J. T. (2007). Examples of consultations with older adults: *Behavioral consultation and primary care: A guide to integrating services.* New York, NY: Springer. (pp. 289–318).

Rockwood, K., Howlett, S., Stadnyke, K., Carver, D., Powell, C., & Stolee, P. (2003). Responsiveness of goal attainment scaling in a randomized controlled trial of comprehensive geriatric assessment. *Journal of Clinical Epidemiology, 56,* 736–743.

Rogers, C. R. (1942). Counseling and psychotherapy; Newer concepts in practice. Boston, MA: Houghton Mifflin.

Rogers, C. R. (1949). The attitude and orientation of the counselor in client-centered therapy. *Journal of Consulting Psychology, 13*(2), 82.

Rogers, C. R. (1957). The necessary and sufficient conditions of therapeutic personality change. *Journal of Consulting Psychology, 21,* 95–103.

Rosenbaum, M. E., Ferguson, K. J., & Lobas, J. G. (2004). Teaching medical students and residents skills for delivering bad news: A review of strategies. *Academic Medicine, 79*(2), 107–117.

Rost, K., & Frankel, R. (1993). The introduction of the older patient's problems in the medical visit. *Journal of Aging Health, 5*(3), 387–401.

Rotar, D. L. (2000). The enduring and evolving nature of the patient–physician relationship. *Patient Education and Counseling, 39,* 5–15.

Roter, D. L., & Hall, J. A. (1989). Studies of doctor–patient interaction. *Annual Review of Public Health, 10,* 163–180.

Salloway, S., & Correia, S. (2009). Alzheimer disease: Time to improve its diagnosis and treatment. *Cleveland Clinic Journal of Medicine, 76*(1), 49–58.

Schaepe, K. S. (2011). Bad news and first impressions: Patient and family caregiver accounts of learning the cancer diagnosis. *Social Science & Medicine, 73*(6), 912–921.

Schonfeld, T. L., Stevens, E. A., Lampman, M. A., & Lyons, W. L. (2012). Assessing challenges in end-of-life conversations with elderly patients with multiple morbidities. *American Journal of Hospice & Palliative Medicine, 29*(4), 260–267.

Schulz, R., & Beach, S. R. (1999). Caregiving as a risk factor for mortality: The Caregiver Health Effects Study. *Journal of the American Medical Association, 282*(23), 2215–2219.

Sleath, B., Rubin, R. H., & Arrey-Wastavino, A. (2000). Physician expression of empathy and positiveness to Hispanic and non-Hispanic white patients during medical encounters. *Family Medicine, 32*(2), 91–96.

Smith, S., Hanson, J. L., Tewksbury, L. R., Christy, C., Talib, N. J., Harris, M. A., et al. (2007). *Evaluation and the Health Professions, 30*(1), 3–21.

Sosa-Ortiz, A. L., Acosta-Castillo, I., & Prince, M. J. (2012). Epidemiology of dementias and Alzheimer's disease. *Archives of Medical Research, 43*(8), 600–608.

Starfield, B., Lemke, K. W., Herbert, R., Pavlovich, W. D., & Anderson, G. (2005). Comorbidity and the use of primary care and specialist care in the elderly. *Annals of Family Medicine, 3*(3), 215–222.

Stepanikova, I., & Cook, K. S. (2004). Insurance policies and perceived quality of primary care among privately insured patients: Do features of managed care widen the racial, ethnic, and language-based gaps? *Medical Care, 42*(10), 966–974.

Street, R. L., Jr, Krupat, E., Bell, R. A., Kravitz, R. L., & Haidet, P. (2003). Beliefs about control in the physician-patient relationship: Effect on communication in medical encounters. *Journal of General Internal Medicine, 18*(8), 609–616.

Szanto, K., Prigerson, H. G., & Reynolds, C. F., III (2001). Suicide in the elderly. *Clinical Neuroscience Research, 1*, 366–376.

Thomas, K. E. (2010). *Dialogue systems, spatial tasks and elderly users: A review of research into elderspeak. SFB/TR 8 Report No. 021-02/2010.* Bremen, Germany: University of Bremen/University of Freiburg.

Toner, M.A., Shadden, B.B., & Gluth, M.D. (2011). Communication and aging. In Communication and Aging: For Clinicians by Clinicians (2nd ed.) Austin, TX.

Tulsky, J. A., Fischer, G. S., Rose, M. R., & Arnold, R. M. (1998). Opening the black box: How do physicians communicate about advance directives? *Annals of Internal Medicine, 129*(6), 441–449.

U.S. Census Bureau (2004). Interim Projections by Age, Sex, Race and Hispanic Origin. Washington, DC. Available at: <www.census.gov/ipc/www/usinterimproj>. Accessed June 20.06.14.

Van Ryn, M., Burgess, D., Malat, J., & Griffin, J. (2006). Physicians' perceptions of patients' social and behavioral characteristics and race disparities in treatment recommendations for men with coronary artery disease. *American Journal of Public Health, 96*(2), 351–357.

Van Vliet, D., de Vugt, M. E., Bakker, C., Pijnenburg, Y. A. L., Vernooij-Dassen, M. J. F. J., Koopmans, R. T. C. M., et al. (2013). Time to diagnosis in young-onset dementia as compared with late-onset dementia. *Psychological Medicine, 43*(02), 423–432.

White, M., Garbez, R., Carroll, M., Brinker, E., & Howie-Esquivel, J. (2013). Is "teach-back" associated with knowledge retention and hospital readmission in hospitalized heart failure patients? *Journal of Cardiovascular Nursing, 28*(2), 137–146.

Williams, K. N., Herman, R., Gajewski, B., & Wilson, K. (2009). Elderspeak communication: Impact on dementia care. *American Journal of Alzheimer's Disease and Other Dementias, 24*(1), 11–20.

Williams, S. L., Haskard, K. B., & DiMatteo, M. R. (2007). The therapeutic effect of the physician–older patient relationship: Effective communication with vulnerable older patients. *Clinical Interventions in Aging, 2*(3), 453–467.

Wispe, L. G. (1968). Sympathy and empathy. *International Encyclopedia of the Social Sciences, 15*, 441–447.

Zeiss, A., & Karlin, B. (2008). Integrating mental health and primary care services in the Department of Veterans Affairs health care system. *Journal of Clinical Psychology in Medical Settings, 15*, 73–78.

5

Culture of Medicine

Willie Underwood III

Roswell Park Cancer Institute, Buffalo, New York, USA

INTRODUCTION

"Is it too late to send all the Niggers back to Africa ... I think we should just kill them all."

I still remember my pain and shock upon discovering the above comment etched on my medical school restroom as a first-year student in the 1990s. I had been so excited to have the opportunity to satisfy my dream of becoming a physician. I believed I would be in the presence of future colleagues who, like me, were prepared to dedicate their entire lives to helping others, a goal I had made plain and clear in my personal statement and without regard to future patients' ethnicity, sex, socioeconomic status, or age. Simply put, my passion was to help heal those most vulnerable.

As time progressed, though, it became increasingly more difficult to ignore similar examples of intolerance. The sting of angry racism was not new, but what made it worse was it came from physicians, my prior image of whom was largely informed by Marcus Welby, M.D., a popular fictional television character during the early 1970s. Dr. Welby was an empathic primary care physician who cared for and truly loved all his patients, doing all he could to improve their health and their lives in general. Now, after more than 20 years of surgical training and practice, most of which centered on cancer, two simple realizations have become clear:

1. Physicians are merely human.
2. Physician behavior is greatly influenced by a deeply warped medical culture.

B. Bensadon (Ed): Psychology and Geriatrics.
DOI: http://dx.doi.org/10.1016/B978-0-12-420123-1.00005-8

HIPPOCRATIC OATH

Physicians have been admired for centuries and medicine has long been considered among the most honorable professions. Much of the public's image of medical practice is consistent with the Hippocratic Oath (Lasagna, 1964) that most of us must pledge during medical school:

"I swear to fulfill, to the best of my ability and judgment, this covenant: I will respect the hard-won scientific gains of those physicians in whose steps I walk, and gladly share such knowledge as is mine with those who are to follow. I will apply, for the benefit of the sick, all measures which are required, avoiding those twin traps of overtreatment and therapeutic nihilism. I will remember that there is art to medicine as well as science, and that warmth, sympathy, and understanding may outweigh the surgeon's knife or the chemist's drug. I will not be ashamed to say 'I know not,' nor will I fail to call in my colleagues when the skills of another are needed for a patient's recovery. I will respect the privacy of my patients, for their problems are not disclosed to me that the world may know. Most especially must I tread with care in matters of life and death. If it is given me to save a life, all thanks. But it may also be within my power to take a life; this awesome responsibility must be faced with great humbleness and awareness of my own frailty. Above all, I must not play at God. I will remember that I do not treat a fever chart, a cancerous growth, but a sick human being, whose illness may affect the person's family and economic stability. My responsibility includes these related problems, if I am to care adequately for the sick. I will prevent disease whenever I can, for prevention is preferable to cure. I will remember that I remain a member of society, with special obligations to all my fellow human beings, those sound of mind and body as well as the infirm. If I do not violate this oath, may I enjoy life and art, respected while I live and remembered with affection thereafter. May I always act so as to preserve the finest traditions of my calling and may I long experience the joy of healing those who seek my help."

This inspiring ethical contract that demands, above all, that physicians do no harm, plays out routinely in medical practice. However, the culture of medicine is both Hippocratic and hypocritical. On one hand, altruism and selflessness abound, yet on the other hand there exists a one-upmanship culture driven by arrogance, ego, and bias. Because the latter leads to discomfort with medicine's limits, geriatric patients, who may be most complex to safely manage, are among the most vulnerable.

PATIENT-CENTEREDNESS

The physician–patient relationship is paramount to the health care system (Epstein & Street, 2011). Recent trends have led to a formal paradigm shift toward patient-centered health care. The Institute of Medicine's 2001 report, *Crossing the Quality Chasm: A New Health System for the 21st Century*, provides a definition of patient-centered care that prioritizes and respects individual patient preferences, needs, and values, above all else. To the layperson, this seems straightforward and rational. In fact, one might wonder, if this is a *new* model of practice, what has been done previously?

In truth, it is not difficult to find evidence that the traditional medical system is actually *physician*-centered. Medical culture shapes this perception in many ways. For starters, there is the white coat. While patients and their families may automatically recognize this as a powerful symbol of doctorhood, they may not know that most first-year medical students are granted their white coat in an elaborate and formal ceremony. Pros and cons of this tradition have been described elsewhere (e.g., Jones, 1999; Russell, 2002; Goldberg, 2008), and evidence of the coat's immense psychological power over patients is clearly demonstrated by white coat hypertension (Pickering et al., 1988). More recently and perhaps not coincidentally, the white coat has been adopted by other health care providers, including nurse practitioners, pharmacists, and even clinical nutritionists. Rarely do clinical psychologists wear white coats.

Attire aside, most hospital parking lots have spaces clearly delineated for physicians only, usually adjacent to similarly labeled physicians-only entrances. Physicians-only lounge areas and cafeterias are common, and usually include access to complimentary food and drink, distinct from the other cafeterias where patients and others must pay. In outpatient offices and clinics, navigating medical visits is often complex. Patients must often report to a front desk, fill out paperwork, and wait for variable lengths of time, before being led by a nonphysician clinician to an examining room to wait again. This process culminates with the physician visiting the patient, be it alone or with trainees, again for a variable length of time, often a fraction of what had transpired heretofore. As discussed elsewhere in this publication, the extent to which the physician communicates directly and effectively with patients and their families varies. Given this context, the novelty of a truly *patient*-centered model becomes clear. Though a crude concept to digest, as depicted in mainstream media (e.g., *The Doctor*) and observable across our nation's health care settings, being relegated to "patient" status is not value-neutral and can even seem like a demotion from human being. The common danger of patient dehumanization has been revealed in psychology experiments (e.g., Rosenhan, 1973), medical education interventions (e.g., Wilkes, Milgrom, and Hoffman, 2002), and my own life (Underwood III, 2012).

TRUST AND RESPECT

Medical culture frequently communicates mixed messages (Wear & Zarconi, 2008) that can confuse trainees, patients, and providers alike.

For example, at the beginning of my surgical residency, senior physicians taught me the following four (incompatible) rules to live by:

1. Trust no one.
2. Feel free to call.
3. If you call I will consider that a sign of weakness.
4. You'd better not make a mistake.

Psychologists have long theorized the negative psychological implications of incongruent (i.e., mixed) messages (Galloway, 1968). They have even hypothesized the resulting "double-bind," where a person cannot win no matter which course of action he or she chooses, as a potential precursor of schizophrenia (Bateson, Jackson, Haley, & Weakland, 1956). Medical trainees are not immune to this perplexing impact. Many physicians themselves recognize that in a dysfunctional system or culture, trust and respect, core to the therapeutic relationship between patients and their clinicians, and equally vital to collaborative practice among colleagues, can suffer (Leape, 2006; Leape et al., 2012a, 2012b).

Medical culture values skepticism, especially when applied to complex diagnostic problem-solving that leads to thorough and accurate differential diagnosis of illness. But when exaggerated beyond productive levels, it can result in pathological distrust and pessimism. In the face of frequent trauma, hope and optimism are distorted and discounted as naïveté, and specialty-specific cliques perpetuate interspecialty (and interdisciplinary) stereotypes: Surgeons are not empathic, family physicians are not knowledgeable, physical medicine is glorified physical therapy, and psychiatrists are not even physicians. Geriatrics, many believe, is not a bona fide subspecialty, and palliative care physicians may be "affectionately" referred to by colleagues as Dr. Death. These are just some of the stereotypes that prevail in a medical culture where trust and consensus are rare, and individuals often demand respect for their logical reasoning rather than elicit it with compassion. Perceived prestige often follows and is frequently wed to salary and reimbursement rates. Of course, these subjective perceptions are fickle. In earlier eras surgeons were generally viewed as mere technicians, whereas currently they rank near the top of the earnings, and therefore prestige, totem pole.

TOUCHY FEELY

As a surgical resident, I earned what appeared to be a laudatory evaluation, receiving 4 out of 5 on all technical and knowledge criteria used to evaluate my performance. Needless to say, I was confused to discover the reviewer's narrative comments, which concluded *"Dr. Underwood does not have what it takes to be a surgeon. I recommend that he go into family medicine."*

This assessment was then justified by pointing out patients and their families connected well with me and these characteristics were not compatible with being an effective surgeon. That was it. Case closed.

Bewildered, I sought greater clarity from the residency program director, but no further explanation was given. Ironically, in the more than 12 years since that pivotal moment, something else did become extremely clear to me. Most patients seem to appreciate my humanity as much as (if not more than) my technical ability. In fact most people can be taught the technical skills necessary to safely perform most operations. For most surgical procedures, undesirable patient outcomes will occur even in the best technical hands. But contrary to what we are taught, and as robust data on litigation and risk management suggest, when this does inevitably occur, it is usually the breakdown of the physician–patient relationship that motivates malpractice suits, not inferior technical skill or degree of patient injury (Beckman, Markakis, Suchman, & Frankel, 1994; Kraman & Hamm, 1999; Penchansky & Macnee, 1994).

By definition, surgery, perhaps more than any other specialty, involves *touching* and *feeling* the patient. Yet sadly, this message is rarely promulgated in training and illustrates a major disconnect between our formally stated goals, daily work, and hidden reality. Instead, relational skills are often devalued as soft, imprecise, and unscientific, and therefore outside the scope of our required professional expertise and responsibility.

ZERO-SUM GAME

The above false dichotomy between interpersonal and technical skill presents a daunting and ongoing challenge to optimal patient care. Historically, instead of fostering an environment that truly embraces empathy, compassion, and shared clinical decision-making (i.e., patient-centeredness), in practice, medical culture continues to reinforce the notion that these attributes are "soft" while technical and problem-solving abilities are "rigorous." Worse yet, they are often viewed as mutually exclusive. For decades many critics with evidence have challenged this "zero-sum game" (Arnold, Povar, & Howell, 1987; Coulter, 2002; Hurwitz & Vass, 2002; Kirch, 2012; Wensing, Jung, Mainz, Olesen, & Grol, 1998), but breaking through related cultural barriers has proven a slow and arduous process. This is especially true in the surgical fields, where trainees are explicitly taught to operate on organs, not people. In fact, it is not uncommon to hear surgeons describe their day by the very organs they've removed (e.g., nephrectomy, colestectomy, prostatectomy).

The Association of American Medical Colleges (AAMC), led by psychiatrist and CEO Darrell Kirch, M.D., has responded by expanding the Medical College Admission Test (MCAT) to include psychological and behavioral science content for the first time ever (AAMC, 2012). Implications are unknown but this is an important step in the right direction (OBGYN. net staff, 2012). The blog post from an obstetrics and gynecology website quoted below is illustrative, as is the fact that it was posted anonymously:

I once fired a doctor for her lousy bedside manner. She was technologically advanced and scientifically up to date; her exam and waiting rooms were lovely; the front office staff was friendly, helpful, and efficient. But she was unable or unwilling to answer questions, address or allay fears, and treat me with compassion. Last Sunday's *New York Times* featured a story on the Association of American Medical Colleges' (AAMC) revision of the MCAT, so that it now incorporates "squishier" subjects including social and behavioral sciences and medical ethics. When AAMC's president, Darrell G. Kirch, announced the changes, he said:

"[In surveys,] the public had great confidence in doctors' knowledge but much less in their bedside manner. The goal is to improve the medical admissions process to find the people who you and I would want as our doctors. Being a good doctor isn't just about understanding science, it's about understanding people."

But a response from *MedPage Today*'s "Dr. Wes" claims that this is preparing medical students for "a health care world that will not exist." He goes on to say:

"Developing selection criteria for medical school based on social and humanitarian coursework without addressing the reality of today's increasingly computer-screen-focused medical practice is whistling in the dark. As it is developing today, the AAMC would be more effective by preparing students with typing lessons and pre-selecting them for unflagging conformity and rule-following skills. ... If the AAMC is truly concerned about patient-centric medicine, it would promote student activism to participate in policy changes that insist on more patient contact."

I find it ironic that he chastises this effort as creating "unflagging conformity and rule-following" while encouraging the AAMC and students to lobby for more rules to follow. Instead of training physicians to assess a patient's emotional and psychological needs and respond accordingly, this approach encourages another layer of bureaucracy, another box to tick, without regard for how each physician interacts with the human sitting in front of them. My former doctor could have checked the "patient contact" box, but she still didn't understand people.

All medicine is, essentially, intimate. Even in the best case scenario – a healthy patient undergoing an annual physical – a patient is submitting his body to a virtual stranger. But this intimacy is especially profound in obstetrics and gynecology. When a patient doesn't feel heard, when she feels judged or embarrassed, she just wants to get out of that office as quickly as possible. If that happens, physicians lose the opportunity to ask and answer questions, to clarify, instruct, and explain. They lose the opportunity to help a patient heal and be healthy. They lose the opportunity to do their job.

We need to stop treating technical adeptness and the ability to understand and communicate with patients as a zero-sum game. I hold no illusion that pre-med students enrolling in medical anthropology courses will solve this issue, but at least it acknowledges that there is one. And that's an important first step.

As illustrated in the next clinical example, this insight is not innately guaranteed, it can be trained, and negative consequences often occur without it.

EMPATHY VS BLAME

As a senior resident working with a competent and caring junior colleague, I recall a young Hispanic woman who arrived with four children, each under the age of 5. My junior trainee performed the initial evaluation and presented the patient's case to me. Symptoms included pain with intercourse, incontinence, post-void dribbling and recurrent urinary tract infections, symptoms consistent with a urethral diverticulum. I asked the resident if this diagnosis matched what he found after performing his pelvic exam. To my surprise, he stated he did not perform the exam. When I asked why not, he became upset and seemed offended. He then explained that the patient brought her children to the clinic, arrived late, and had missed her two prior clinic appointments. I remained unclear about the connection between her late arrival, attendance history, and his decision not to perform this necessary diagnostic exam.

Given my trainee's aroused emotional state, I simply suggested we talk to the patient together. On the way to her room, I asked the staff to watch the children while we examined the patient. I introduced myself, assessed the clinical situation, and repeated my understanding of her chief complaint. I then asked her how she got to the clinic, to which she replied the following:

"Doctor, I'm sorry for bringing my children. I waited as long as I could for my friend who agreed to watch my children. But when she didn't arrive, I decided to bring them. I missed the last two appointments because the sitter didn't show up, and I know that if you miss or reschedule three appointments, you will be kicked out of the clinic. Honestly, I would have been on time, but I had to catch three buses. I missed the second bus because we had to walk a few blocks to catch it and the three-year-old doesn't walk fast. Since we missed the second bus we had to wait another 20 minutes for the next one."

By the time she finished her story, my junior resident understood that she was not as he had assumed. She was not someone who didn't care about herself and therefore somehow unworthy of his time and improvement in her health. On the contrary, she worried so much about her health that she spent hours on several buses with four young children in tow, in order to see a medical specialist. Armed with this psychological insight, the resident was apologetic and asked if he could perform the exam and appropriately complete her work-up. He later shared privately that he finally understood the point behind my frequent comment that it is not our job to judge, but it is our duty to help. We cannot and must not try to determine whether our patients are "good" or "bad" people, but we can and must treat them with compassion.

Understanding context is inseparable from quality patient-centered care. People do not become sick in a vacuum. Illness affects multiple aspects of life, and multiple factors can contribute to illness. Physicians who display warmth, friendliness, and a reassuring manner have been found to be more effective than those who do not (Di Blasi, Harkness, Ernst, Georgiou, & Kleijnen, 2001). Clinical empathy, touted by clinical psychologists for more than half a century (e.g., Rogers, 1949, 1957), is a core contributor to accurate diagnosis, humane practice, and positive patient outcomes (Halpern, 2001; Larson & Yao, 2005). But unlike clinical psychology training, medical education has traditionally lacked a formal process to positively shape learners' perceptions and self-awareness so they are more likely to accurately empathize and less likely to inappropriately blame.

Clearly, one could argue that any patient should be punctual and make necessary arrangements for child care. But when patients do not meet our expectations, we physicians must decide as an industry how to perceive their behavior and subsequently respond. Do we blame them for audaciously showing us too little respect and deference, or do we seek to understand them and their behavior in the context of illness and vulnerability? A formal patient-centered model provides a clear answer and structure. But if the medical profession truly desires a more empathic physician workforce, it must confront a very real subculture that is consistently and painfully revealed by the "hidden curriculum" literature described in the following. To date, while counterintuitive and in violation of the admirable Hippocratic Oath described earlier, the evidence shows traditional medical culture actually grooms trainees to be *less, not more*, empathic.

Hidden Curriculum

In medicine, the hidden curriculum refers to the distinction between what future physicians are taught and what they actually learn (Hafferty, 1998).

Consistent with Bandura's social learning theory and focus on imitation and modeling (e.g., Bandura, Ross, & Ross, 1961; Bandura, 1962; Bandura & Walters, 1963), evidence continues to show that medical trainees, like anyone else, do what others *do*, not what they *say*. Faulty professional models contribute to medical resident burnout and cynicism (Billings et al., 2011). Gaufberg, Batalden, Sands, and Bell (2010) identified specifics by combing through third-year Harvard medical student narratives. Students were given the following prompt:

The "hidden curriculum" is the set of influences on one's development as a physician that is not explicitly taught. It is transmitted through interpersonal interactions on the wards or in other clinical settings, through positive or negative role model behaviors, and through the culture and hierarchy of medicine. Examples of what might be imparted through the hidden curriculum include implicit "rules to survive" at a particular institution, the accepted manner of interacting with patients or colleagues, attitudes toward and treatment of difficult or marginalized patients, choices about personal/professional balance, and ways of coping with suffering/loss/death. The hidden curriculum influences the values, roles, and identity a physician develops over the course of training. The hidden curriculum is a strong socializing force, and its influence can be positive, negative, or mixed.

Please write a two-page paper reflecting on the hidden curriculum as you have observed it during your clerkship experience. We suggest that you start out with a personal anecdote or story that epitomizes some aspect of the hidden curriculum and use this anecdote as a starting-off point for your reflection.

The authors found four overarching concepts across virtually all students – medicine as culture, importance of haphazard learning, role modeling, and the tension between real medicine and prior idealized notions. Half the reflections focused on power-hierarchy issues in training, and nearly one-third described patient dehumanization, hidden assessment of their performance, suppression of their own normal emotional responses, and struggling with the limits of medicine.

One student wrote: "I always thought my first time would be different. I took extra time through first and second year to hear about what it was like to have dying patients, going to seminars, hearing from professors, even researching music in palliative care. But when a 42-year-old man with terminal Gardner syndrome was admitted to my surgery team, I followed everyone else's lead and avoided him."

A different student wrote: "It was during the physical exam that I became most uneasy because I usually had no idea what the attending was going to say or do next. There were several times when a patient was called 'demented' or 'frontal' without having any explanation given to them ... The most horrific thing I saw was when the attending asked the patient to turn over and then proceeded to demonstrate the anal wink reflex to us without warning the patient of what he was going to do."

GOD COMPLEX

In 1978 psychiatrist Stephen Bergman (pseudonym Samuel Shem) published *The House of God*, a satirical novel describing the dehumanization and psychological harm of medical internship in the 1970s (Shem, 1978). Medical slang shorthand is referenced throughout, including derogatory terms frequently used to describe geriatric patients today: GOMER (get out of my emergency room) and LOLNAD (little old lady in no apparent distress). By the author's own admission, though technically fictional, much of the content was rooted in his own residency experience, and it is easy to identify commonality with the harsh realities alluded to above. The book has sold over 2 million copies and has likely validated the psychologically traumatic experiences endured by many if not all medical trainees during residency (Markel, 2008). Some physicians have criticized it for being outdated (Hood, 1996) while medical educators from the behavioral sciences have defended its current relevance and advocate for its use as a tool for reflection (Wear, 2002).

Undoubtedly the 36 years since its original publication have included changes in health care and medicine, yet hidden curriculum research is a reminder of what remains the same. Some physicians relish the hero role and seek opportunities to do what they believe colleagues could not or would not do. This brazen mentality is a double-edged sword. On one hand, pushing the envelope has resulted in many advances in health care delivery and positive patient outcomes. Performing open heart surgery, transplantation surgery and more recently laparoscopic and robotic surgery are a few examples of how physicians have challenged preexisting limits in knowledge and understanding. Of course, just because something can be done does not mean that it should be done. As in the case example below, sometimes it is as simple as an individual physician's ego and desire to play "God" that drives risky clinical decision-making with patients for whom there may be little to no benefit.

A 77-year-old male presented with several enlarged lymph nodes and a large renal mass, in addition to comorbid chronic conditions including diabetes, hypertension, and atrial fibrillation. This patient, who also wore a pacemaker, was later diagnosed with small cell lymphoma. One urologist informed him that partial nephrectomy would put him at risk for urinary leak and postoperative bleeding since he would require anticoagulation immediately afterward. Therefore, a total nephrectomy would be safest. But another colleague, apparently desiring to set himself apart from the other kidney surgeons in the area, provided a second opinion, which included a partial nephrectomy done robotically, a new and technologically advanced procedure. The patient agreed. Postoperatively, the patient had several surgery-related complications, including urinary leak, life-threatening postoperative bleeding, and 45 days later, death.

It is difficult to know the thought process of the second surgeon. In hindsight, the first urologist was correct in assessing the risk and probable outcome for the patient. An important question is whether the second surgeon's personal desire to demonstrate his superiority directly or even indirectly influenced his clinical decision-making. An even more important question is why this case was not submitted for peer-review, especially since the patient was readmitted to the hospital twice following surgery, including another stint in the operating room. Readmissions coupled with three postsurgery complications and the fact that this case was not submitted for peer review suggest that more than the patient's best interest was at play.

FUTURE SOLUTIONS

Culture transformation is difficult and slow. It requires tremendous courage and persistence. Many of the cultural elements addressed above have contributed to the nation's impressive shift toward an explicit emphasis on *patient*-centered health care. To accomplish this paradigmatic culture change, physicians must develop, and demonstrate, greater psychological insight into their patients, themselves, and each other. How might this occur?

One promising trend is the implementation of Schwartz Rounds®, an interdisciplinary forum for clinicians to debrief and process emotionally and/or ethically challenging experiences ("cases"). According to The Schwartz Center's website (The Schwartz Center, 2014), the program occurs in more than 350 facilities nationwide. For a fee, the organization provides structured tools and implementation guidance, once an interested facility has identified a physician leader. Clinical psychologists, all of whom receive training in group psychotherapy, can facilitate similar programs, and when integrated, they often do, as in Balint groups (American Balint Society, 2014). Founded in the 1950s by psychoanalysts Michael and Enid Balint, these weekly or biweekly groups aim to assist physicians with the psychological aspects of medical care. The organization is now international in scope and its popularity has spread beyond its original roots in family medicine (e.g., Abeni et al., 2014).

Quality and impact of these promising interventions depend on how they are led (Johnson, Nease, Milberg, & Addison, 2004). The logical approach is to integrate health professionals with appropriate expertise in these leadership roles. By definition, depth of training, and scope of practice, clinical psychologists meet that criterion. Yet in medical culture, the need to fill this role seems clearer than perceptions of which health care professionals are most qualified to fill it. Some physicians have explicitly advocated for psychologist inclusion in medical training (e.g., Wilkes, Hoffman, Slavin, & Usatine, 2013). But as discussed throughout this publication, that voice is the exception, not the rule.

Unlike the Schwartz Rounds model, Balint groups do not require leaders to be physicians. However, a national survey of 381 family medicine residencies where they were implemented revealed 32% were physician-led, 25% psychologist-led, and 19% were led by social workers (Brock & Stock, 1990). Criteria for choosing these leaders is unknown but may be explained, in part, by the absence of clinical psychologists in most medical settings outside the Veterans Administration (VA). For the culture to truly change, integration of psychology and medicine disciplines must occur.

Epstein and Street Jr. (2011) suggest physicians should be trained to be more mindful, informative and empathic; thus they may perceive their role as partner rather than authority figure. Modifying this perception is possible, though as history has shown, not an easy process.

In the current medical culture, clinical psychologists are rarely considered, and many physicians are uncomfortable with their inclusion. At the same time, psychologists, also bound by their own disciplinary culture, have not articulated their clinical value in a compelling fashion. In many ways psychologists and physicians have much in common. But their similarities are rarely highlighted and their true differences perhaps exaggerated. In fact, the greatest differences between them may be cultural. While medicine may be defined by confidence and action, psychology may be defined as observation and reflection. Physicians are often eager to demonstrate the uniqueness of what they do, while psychologists, often in the spirit of inclusiveness, inadvertently downplay their own unique expertise. It is not surprising, therefore, that in medicine, where pressure and stakes are high and available time is not, those professionals already included in today's health care system – lesser trained social workers, along with nurses and physicians – continue to occupy the role of behavioral expert. The cultural landscape described throughout this chapter underscores why changing this trend is not only challenging, but vital.

References

Abeni, M. S., Magni, M., Conte, M., Mangiacavalli, S., Pochintesta, L., Vicenzi, G., et al. (2014). Psychological care of caregivers, nurses and physicians: A study of a new approach. *Cancer Medicine*, 3(1), 101–110.

American Balint Society Website. Available at: <http://www.americanbalintsociety.org/content.aspx?page_id=22&club_id=445043&module_id=123024>.

Arnold, R. M., Povar, G. J., & Howell, J. D. (1987). The humanities, humanistic behavior, and the humane physician: a cautionary note. *Annals of Internal Medicine, 106*(2), 313–318.

Association of American Medical Colleges. New Medical College Admission Test® Approved Changes Add Emphasis on Behavioral and Social Sciences. Washington, D.C., February 16, 2012. Available at: <www.aamc.org/newsroom/newsreleases/273712/120216.html>. Accessed 01 08 14.

Bandura, A. (1962). Social learning through imitation. In M. R. Jones (Ed.), *Nebraska symposium on motivation*. Lincoln, Nebraska: University of Nebraska Press.

Bandura, A., Ross, D., & Ross, S. A. (1961). Transmission of aggression through imitation of aggressive models. *The Journal of Abnormal and Social Psychology, 63*(3), 575.

Bandura, A., & Walters, R. H. (1963). *Social learning and personality development*. New York: Holt, Rinehart and Winston.

Bateson, G., Jackson, D. D., Haley, J., & Weakland, J. (1956). Toward a theory of schizophrenia. *Behavioral Science, 1*(4), 251–264.

Beckman, H. B., Markakis, K. M., Suchman, A. L., & Frankel, R. M. (1994). The doctor–patient relationship and malpractice lessons from plaintiff depositions. *Archives of Internal Medicine, 154*(12), 1365–1370.

Billings, M. E., Lazarus, M. E., Wenrich, M., Curtis, J. R., & Engelberg, R. A. (2011). The effect of the hidden curriculum on resident burnout and cynicism. *Journal of Graduate Medical Education, 3*(4), 503–510.

Brock, C. D., & Stock, R. D. (1990). A survey of Balint group activities in US family practice residency programs. *Family Medicine, 22*(1), 33–37.

Coulter, A. (2002). Patients' views of the good doctor. *British Medical Journal, 325*(7366), 668–669.

Di Blasi, Z. D., Harkness, E., Ernst, E., Georgiou, A., & Kleijnen, J. (2001). Influence of context effects on health outcomes: A systematic review. *Lancet, 357*, 757–762.

Epstein, R. M., & Street, R. L., Jr (2011). The values and value of patient-centered care. *Annals of Family Medicine, 9*(2), 100–103.

Galloway, C. (1968). *Nonverbal communication: A needed focus*. Washington, DC: ERIC Clearinghouse, US Dept of Education.

Gaufberg, E. H., Batalden, M., Sands, R., & Bell, S. K. (2010). The hidden curriculum: What can we learn from third-year medical student narrative reflections? *Academic Medicine, 85*(11), 1709–1716.

Goldberg, J. L. (2008). Humanism or professionalism? The white coat ceremony and medical education. *Academic Medicine, 83*(8), 715–722.

Hafferty, F. W. (1998). Beyond curriculum reform: Confronting medicine's hidden curriculum. *Academic Medicine, 73*(4), 403–407.

Halpern, J. (2001). *From detached concern to empathy: Humanizing medical practice*. New York, NY: Oxford University Press.

Hood, R. R. (1996). The house of God. *New England Journal of Medicine, 335*, 1165–1166.

Hurwitz, B., & Vass, A. (2002). What's a good doctor, and how can you make one? By marrying the applied scientist to the medical humanist. *British Medical Journal, 325*(7366), 667.

Institute of Medicine (2001). *Crossing the quality chasm: A new health system for the 21st century*. Washington, DC: National Academy Press.

Johnson, A. H., Nease, D. E., Milberg, L. C., & Addison, R. B. (2004). Essential characteristics of effective Balint group leadership. *Family Medicine – Kansas City, 36*(4), 253–259.

Jones, V. A. (1999). The white coat: Why not follow suit? *Journal of the American Medical Association, 281*(5), 478.

Kirch, D. G. (2012). Transforming admissions: The gateway to medicine. *Journal of the American Medical Association, 308*(21), 2250–2251.

Kraman, S. S., & Hamm, G. (1999). Risk management: Extreme honesty may be the best policy. *Annals of Internal Medicine, 131*, 963–967.

Larson, E. B., & Yao, X. (2005). Clinical empathy as emotional labor in the patient–physician relationship. *Journal of the American Medical Association, 293*, 1100–1106.

Lasagna, L. (1964). Would hippocrates rewrite his oath? after 2,000 years, the greek pledge traditionally taken by doctors is falling into disuse. A professor of medicine here stresses the need for a new declaration of ethics. *New York Times Magazine, 11*, 40–43.

Leape, L. (2006). When good doctors go bad: A systems problem. *Annals of Surgery, 244*(5), 649–652.

Leape, L. L., Shore, M. F., Dienstag, J. L., Mayer, R. J., Edgman-Levitan, S., Meyer, G. S., et al. (2012a). Perspective: A culture of respect, Part 1: The nature and causes of disrespectful behavior by physicians. *Academic Medicine: Journal of the Association of American Medical Colleges, 87*(7), 845–852.

Leape, L. L., Shore, M. F., Dienstag, J. L., Mayer, R. J., Edgman-Levitan, S., Meyer, G. S., et al. (2012b). Perspective: A culture of respect, Part 2: Creating a culture of respect. *Academic Medicine: Journal of the Association of American Medical Colleges, 87*(7), 853–858.

Markel, H. (2008). The House of God 30 years later. *Journal of the American Medical Association, 299*(2), 227–229.

OBGYN.net Staff. The New MCAT incorporates the "softer" side of medicine. And that's a good thing. April 21, 2012. Available at: <www.obgyn.net/articles/new-mcat-incorporates-softer-side-medicine-and-thats-good-thing>. Accessed 01.08.14.

Penchansky, R., & Macnee, C. (1994). Initiation of medical malpractice suits: a conceptualization and test. *Medical Care, 32*, 813–831.

Pickering, T. G., James, G. D., Boddie, C., Harshfield, G. A., Blank, S., & Laragh, J. H. (1988). How common is white coat hypertension? *Journal of the American Medical Association, 259*(2), 225–228.

Rogers, C. R. (1949). The attitude and orientation of the counselor in client-centered therapy. *Journal of Consulting Psychology, 13*(2), 82–94.

Rogers, C. R. (1957). The necessary and sufficient conditions of therapeutic personality change. *Journal of Consulting Psychology, 21*, 95–103.

Rosenhan, D. L. (1973). On being sane in insane places. *Science, 179*(4070), 250–258.

Russell, P. C. (2002). The white coat ceremony: Turning trust into entitlement. *Teaching and Learning in Medicine, 14*(1), 56–59.

Shem, S. (1978). *The House of God: A novel.* New York, NY: R. Marek Publishers.

The Schwartz Center (2014). Schwartz Center Rounds® Website. Available at: <http://www.theschwartzcenter.org/supporting-caregivers/schwartz-center-rounds/>.

Underwood, W., III (2012). A physician's perspective on health care discrimination. *American Journal of Public Health, 102*(5), 779.

Wear, D. (2002). The house of God: Another look. *Academic Medicine, 77*(6), 496–501.

Wear, D., & Zarconi, J. (2008). Can compassion be taught? Let's ask our students. *Journal of General Internal Medicine, 23*(7), 948–953.

Wensing, M., Jung, H. P., Mainz, J., Olesen, F., & Grol, R. (1998). A systematic review of the literature on patient priorities for general practice care. Part 1: Description of the research domain. *Social Science and Medicine, 47*(10), 1573–1588.

Wilkes, M., Milgrom, E., & Hoffman, J. R. (2002). Towards more empathic medical students: A medical student hospitalization experience. *Medical Education, 36*(6), 528–533.

Wilkes, M. S., Hoffman, J. R., Slavin, S. J., & Usatine, R. P. (2013). The next generation of doctoring. *Academic Medicine, 88*(4), 438–441.

Psychology Consult: When and Why

Robert J. Maiden[1], Peter Lichtenberg[2], and Benjamin A. Bensadon[3]

[1]Alfred University, Alfred, New York, USA; [2]Wayne State University, Detroit, Michigan, USA; [3]Charles E. Schmidt College of Medicine, Florida Atlantic University, Boca Raton, Florida, USA

Old age ain't no place for sissies.

—Bette Davis

INTRODUCTION

Geriatric patients have a lot to say. Often overwhelmed with multiple chronic diseases, wide-ranging physical limitations, a narrowing social network, and limited life expectancy, they have much to cover – all in a brief encounter with a busy physician. How does the nation's health care system respond? Medical trainees chuckle about how to structure such encounters, cut off patients who "ramble," and worry about their own need to get to the point and move on. More experienced physicians may quickly assess their patients' physical and mental health with confidence and clarity, yet, untrained in the subtleties of effective communication, fail to accurately "read" and hear their older patients. And this is vital. Effective communication and accurate assessment can save lives.

With the help of appropriate geropsychology consultation, this failure is not inevitable. Psychologists can enhance communication – both verbal and nonverbal – to maximize efficiency when obtaining information from patients. Consultation can identify and help correct patient nonadherence (Roter et al., 1998), differentiate unexplained symptoms of pain (Henningsen, Zimmermann, & Sattel, 2003), and manage family dysfunction (Blount, 1998; Glenn, 1987). From a practical standpoint, consultation

B. Bensadon (Ed): Psychology and Geriatrics.
DOI: http://dx.doi.org/10.1016/B978-0-12-420123-1.00006-X

can directly and immediately benefit physicians, who, short on time, may be overwhelmed by a patient's emotional needs and/or disturbing behaviors. Not only can psychologists save physicians' time, they can expand physician understanding of their patients' needs by stepping in to engage patients in psychosocial talk (Morriss et al., 2010), particularly relevant to older patients (Greene & Adelman, 1996; Greene, Hoffman, Charon, & Adelman, 1987) and consistently correlated with patient satisfaction (Bertakis, Roter, & Putnam, 1991; Roter et al., 1997), yet inadequately used in standard medical practice (Ring, Dowrick, Humphris, Davies, & Salmon, 2005). Insights psychologists glean from such psychosocial talk with patients can then provide physicians with data crucial to customizing and delivering patient-centered care. As illustrated here, psychologists' insights can include detection of acute, albeit hidden, emotional distress that, when unrecognized, can lead to dangerous outcomes.

CASE EXAMPLE: LATE LIFE DEPRESSION AND SUICIDE RISK

A 77-year-old recently widowed white male was on the rehabilitation unit for his third stay in 6 months following a hunting accident. He had fallen from a tree, suffering multiple leg fractures and torn knee cartilage. An executive in the auto industry, he had retired 5 years earlier. One year after his retirement he became a caregiver for his wife who was diagnosed with stage IV pancreatic cancer and died 9 months later. He had two adult daughters who lived nearby and with whom he had a good relationship. The patient was energetic and independent following his wife's death, and continued to pursue his personal interests, which included fishing, hiking, camping, and hunting.

It was common practice that new admissions to the rehabilitation unit be interviewed by a psychologist. In this case, however, the attending physician asked the psychologist *not* to interview the patient because, he said, the patient was used to being treated as a high-functioning executive and would be insulted by having an appointment with a psychologist. The psychologist reacted with curiosity and wondered who this high-powered executive was who intimidated the attending physician.

While on daily rounds with the physician and his residents, something in the patient's manner troubled the psychologist, who asked the attending to reconsider his initial worry about potentially embarrassing the patient. The physician refused to do so. At team rounds the next day, the occupational and physical therapy reports and social work discharge plans were set. The team estimated an inpatient stay of approximately 3 weeks. No one on the team expressed concern. The patient was highly functioning, progressing well in his therapies, and had a supportive family.

Because the scheduler was accustomed to the psychologist interviewing and assessing each patient, the patient appeared on the schedule a few days later in spite of the attending physician's discomfort. During the encounter the patient presented as an engaging and likable individual, relaxed and at ease. But suddenly his demeanor changed when discussing the functional limitations caused by his medical condition.

He told the psychologist that he had never in his life been physically limited and that he viewed any permanent disabling condition as a serious threat to his independence. Administration of the Geriatric Depression Scale (GDS) revealed 26 out of 30. GDS criteria classify a score of 20 or greater as "severely depressed." These data confirmed that he was devastated by the abrupt and permanent changes his condition had caused. When the psychologist assessed him for suicidal ideation, he stated clearly that he was planning to kill himself with a shotgun once he left the facility unless he saw a dramatic improvement in his condition. He confided that he had yet to grieve over his wife's death and instead had thrown himself into his outdoor hobbies to the fullest extent possible. He and his late wife had shared a happy life together, and he was sure that once he slowed down he would miss her tremendously. He described feeling deep helplessness and hopelessness. This patient had raised no obvious red flags; he did not drink alcohol, had few other preexisting medical conditions, and demonstrated significant strength in all areas of cognitive functioning.

The next morning the psychologist spoke with the attending physician about the encounter. The physician was astounded and expressed relief that the patient's true emotional state had been uncovered. The psychologist described for the physician the classic risk factors with which the patient presented – white male over age 75, recently widowed, burdened for the first time ever with significant medical problems that limited his usual activities – and a self-described avid hunter with easy access to guns. Review of the GDS with psychologist's clinical notes enabled the physician to see for the first time that below the patient's social presentation lay an acutely tortured, dangerously depressed, suicidal man.

Going forward, both the attending physician and consulting psychologist worked with the patient and his daughters. They obtained permission to have the patient's guns removed from the house, and he agreed to start a treatment regimen of antidepressant medication and psychotherapy. Fortunately the team had two additional weeks to work with him on an inpatient basis, so that even though he was still limited *physically*, having reduced mobility and strength, he improved *psychologically*, gaining a sense of progress, building his self-efficacy, and combatting his hopelessness. Through psychotherapy, the patient and psychologist identified additional avenues of social support and made concrete plans for the patient to teach his grandchildren how to fish. Both physical and psychotherapy were continued on an outpatient basis and the patient continued to improve. Within 6 months he returned to many of his outdoor activities.

Integrating psychology and medicine, as illustrated in this example, has long been challenged by interprofessional bias and a *discipline-* rather than *patient-*centered focus. But when bias is minimized and collaboration ensues, it can, as noted, save patient lives.

While it remains impossible to predict suicide completion with 100% accuracy, consistent data show that many older adults who commit suicide have seen their primary care provider within the month prior to ending their life (e.g., Luoma, Martin, & Pearson, 2002). Is this a missed opportunity for intervention? Though there are many plausible interpretations for the relationship between primary care visits and suicides, the well-documented links between depression, suicidal ideation, and suicide completion (Conwell, Olsen, Caine, & Flannery, 1991; Kuo, Gallo, & Eaton, 2004; Tsoh et al., 2005) underscore the need for improved vigilance among physicians.

Physicians must be schooled in recognizing signs of psychological distress, often too subtle to attract the untrained eye. Too frequently, patients' hopelessness and sense of a bleak future go unrecognized during routine physician appointments. Indeed, older people are less likely than their younger counterparts to openly communicate their suicidal intent or attempt suicide as a cry for help or attention. This pattern is nothing new and has held in the United States (U.S.) for as long as suicide data have been collected by the government (Osgood & Thielman, 1990). In contrast to physicians, clinical psychologists are specifically trained to look for and identify the subtle cues of emotional pain and mental illness, and to respond accordingly.

In the case described here, psychology consultation revealed the patient's identity crisis: Who would he be now that he could no longer engage in the physical activities that defined him and his life? Psychological counseling was clinically indicated to uncover, manage, and move beyond this root problem. Tragically though, while suicide among geriatric patients is increasingly common, psychologist consultation in standard health care is not. Indeed, behavioral approaches are infrequently considered as a viable management option. Even when underlying mood and related difficulties are detected, when it comes to interventions, national data highlight a major disconnect between what older patients prefer – psychotherapy – and what they actually receive – medication (Alvidrez & Areán, 2002; Wei, Sambamoorthi, Olfson, Walkup, & Crystal, 2005).

As addressed in Chapter 8, managing suicide is complex and includes intense psychological discomfort for all involved – clinicians, as well as patients and their loved ones. Though seldom admitted openly within the culture of medicine, physicians and other health care professionals are not immune to discomfort with death. This extends beyond suicide and characterizes communication of bad news and end-of-life discussions as well.

Nearly 50 years ago psychologist Ezra Saul revealed disclosure of a terminal diagnosis and communicating a patient's death to his or her family were the two most anxiety-inducing clinical scenarios imaginable for first-year medical students at Tufts University (Saul & Kass, 1969). How have medical educators responded?

Orlander and colleagues (2002) found 73% of practicing physicians first delivered bad news as a medical student or first-year resident. Of these, 95% did so alone, without the support or guidance of an attending physician present. Litauska and Colleagues (2014) sampled 280 physicians about barriers to hospice referral and found that, while more than a third feared an angry response from patients and families, 96% reported *never*, *sometimes*, or *rarely* actually receiving such a response when they did mention it. Subjective fear is understandable and "valid" even though it may not be rooted in objective evidence. Consulting psychologists are specifically trained to recognize and validate fear and anxiety. They are also trained in specific techniques to manage them and to maximize therapeutic communication even in challenging circumstances. Psychological facets of medical communication include empathic responding to patient and family emotion, effectively involving patient and family in decision making, managing stress created by the expectation of cure, and the ability to enable patients and family members to feel included and cared for.

Many physicians care for older patients. And all clinicians would likely state they listen to them. But as shown in Chapter 4, how effectively this is done in clinical practice varies. As noted by some physicians themselves (e.g., Meier, Back, & Morrison, 2001; Novack et al., 1997), greater self-awareness is likely the optimal response, but national data suggest without integration, avoidance is more common.

DEALING WITH DEATH

By definition, geriatricians and geropsychologists recognize and differentiate uniquely geriatric aspects of illness and care. In contrast, untrained clinicians working with older patients often view problems by individual diagnosis (e.g., stroke or hip fracture) or disability (e.g., walking or other activities of daily living) rather than holistically. As illustrated in the following example, without training, geriatric syndromes like sarcopenia (weakness) and frailty, often representative of a final pathway toward the end of life, are rarely considered.

Case Example: Frailty and End of Life

An 88-year-old woman with hypertension entered a subacute rehabilitation unit with pelvic fractures after driving her car into a pole in a parking garage. Overall the patient was cheerful and cooperative, though the rehabilitation team noted some physical weakness. One week into her stay the team became confused. The patient had visited the emergency room twice for unexplained breathing difficulty, and she appeared increasingly disoriented upon return to the rehab unit. Striking behavioral observations were made during a neuropsychological evaluation. The patient was very weak, easily exhausted, and began to either refuse or prematurely discontinue her physical and occupational therapies. She also experienced substantial loss of appetite and weight loss and demonstrated significant memory and executive functioning problems of relatively new onset. Her condition was a classic frailty syndrome indicative of multiple system dysfunctions. After factoring in her breathing difficulty, a family meeting was arranged to discuss end-of-life options.

Not every provider was on board with this decision. The director of nursing (DON) was outraged when, a few days after the team met, the neuropsychologist recommended to the patient's children that they begin considering the possibility that their mother would not survive much longer. The DON immediately informed the children that the neuropsychologist was grossly mistaken and any discussion of their mother's demise was premature. In fact, several members of the treatment team showed similar disapproval that such "negative" messages (i.e., dying) were expressed to the patient's family. Notably, the attending physician remained quiet throughout these discussions. A week later the patient was discharged to the long-term care unit because she could no longer participate in her therapies. She died 10 days later. Her daughters were extremely grateful that "at least someone" had prepared them for their mother's death.

In this case, the psychologist was both *prognostically* accurate and *psychologically* able to recognize "the bigger picture" and address with the family something other clinicians had not – namely, the patient's end of life. In medicine death and dying are often regarded by the health care team as "failure." But it is precisely this mindset, ironically, that can lead to clinicians' insensitivity and older patients' unmet needs and related despair. Geropsychology consultation can and must empower patients, families, and clinicians to confront the end of life by promoting an open, trusting, and understanding atmosphere in which death and dying are viewed as a difficult process of acceptance, not a taboo topic to be avoided.

These examples should not be surprising. Medical rehabilitation placement is linked to the goal of recovery. When functional ability is restored, so too is patient independence. But as many psychologists can attest, it is painfully difficult for people to let go of hope – physicians included. Thus, many admissions for "rehabilitation" occur even when end-of-life care is the more appropriate option. By admitting geriatric patients to rehabilitation units, even when they can no longer participate in physical or occupational therapies, providers send an unrealistic message of recovery to both patient and family. In the case above, breathing difficulties and frailty signaled the end of life was near. Decline, not rehabilitation, was the more likely outcome. Why does this matter? Empirical evidence has shown that psychosocial suffering (e.g., guilt, complicated grief) is exacerbated and risk for morbidity (e.g., depression) elevated in families who are unprepared for the death of their parent or partner (Apatira et al., 2008; Barry, Kasl, & Prigerson, 2002; Hebert, Schulz, Copeland, & Arnold, 2009).

Geropsychologists can demonstrate how to continue engaging the older adult who is still very much alive, and begin to prepare loved ones for shortened survival time, when aggressive intervention options are no longer feasible. This is rarely straightforward since accurate prognostication of decline, including timing and duration, is complex, imprecise, and an area where physicians lack training. But transparently and supportively educating families about frailty and the end of life is critical. It helps them better understand what their loved one is experiencing and enables them to more adequately prepare for their impending loss. The concept is discussed to some degree in year-long hospice and palliative medicine fellowships. But the necessary skills to implement that concept – to facilitate, enhance, recognize and confirm such understanding and awareness – are the essence of clinical psychology training. Both disciplines must learn from each other.

WHO IS THE EXPERT?

Generally, when integrated into rehabilitation, long-term care, or hospital settings, psychological services include neurocognitive and mental health assessment and intervention, consultation, and psychoeducation as part of a larger interdisciplinary approach that may include a team of physicians, nurses, social workers, physical and occupational therapists, chaplains, and speech language pathologists. Given that colleagues from these and most other health care disciplines claim behavioral expertise, it is crucial that psychologists differentiate their own roles more precisely and confidently. This has yet to occur. As a result, a plethora of self-described behavior and mental health "specialists" (e.g., social workers, chaplains, coaches) continue to surface. Oddly, though all have significantly less clinical training and education, they have nevertheless been able to integrate within medical care more effectively than psychologists have. Table 6.1 provides a brief comparison of their respective credentials and expertise.

CONSULTATION WITH OCCUPATIONAL AND PHYSICAL THERAPIES

Psychologist observation of the patient during occupational or physical therapy (OT or PT) can be useful in consultation to improve the

TABLE 6.1   Nonphysician Behavioral Health Providers

Provider type	Required degree (minimum)	Formal training (years)	Required supervised clinical hours (minimum)	State license
Clinical Psychologist	Doctorate	5–7	4000	Y
Social Worker	Master's	2 + 2 post-master's	1500	Y
Mental Health Counselor	Master's	2 + 2 post-master's	1500	Y
Marriage and Family Therapist	Master's	2 + 2 post-master's	1500	Y
Hospital Chaplain	Master's	Variable	Variable	N
Coaches	None	Variable	Variable	N
Pastoral Counselor	GED/High School Diploma	Variable	Variable	N

rehabilitation process. When older patients demonstrate subpar improvement, clinically what must be differentiated is: Why? Psychologists are frequently the first to recognize lackluster performance may be related to a patient's mood or cognitive dysfunction such as anxiety, depression, or cognitive impairment. By sensitizing providers from other disciplines to the more prevalent cognitive and affective comorbidities, consulting psychologists can equip them to provide related screening and assessment themselves (e.g., Lysack, Leach, Russo, Paulson, & Lichtenberg, 2013).

Clinical observation of sessions at the therapy gym enables psychologists to identify ways for the rehabilitation therapists and patients to work together more effectively. This commonly includes behavioral and communication tips such as reducing the complexity of task instruction, pacing the therapy, attending to issues of rapport, breaking down complex behaviors into component parts, and repetition. These details may seem intuitive but without behavioral sensitivity, it is difficult to differentiate whether struggling patients are unmotivated, unable to follow directions, in pain, depressed, apathetic, or even sleep-deprived. Psychologists are specifically trained to attend to this level of detail so they can accurately interpret the patient's behavior and formulate an effective response or modification to ensure quality, patient-centered care and optimal clinical outcome.

As mentioned later, a particularly important target of intervention is the older patient's sense of personal control. Rehabilitation success is optimized when the patient-therapist relationship can be defined as a collaborative working partnership. Perceived loss or lack of control often contributes to depression and anxiety, each prevalent in older medical rehabilitation patients but rarely assessed and often unrecognized in the absence of a psychologist.

PSYCHIATRY VS PSYCHOLOGY

Clinical geropsychologist consultation is appropriate for geriatric patients across all levels of illness and care settings (e.g., retirement and independent living communities, assisted living, skilled nursing, hospice, inpatient hospitals, outpatient clinics). Like psychiatrists, clinical psychologists are often consulted to help manage behavior and determine decision-making capacity. Does the older adult retain the capacity to make health and financial decisions or select his or her own placement? A recent collaboration between the American Bar Association and the American Psychological Association has resulted in a handbook to assist psychologists in performing such assessment (ABA/APA, 2008).

Unlike psychiatrists, clinical psychologists focus more on helping patients to modify their behavior than on medication as first-line treatment. Accordingly, psychologists implement a wide range of drug-free strategies proven to be effective and safe. This distinction is increasingly important as the dwindling national supply of psychiatrists continues to shift therapeutic focus – from less talking to more prescribing – in contrast to what older patients want (Unützer, Katon, Callahan, Williams, Hunkeler, Harpole, et al. 2003; Gum, Areán, Hunkeler, Tang, Katon, Hitchcock, et al., 2006; Raue, Schulberg, Heo, Klimstra, & Bruce, 2009). For example, national data reveal a consistent trend toward antidepressant medication to manage depression. Between 1987 and 1997 the rate of such outpatient prescriptions nearly doubled from 37.3% to 74.5% while psychotherapy utilization declined significantly from 71.1% to 60.2% (Olfson et al., 2002). Between 1996 and 2005 the rate of antidepressant prescriptions nearly doubled again, making them the most commonly prescribed class of medication in the nation (Olfson & Marcus, 2009). Though medicating mood is controversial (Breggin, 1994; Kirsch, 2010), many physicians continue to automatically call upon psychiatry rather than clinical psychology (e.g., Meier & Beresford, 2010), even though the latter may be best able though not necessarily integrated medically to provide nonpharmacologic (i.e., behavioral) intervention.

Turf

Competition between psychiatry (medical) and psychology (nonmedical) for authority over clinical care provision is not new. Clinical psychologists have fought to practice independently outside the umbrella of medical supervision for decades (Dickel, 1966). Until recently, psychological services, including assessment and psychotherapy, had to be ordered by physicians to be covered under Medicare Part A. Now, clinical psychologists may bill for services directly under Medicare Part B. Physicians generally trust psychologists to carry out their responsibilities and many, including psychiatrists, recognize they have little expertise or desire to engage in psychotherapy or administration and interpretation of psychological and neuropsychological tests. Related power struggles tend to be the priority of professional organizations rather than individual health care providers. Indeed, numerous studies have documented that partnerships between clinical psychologists and physicians achieve medical and therapeutic goals better than either alone (Bartels et al., 2004; Blount et al., 2007; Cummings, 1998; O'Malley, 1998; Pomerantz et al., 2010). The Institute of Medicine (IOM) Board on Health Care Services (2006) echoed a similar sentiment in its report concluding physical and mental health concerns were inseparable and the two types of care provision should therefore be integrated.

CO-LOCATION

In the late 1970s, Medicare Part A required psychology services to be co-located with other (i.e., medical) services. Psychologists and the admitting physician saw patients in the same general location. Currently though, such co-location is primarily found only in the Veteran's Administration (VA) health care system, which employs a payment structure that is *not* based on the nationally predominant fee for service model (Kathol, Butler, McAlpine & Kane, 2010; Pomerantz et al., 2010). Instead of depending upon volume, that is, *quantity* of patient encounters, the focus is *quality*, in terms of streamlined communication among team members in developing shared treatment plans and decision making to provide truly integrated biopsychosocial care. Unsurprisingly, the VA health system employs the largest number of clinical psychologists in the nation and has mandated clinical psychology presence, nationally, as part of its primary care mental health integration and collaborative care model (see Dundon, Dollar, Schohn, & Lantinga, 2011).

In-hospital co-location is particularly advantageous when caring for older patients with multiple chronic conditions (Burling, 2014), some of which (e.g., depression) might not otherwise be detected (Zivin et al., 2010). Co-located models allow patients to be seen immediately as part of the medical routine rather than be referred to separate, often distant specialty care settings where wait time can be high and likelihood of follow-up low.

THE MEDICAL MODEL OF HEALTH CARE

Any new model of care takes time to coalesce. Traditionally, the organic disease model guided care, with physicians heading health care teams and taking full responsibility for patient care. Although psychologists provided input, it was limited and generally considered to be of less importance. In the past decade, however, this traditional medical model has been challenged. Effective management of the biopsychosocial impact of chronic disease and unprecedented life expectancy, while critical, is hampered by a model organized by discrete organ systems and guided by cost containment. Department of Defense research has shown that ambiguity about the psychologist's role has led to increased chronic suffering and decreased patient satisfaction (Hunter, Goodie, Dobermeyer & Dorrance, 2014). In contrast, integrated psychological care and better communication reduced the need for extensive assessment; and not surprisingly, agreement between physician and clinical psychologist (i.e., being "on the same page") enhanced its effectiveness (Blount & Miller, 2009). Hunter and colleagues (2014) found that a blended model, in which primary care physicians and behavioral health providers (i.e., clinical psychologists) share information and communicate, redresses the shortcomings and limitations of the traditional medical model, improves patient care, and reduces cost.

Although the concomitant role of psychopathology and medical illness, now well-established empirically (Ogden, 2012; Straub, 2012), has been apparent to practicing psychologists for decades, this recognition is still not standard among physicians and other medical practitioners.

Case Example: Differential Diagnosis

An 83-year-old man arrived for admission to a tertiary hospital. Presenting symptoms included disorientation, disorganization, and floridly psychotic visual hallucinations. His verbalizations were nonsensical and illogical. His family noted personality changes in the past few months and that he had become unpleasant and prone to agitated outbursts. The preliminary diagnosis by the medical team was that he suffered from Alzheimer's disease (AD) and that nothing could be done for him medically. But after a neuropsychological evaluation was performed by a psychologist, it was apparent that he most likely did *not* have AD but rather normal pressure hydrocephalus (NPH), a neurodegenerative disorder known to be reversible in certain cases (Fife, 2003). Further tests by medical staff corroborated the NPH diagnosis. Surgery was performed and a shunt implanted to drain off excess fluid, causing the ventricle in the patient's brain to decrease in volume, removing the pressure on the surrounding brain tissue. Following surgery, the patient's psychological functioning returned to normal within a short period of time, and he engaged in reality-oriented, coherent conversations. In due course, he made a full recovery. Impressed that a psychologist had made this differential diagnosis, the primary care physicians began referring to him for the first time as "Doctor."

LONG-TERM CARE

Concomitant psychological and medical conditions are especially characteristic of patients in long-term care (LTC) facilities. Approximately two-thirds of LTC residents have been diagnosed with comorbid mental disorders (Rosowsky, Casciani, & Arnold, 2009). This percentage increases to 80% of those receiving nursing-level care (Hyer and Shah, 2009). Karel and colleagues (2012) reported that such concomitant conditions appear to be most prevalent among those with neurodegenerative disorders, frequent among nursing home residents, and that more than half of older patients with dementia experience depression, anxiety, or other behavioral disturbances such as agitation. Kaskie (2013) noted that depression may be more prevalent among individuals with diabetes, cancer, or behavioral disturbances, further complicated by the fact that they may also have cognitive impairment or a history of anxiety or substance abuse. Mental health problems are more likely to be found among those who suffer from serious medical illnesses, are frail, exposed to prolonged pain, and experience the many, often psychological, losses associated with LTC placement. These include the loss of personal belongings, home, family, finances, health, control, self-efficacy, independence, and privacy. In addition to needing to adapt to new rules and regulations, frequently LTC residents must also adapt to living with a roommate.

Not surprisingly, psychological services in LTC settings, though not standard care, have been found to enhance patients' emotional and cognitive function. Such interventions may also reduce the likelihood of negative outcomes, including increased mortality and higher suicide rates found in individuals with comorbid diagnoses (Lin, Zhang, Leung & Clark, 2011). Nevertheless, "the most applied model in LTC is medical" (Hyer & Shah, 2009, p. 66). Without integration, the recognition of the need for psychological care and the provision of such services depend on nonspecialists such as primary care physicians and hospitalists, who are neither trained nor incentivized to provide it (Noel et al., 2004).

LIVING OLD

Chronic Disease

Many older adults are painfully aware that living longer means living sicker. Dramatic increases in life expectancy in the U.S. are accompanied by increased infirmity, illness, and chronic disease prevalence. According to the Centers for Disease Control and Prevention about 80% of older adults live with at least one chronic condition and 50% with at least two. The resulting demands and lifestyle adjustments caused by chronic conditions often exert a powerfully negative psychological impact on quality of life, both for patients and their caregivers (generally spouses or other family members). Effective health care, in turn, demands disease self-management and other lifestyle and behavioral changes (Clark et al., 1991), areas inadequately discussed in medical training and practice (Darer, Hwang, Pham, Bass, & Anderson, 2004).

Regardless of the nation's unprecedented aging, system-level patient support remains inadequate when it comes to chronic disease because U.S. health care has traditionally focused on acute care. This societal scotoma (Leipzig, Hall, & Fried, 2012) is exacerbated and exemplified by the system's absence of clinical psychologists who, by definition, are most thoroughly trained in understanding and managing human behavior. As a result, older patients and their families often confront the daily battle of chronic disease feeling poorly understood and alone. For patients without close family ties, isolation can be both geographic and psychological. The clinical relevance is high for illness-related behavioral and psychological correlates such as health literacy (Cavanaugh et al., 2010), adherence (Bensadon, 2014; Pasina et al., 2014), perceived stigma and intrusiveness (e.g., Hundt et al., 2013) and self-efficacy (see Chapter 3). Unfortunately, related training and subsequent insights in care delivery are low. Not surprisingly, some of the most common ailments affecting geriatric patients are depression and anxiety (Mehta et al., 2003), both of which have been shown to benefit from psychological intervention.

Loss of Personal Control

Chronic disease is a powerful example of the undesirable yet unavoidable changes aging often imposes. Rarely does one advance through old age without enduring the cumulative impact of loss. In addition to changes in one's own physical and mental functioning, previously intimate relationships with others change or end due to illness or death. Psychologists have described for decades the cumulative traumatic result of a diminished sense of control of one's life. One noteworthy example is the work of Drs. Ellen Langer and Judith Rodin (1976), who measured the health-related impact of encouraging nursing home residents to feel more personal control and responsibility in their daily living. In their seminal study, the facility administrator provided the intervention group with plants to care for and emphasized the group's autonomy and responsibility for themselves. The control group received a message emphasizing the staff's responsibility for residents' well-being, and while these residents were also given plants, they were told staff would water them. Following the intervention, the group with more responsibility showed significant improvement in alertness, was more involved in social activities, and reported being happier than the comparison group did.

Rodin and Langer (1977) conducted a follow-up study 18 months later and found those in the responsibility group were judged by clinicians to be significantly more interested in their environment, more sociable and self-initiating, and more vigorous than the residents in the control group. Most striking, however, was the difference in mortality rates compared to the nursing home's average during the 18 months prior to the original study, which was 25%. At follow-up 18 months postintervention, 7 of the 47 residents in the responsibility group (15%) had died, compared to 14 of 44 residents in the control group (30%).

Dr. M. Powell Lawton (1999) and other geropsychologists (e.g., Baltes & Baltes, 1990) continue to address the important psychological changes associated with aging, including the link between older adults' perceived competence and mastery over one's environment with quality of life (Maiden, 1987). Some have shown that encouraging a schedule of positive activities can increase an older patient's sense of personal control 18 months later (Teri & Gallagher, 1991; Teri & Logsdon, 1991).

More recently Dr. Jutta Heckhausen and colleagues (Heckhausen & Schulz, 1995; Heckhausen, Wrosch, & Schulz, 2010) differentiated between primary and secondary control, the former being attempts to mold the external environment to fit one's needs and desires, the latter focusing internally to minimize losses of primary control and maintain or expand existing levels of control. According to their theory of human motivation and goals throughout the lifespan, as primary control becomes objectively less attainable with age, people continue striving to maintain it, often by employing secondary control strategies such as adjusting expectations, values, and attributions.

Dr. Laura Carstensen and colleagues (1999) have theorized that aging is characterized by a priority shift away from knowledge acquisition toward emotional goals (Carstensen et al., 1999) and have provided some empirical support for this concept (e.g., Carstensen, 2006).

Loss of Independence and Confidence

As chronically ill geriatric patients suffer diminished functional ability, they consequently experience loss of independence and confidence. For example, sensory impairment (e.g., vision or hearing) can make driving hazardous and frightening (Owsley & McGwin Jr., 2010; Taylor, Alpass, Stephens, & Towers, 2011; Taylor, Deane, & Podd, 2002). Depending on geographic region, this can significantly limit access to essential services at pharmacies, supermarkets and banks, not to mention limiting opportunities for social engagement with friends and family. Older adults who are physically frail and/or living with chronic joint or muscle pain are at increased risk for incontinence, malnutrition, or falls, the leading cause of injury and death among adults aged 65 and older (Boyd & Stevens, 2009). Shortness of breath, insomnia, fatigue, sexual dysfunction, diarrhea, constipation, all common symptoms of chronic disease, challenge geriatric patients' trust in their body and confidence in themselves on a daily basis.

The devastating physical impact of these and other chronic ailments is well documented and often recognized by physicians and nurses caring for geriatric patients. Much less obvious to these clinicians, however, is the concomitant psychological pain of physical disability, especially since many older patients attempt to maintain personal pride and dignity by minimizing or hiding their problems and concerns. Psychologists have examined these areas of "self-presentation" and "impression management" in relation to health and well-being (Martin, Leary, & Rejeski, 2000). Social stigma, shame, and embarrassment that accompany aging and illness are harmful in their own right and can elicit a negative impact on both psychological and biological health (Dickerson, Gruenewald, & Kemeny, 2004). Familial (informal) caregivers face similar consequences. (See Chapter 2.)

Burden

Limited empirical inquiry has targeted chronic disease patients' own, self-perceived burden. Yet when directly examined, such burden appears common. Data consistently reveal a stronger correlation of self-perceived burden with distress related to coping and psychological and existential factors than with physical symptoms. Common contributors to patients' self-perceived burden include guilt, shame, medical uncertainty, death anxiety, and reduced hope (McClement et al., 2007; McPherson, Wilson, Chyurlia, & Leclerc, 2010; Wilson, Curran, & McPherson, 2005). Consistent with Dr. Carstensen's socioemotional selectivity theory cited previously, self-perceived burden is particularly intense near the end of life (McPherson, Wilson, & Murray, 2007). As highlighted in Chapter 8, burden is also associated with suicidal ideation (Kowal, Wilson, McWilliams,

Péloquin, & Duong, 2012) and requests for physician-assisted suicide (Sullivan, Hedberg, & Hopkins, 2001).

Case Example: Postoperative Reassurance and Follow-up

An 87-year-old Russian widow was seen while recovering in the hospital from ileus following abdominal surgery 2 days prior. The psychologist and medical resident listened to the patient's frustration. She described a sleepless night due to vomiting nine times, and a difficult morning of incessant diarrhea after enema treatment. She expressed anger that she had been talked into surgery and exhibited passive suicidal ideation (e.g., "Nothing matters anymore, I've had enough, I can't do anything"). The resident responded by pointing out that it was, in fact, she, who requested the surgery due to acute gastrointestinal discomfort, and that her recent ability to pass gas was a positive sign in the right direction. This did not console her. The patient continued discussing her situation and concern that she might never improve. At this point the psychologist identified and reflected her *fear*, asking directly, "Are you scared?" The patient stopped speaking. Her eyes widened, she paused, lowered her voice, and said, "You know, yes, yes, I am." She then elaborated that she was terrified of eating and did not *trust* that she would ever be able to tolerate food again. The resident and psychologist reassured her that she was, in fact, making progress and together they outlined for her a clear course of events that she could expect with regard to timing and gradual food intake.

Following discharge to rehabilitation, and in consultation with the attending physician, the psychologist planned a follow-up encounter with the patient, again accompanied by the resident. The patient was pleasantly surprised by the unannounced visit. The next 45 minutes were characterized primarily by the patient repeatedly describing how excited the visit made her and how lonely she was otherwise. She proudly displayed pictures of her children and grandchildren, all of whom lived at a great distance. She discussed international politics and her personal experiences immigrating to the U.S. When it was time to part ways, the patient requested assistance in standing up. After rising out of her bed, and with tears in her eyes, she asked permission to hug the psychologist and resident. She embraced each and thanked them for providing her "this gift." The patient progressed and was soon discharged home. During a follow-up appointment with her primary care physician 3 months later, she was still discussing the impact of the visit.

PATIENT SAFETY

If ranked as a disease, adverse drug reactions would be the fifth leading cause of death in America (Petrone & Katz, 2005, p. 757–758). Iatrogenic impact of potentially inappropriate prescribing is a major threat to patient safety, increasingly a national priority according to an IOM report in 2000, *To Err Is Human: Building a Safer Health System* (Kohn, Corrigan, & Donaldson, 2000).

Geriatric patients are particularly vulnerable to medication-related error involving polypharmacy and nonadherence. Older adults are the greatest consumers of medication, with more than 94% of women over the age of 65 taking at least one daily prescription medication and 12% taking 10 or more (Kaufman, Kelly, Rosenberg, Anderson, & Mitchell, 2002). Not only do elderly patients consume more medication than their younger counterparts, but aging-associated pharmacokinetic and pharmacodynamic changes increase susceptibility to drug-drug and drug-disease interactions that often are not considered until it is too late (Mallet, Spinewine, & Huang, 2007). Research has found 35% of ambulatory older adults experience adverse drug reactions on a yearly basis and 29% of these require physician evaluation in an emergency room or hospital (Petrone & Katz, 2005).

Geriatricians have identified pharmaceutical risks to guide prescribing clinicians regarding potentially inappropriate medications, particularly for nursing home residents, via the "Beers Criteria" (Beers et al., 1991; Fick et al., 2003). But while this guide may help safeguard against *physician* prescription-related errors, it cannot sufficiently prevent *patient* error, such as that caused by misunderstanding directions and subsequent failure to take medications as prescribed, a critical behavioral component of effective medical treatment. The clinical relevance and poor management of patient adherence has been discussed by psychologists for decades (DiMatteo, 2004a), as has the key benefit conferred by social support (DiMatteo, 2004b). Multimorbid older patients are especially vulnerable and may be seriously challenged by complex medication regimens and/or adverse side effects. For some chronic diseases, in which the presence and severity of symptoms may fluctuate or go unnoticed (e.g., hypertension), ensuring appropriate adherence can be extremely difficult for any clinician, especially since standard frequency of ambulatory outpatient contact with primary care physicians is 1–3 visits per year. Some have estimated that only 29–59% of elderly patients are able to take their medications as prescribed (Stewart & Caranasos, 1989). In response, many geriatric physicians (e.g., Rayner, O'Brien, & Schoenbachler, 2006) advocate the "start low and go slow" approach.

In some cases patients may not feel motivated to adhere to their medication regimen or adjust their lifestyle (e.g., diet, exercise). As described elsewhere in this publication, motivational interviewing (MI), a behavioral intervention created by psychologists and most often used by psychologists, has proven effective for negotiating patient ambivalence about behavior change related to health and illness. Rubak and colleagues (2005) conducted a systematic review and meta-analysis of 72 randomized control trials that revealed a significant, clinically relevant effect of MI in 75% of studies reviewed. Impact was comparable on both physiologic and psychological conditions and more likely to be achieved when MI was conducted by physicians and psychologists than by other professionals (80% vs. 46%). Consulting psychologists can conduct such interventions and train other providers to do so.

Harvard surgeon Atul Gawande has described the enormous human and financial costs associated with adhering solely to a medical model of geriatric care (Gawande, 2014). Others have also shown that lack of mental health input leads to higher health care utilization and costs, greater functional impairment, increased utilization of staff time, patient non-adherence, increased mortality, and reduced quality of life (Hyer and Shah, 2009; Ormel et al., 1998; Rodriguez, 2013). A growing number of physician and nonphysician geriatric specialists (e.g., Bensadon & Odenheimer, 2014; George & Whitehouse, 2014; Kathol, deGray, & Rollman, 2014) have therefore recommended psychosocial interventions as appropriate first-line treatment of conditions for which unnecessary medical and surgical services continue to be used at an annual cost approaching 350 billion dollars. Even among the most seriously mentally ill, "two-thirds of the patients receive no care at all, and those who do, receive care in the medical and not the behavioral care sector" (Hyer & Shah, 2009, p. 172).

Kathol and colleagues (2014) propose the following patient-centered LTC model: 1. The focus should be on complex medical illnesses such as diabetes, asthma, heart disease and patients with high health care costs rather than on screening everyone for behavioral problems; 2. Resources should be administered using a fully integrated model; 3. Behavioral health practitioners (i.e., psychologists) should be well trained in evidence-based methods; and 4. The latest technology should be employed, including telecommunications.

Targeting medically complex and high-utilization patients has led to functional and cost improvements, consistent with the triple aim of enhanced patient experience, population health, and lower per capita cost.

Case Example: The Pink Giraffe

A psychologist was consulted to engage a patient who was convinced she was psychotic after seeing a pink giraffe in her hospital room. Physician response was to simply increase her medication. But only after spending time listening to her narrative did it become clear she had already been prescribed too much amitriptyline and had suffered an adverse reaction. With continued discussions, the patient was able to work through her fears and finally accept that her hallucinations were prompted by an allergic reaction to her medicine, which had caused her delirium. Psychologist consultation was ideal for several reasons. Training and experience enabled the psychologist to avoid prematurely judging the patient's report of hallucinations as evidence of psychosis. Instead, the patient was given a chance to share her story with a nonjudgmental doctor well-trained in active listening. The more the patient was reassured and felt understood, the more she trusted, and subsequently the more details she shared about her unsettling symptoms and related fear. This non-pharmacologic intervention, characterized by health literacy information exchange and nonjudgmental empathic listening, successfully broke the all too frequent cycle of harmful and ineffective but ongoing medication administration (see Campanelli, 2012).

PSYCHOTHERAPY

Many of the challenges identified here can be addressed with psycho-therapy. Since the introduction of cognitive-behavioral therapy (CBT) and interpersonal psychotherapeutic interventions approximately half a cen-tury ago (Beck, 1976; Ellis, 1962; Klerman, DiMascio, Weissman, Prusoff, & Paykel, 1974; Klerman, Weissman, Rounsaville, & Chevron, 1984), out-comes research has yielded a robust evidence base. A meta-analysis of 106 meta-analyses conducted by Hofmann and colleagues (2012) suggests CBT is the most well-supported behavioral treatment modality regardless of patient age and illness type. Specific to the geriatric patient population, most of the earlier efficacy studies of CBT targeted "mental" health distur-bances, particularly depression (Dobson, 1989) and anxiety (Ayers et al., 2007; Hofmann & Smits, 2008; Stanley, Beck & Glassco 1996).

Problem-solving therapies (e.g., Alexopoulos et al., 2011) and other types of outpatient group therapy have also shown effectiveness with older patients for half a century (Liederman & Green, 1965; Steuer et al., 1984). Data consistently reveal that older patients prefer psychotherapy to medication for managing mood (Gum et al., 2006; Mohlman, 2012; Unützer et al., 2003).

The mechanism of action of psychotherapy is multifaceted and consists first and foremost of establishing an intimate connection with an inter-ested, concerned, and caring doctor. Though related benefit is intuitively clear and rational, evidence suggests such opportunities are increasingly rare as people navigate life's last decades, leading to feelings of invisibil-ity, even among highly functioning older community dwellers (Fennell & Davidson, 2003; Monk, 1988). As mentioned earlier, older patients' prefer-ence for psychotherapy has not led to routine referral for and utilization of such services (Alvidrez & Areán, 2002; Wei et al., 2005). Only after these changes can care truly be considered patient-centered.

Psychotherapeutic intervention for older adults is clinically effective for managing common emotional difficulties such as isolation, loneliness, depression, diminished confidence and independence, and feelings of helplessness. The efficacy of psychotherapy has been established for "mental" or affective sequelae (e.g., anxiety or depression) of impaired physical function, including chronic conditions prevalent among geriatric patients such as nocturia (Breyer et al., 2013), cardiopulmonary disease (Yohannes, Willgoss, Baldwin & Connolly 2010), insomnia (Morin, Colecchi, Stone, Sood, & Brink, 1999), and pain (Kerns, Sellinger, & Goodin, 2011).

DEMENTIA

Cognitive-behavioral interventions can also benefit individuals diagnosed with AD. Unlike policies of the past, which incorrectly assumed degenerative disease automatically precluded utility of psychotherapy, Medicare now provides coverage for behavioral intervention to maintain function or slow the rate of decline. Yet even in geriatric practice, in the absence of integration, an automatic, "knee jerk" reliance on antidementia or antipsychotic medication is generally the preferred first line of treatment, especially for behavioral and psychological problems. Though this may be understandable, without integration its benefit is limited, and reduced quality of life and risk of serious adverse effects, including death (Schneider, Dagerman, & Insel, 2005), are well documented (Ballard & Howard, 2006; Sink, Holden, & Yaffe, 2005). In fact, these data have led some to conclude "adverse effects offset advantages in the efficacy of atypical antipsychotic drugs for the treatment of psychosis, aggression, or agitation in patients with Alzheimer's disease" (Schneider et al., 2006, p. 1525).

Dementia is not a black and white disease. Depending on subtype, the dementing process often occurs in phases. Early on, behavioral psychotherapy can be effective in helping patients problem-solve, accept their illness, and adjust to the disease-associated limitations. This is vital, since most people with dementia who commit suicide do so shortly after diagnosis (Seyfried, Kales, Ignacio, Conwell, & Valenstein, 2011). Psychotherapy can boost morale and help patients maintain function. It can also educate and support informal caregivers. Of course, as is true with psychotherapy for any patient, behavioral therapy with dementia requires careful monitoring, documentation, and frequent outcome evaluation to measure clinical benefit. Psychologists are trained to recognize that underlying attention-seeking behaviors often reflect patients' unmet needs related to fear. This can include the threat of isolation and acute loneliness, death, or the perception of being ignored. In patients with dementia behavioral outbursts may signify constipation or other physical pain. Enhanced understanding can positively impact the patient and their care providers. But without it, clinical attention will only be directed toward the more obvious, overt behaviors rather than the subtler symptoms at their root. Standard care that aims to merely control patients with medication inefficiently "treats" the former and ignores the latter.

The Centers for Medicare and Medicaid Services recently launched a national campaign to improve dementia care (Centers for Medicare and Medicaid Services, 2014). Specifically, the goal is enhancing behavioral health while reducing unnecessary medication. Less specific, however, is *who* determines whether medication is necessary and *who* will provide behavioral intervention if it is not.

MANAGING FAMILY CONFLICT

Strained family dynamics can present a major challenge in a system where caregivers are often relied upon for clinical decision-making. Psychology consultation can enable more effective mutual understanding among patients, their families, and clinicians. Terminal or end-stage illness is frequently accompanied by volatile emotion. Consistent with the tenets of interpersonal therapy (Klerman et al., 1984; Nemade, Riss & Dombeck, 2007; Weissman, Markowitz, & Klerman, 2000) and systems approaches to family therapy (e.g., Bowen, 1966, 1978; Minuchin, 1974), psychologist intervention can focus on the specific language and behaviors used to describe feelings about "hot-button issues" through a realistic and positive lens. Psychoeducation can equip family members with communication techniques to maximize respect, minimize blame, and strive for acceptance, painful as it may be (Doherty & McDaniel, 2014; Greenberg & Safran, 1987).

As described in Chapter 2, intervention can help identify, address, and provide closure to longstanding but generally avoided "unfinished business." Imagined insults, jealousy, resentment, perceived exploitation, each potentially relevant to clinical decision-making, can all be exposed and reframed once trust is established. Examination of meta-communications (Tannen, 2002) and alliance formation with each family member (Friedlander, Lee, Shaffer, & Cabrera, 2014) encourages bonding and respect of personal boundaries. This allows family members to gain closure and slowly resolve enduring issues of hurt and pain. As families gain insight and develop new understanding of each other, healing takes place (Hayslip, Maiden, Pate, & Doblin-Macnab, 2015).

SUMMARY

Psychology consultation is an overdue concept whose time has come. By definition, geriatric patients have multiple needs of both mind and body as they age. To treat older adults effectively and safely, medical teams must employ an integrated biopsychosocial care approach. As collaborative care models, such as the patient-centered medical home (Kathol, deGruy, & Rollman, 2014), are implemented nationally (Butler et al., 2008; Miller, Petterson, Burke, Phillips & Green 2014), psychologist integration is increasingly feasible and necessary (Blount, DeGirolamo, & Mariani, 2006). This chapter illustrates that the absence of psychology in standard practice contributes to and perpetuates many long-standing, well-documented gaps in care. In an inadequate and inefficient health care system, appropriate consultation confers benefit to patients, their families, and physicians alike.

References

Alexopoulos, G. S., Raue, P. J., Kiosses, D. N., Mackin, R. S., Kanellopoulos, D., McCulloch, C., et al. (2011). Problem-solving therapy and supportive therapy in older adults with major depression and executive dysfunction: effect on disability. *Archives of General Psychiatry, 68*(1), 33–41.

Alvidrez, J. E., & Areán, P. A. (2002). Physician willingness to refer older depressed patients for psychotherapy. *The International Journal of Psychiatry in Medicine, 32*(1), 21–35.

American Bar Association Commission on Law and Aging and American Psychological Association (2008). *Assessment of older adults with diminished capacity: A handbook for psychologists.* Washington, DC: American Bar Association.

American Psychological Association (2014). *Guidelines for psychological practice with older adults* (69). American Psychological Association. (pp. 34–65).

Apatira, L., Boyd, E. A., Malvar, G., Evans, L. R., Luce, J. M., Lo, B., et al. (2008). Hope, truth, and preparing for death: Perspectives of surrogate decision makers. *Annals of Internal Medicine, 149*(12), 861–868.

Ayers, C. R., Sorrell, J. T., Thorp, S. R., & Wetherell, J. L. (2007). Evidence-based psychological treatments for late-life anxiety. *Psychology and Aging, 22*(1), 8–17.

Ballard, C., & Howard, R. (2006). Neuroleptic drugs in dementia: benefits and harm. *Nature Reviews Neuroscience, 7*(6), 492–500.

Baltes, P. B., & Baltes, M. M. (1990). Psychological perspectives on successful aging: The model of selective optimization with compensation. *Successful aging: Perspectives from the Behavioral Sciences, 1*, 1–34.

Barry, L. C., Kasl, S. V., & Prigerson, H. G. (2002). Psychiatric disorders among bereaved persons: The role of perceived circumstances of death and preparedness for death. *The American Journal of Geriatric Psychiatry, 10*(4), 447–457.

Bartels, S. J., Coakley, E. H., Zubritsky, C., Ware, J. H., Miles, K. M., Areán, P. A., et al. (2004). Improving access to geriatric mental health services: A randomized trial comparing treatment engagement with integrated versus enhanced referral care for depression, anxiety, and at-risk alcohol use. *American Journal of Psychiatry, 161*(8), 1455–1462.

Beck, A. T. (1976). *Cognitive therapy and the emotional disorders.* New York: Meridian.

Beers, M. H., Ouslander, J. G., Rollingher, I., Reuben, D. B., Brooks, J., & Beck, J. C. (1991). Explicit criteria for determining inappropriate medication use in nursing home residents. *Archives of Internal Medicine, 151*(9), 1825–1832.

Bensadon, B. A. (2014). Maximizing treatment adherence: physician-patient partnerships vs. procedures. *Hypertension, 63*(2), e7.

Bensadon, B. A., & Odenheimer, G. L. (2014). Current management decisions in mild cognitive impairment. *Clinics in Geriatric Medicine, 29*(4), 847–871.

Bertakis, K. D., Roter, D., & Putnam, S. M. (1991). The relationship of physician medical interview style to patient satisfaction. *Journal of Family Practice, 32*(2), 175–181.

Blount, A. (1998). *Integrated primary care: The future of medical & mental health collaboration.* New York: Norton.

Blount, A., DeGirolamo, S., & Mariani, K. (2006). Training the collaborative care practitioners of the future. *Families, Systems, & Health, 24,* 111–119.

Blount, A., Kathol, R., Thomas, M., Schoenbaum, M., Rollman, B., & O'Donohue, W. (2007). The economics of behavioral health services in medical settings: A summary of the evidence. *Professional Psychology: Research and Practice, 38,* 290–297.

Blount, A., & Miller, B. F. (2009). Addressing the workforce crisis in integrated primary care. *Journal of Clinical Psychology in Medical Settings, 16,* 113–119.

Bowen, M. (1966). The use of family theory in clinical practice. *Comprehensive Psychiatry, 7*(5), 345–374.

Bowen, M. (1978). Society, crisis, and systems theory. *Family Therapy in Clinical Practice,* 413–450.

Boyd, R., & Stevens, J. (2009). Falls and fear of falling: Burden, beliefs and behaviours. *Age and Ageing, 38*(4), 423–428.

Breggin, P. R. (1994). *Toxic psychiatry: Why therapy, empathy and love must replace the drugs, electroshock, and biochemical theories of the new psychiatry.* Macmillan.

Breyer, B. N., Shindel, A. W., Erickson, B. A., Blaschko, S. D., Steers, W. D., & Rosen, R. C. (2013). The association of depression, anxiety and nocturia: A systematic review. *The Journal of Urology, 190*(3), 953–957.

Burling, S. (2014). The Philadelphia Inquirer, June 20, (p. A2).

Butler, M., Kane, R. L., McAlpine, D., Kathol, R. G., Fu, S. S., Hagedorn, H., et al. (2008). Evidence report/technology assessment number 173; Integration of mental health/substance abuse and primary care (AHRQ Pub. Nl. 09-E003). Rockville, MD: Agency for Healthcare Research and Quality.

Campanelli, C. M. (2012). American geriatrics society updated beers criteria for potentially inappropriate medication use in older adults: The american geriatrics society 2012 beers criteria update expert panel. *Journal of the American Geriatrics Society, 60*(4), 616–631.

Carstensen, L. L., Isaacowitz, D. M., & Charles, S. T. (1999). Taking time seriously: A theory of socioemotional selectivity. *American Psychologist, 54*(3), 165–181.

Carstensen, L. L. (2006). The influence of a sense of time on human development. *Science, 312*(5782), 1913–1915.

Cavanaugh, K. L., Wingard, R. L., Hakim, R. M., Eden, S., Shintani, A., Wallston, K. A., et al. (2010). Low health literacy associates with increased mortality in ESRD. *Journal of the American Society of Nephrology, 21*(11), 1979–1985.

Centers for Disease Control and Prevention. (2011). Available at: <http://www.cdc.gov/chronicdisease/resources/publications/aag/aging.htm>.

Centers for Medicare & Medicaid Services (2014). Available at: <http://www.cms.gov/Medicare/Provider-Enrollment-and-Certification/SurveyCertificationGenInfo/Downloads/Survey-and-Cert-Letter-14-19.pdf>.

Clark, N. M., Becker, M. H., Janz, N. K., Lorig, K., Rakowski, W., & Anderson, L. (1991). Self-management of chronic disease by older adults. *Journal of Aging and Health, 3,* 3–27.

Conwell, Y., Olsen, K., Caine, E. D., & Flannery, C. (1991). Suicide in later life: Psychological autopsy findings. *International Psychogeriatrics, 3*(1), 59–66.

Cummings, N. A. (1998). Approaches to preventative care Hartman-Stein (Ed.), *Innovative behavioral healthcare for older adults* (pp. 1–17). San Francisco: Jossey-Bass Publishers.

Darer, J. D., Hwang, W., Pham, H. H., Bass, E. B., & Anderson, G. (2004). More training needed in chronic care: A survey of US physicians. *Academic Medicine, 79*(6), 541–548.

Dickel, H. A. (1966). The physician and the clinical psychologist. *Journal of the American Medical Association, 195,* 365–370.

Dickerson, S. S., Gruenewald, T. L., & Kemeny, M. E. (2004). *Journal of Personality, 72*(6), 1191–1216.

DiMatteo, M. R. (2004a). Variations in patients' adherence to medical recommendations: A quantitative review of 50 years of research. *Medical Care, 42*(3), 200–209.

DiMatteo, M. R. (2004b). Social support and patient adherence to medical treatment: A meta-analysis. *Health Psychology, 23*(2), 207–218.

Dobson, K. S. (1989). A meta-analysis of the efficacy of cognitive therapy for depression. *Journal of Consulting and Clinical Psychology, 57*(3), 414–419.

Doherty, W. J., & McDaniel, S. H. (2014). Family therapy process. In G. R. Vanderbos, E. Meidenbauer, & J. Frank-McNeil (Eds.), *Psychotherapy theories and techniques: A reader.* Washington DC: American Psychological Association.

Dundon, M., Dollar, K., Schohn, M., & Lantinga, L. J. (2011). Primary care mental health integration-Co-located, collaborative care: An operations manual. Available at: <http://www.mentalhealth.va.gov/coe/cihvisn2/Documents/Clinical/Operations_Policies_Procedures/MH-IPC_CCC_Operations_Manual_Version_2_1.pdf>. Retrieved November 23, 2014.

Ellis, A. (1962). *Reason and emotion in psychology.* New York: Lyle Stuart.

Fennell, G., & Davidson, K. (2003). "The invisible man?" Older men in modern society. *Ageing International, 28*(4), 315–325.

Fick, D. M., Cooper, J. W., Wade, W. E., Waller, J. L., Maclean, R., & Beers, M. H. (2003). Updating the Beers criteria for potentially inappropriate medication use in older adults. *Archives of Internal Medicine, 163,* 2716–2724.

Fife, T. D. (2003). Clinical Features of Normal Pressure Hydrocephalus. *Barrow Quarterly, 19*(N. 2), 1–9.

Friedlander, M. L., Lee, H. H., Shaffer, K. S., & Cabrera, P. (2014). Negotiating therapeutic alliances with a family at impasse. *Psychotherapy, 51*(1), 41–52.

Gawande, A. (2014). Being mortal: Medicine and what matters in the end: *Metropolitan books.* New York: Henry Holt & Company.

George, D. R., & Whitehouse, P. J. (2014). Chasing the white whale of Alzheimer's. *Journal of the American Geriatrics Society, 62*(3), 588–589.

Glenn, M. L. (1987). *Collaborative health care: A family oriented approach.* New York: Praeger.

Greenberg, L. S., & Safran, J. D. (1987). *Emotion in psychotherapy: Affect, cognition, and the process of change.* New York, NY: Guilford Press.

Greene, M. G., & Adelman, R. D. (1996). Psychosocial factors in older patients' medical encounters. *Research on Aging, 18*(1), 84–102.

Greene, M. G., Hoffman, S., Charon, R., & Adelman, R. (1987). Psychosocial concerns in the medical encounter: A comparison of the interactions of doctors with their old and young patients. *The Gerontologist, 27*(2), 164–168.

Gum, A. M., Areán, P. A., Hunkeler, E., Tang, L., Katon, W., Hitchcock, P., et al. (2006). Depression treatment preferences in older primary care patients. *The Gerontologist, 46*(1), 14–22.

Hayslip, B., Jr., Maiden, R. J., Pate, K. S., & Doblin-Macnab, M. C. (2015). Grandparenting. In P. A. Lichtenberg & B. T. Mast (Eds.), *APA Handbook of Clinical Geropsychology.* Washington, D.C.: The American Psychological Association.

Hebert, R. S., Schulz, R., Copeland, V. C., & Arnold, R. M. (2009). Preparing family caregivers for death and bereavement. Insights from caregivers of terminally ill patients. *Journal of Pain and Symptom Management, 37*(1), 3–12.

Heckhausen, J., & Schulz, R. (1995). A life-span theory of control. *Psychological Review, 102,* 284–304.

Heckhausen, J., Wrosch, C., & Schulz, R. (2010). A motivational theory of life-span development. *Psychological Review, 117*(1), 32.

Henningsen, P., Zimmermann, T., & Sattel, H. (2003). Medically unexplained physical symptoms, anxiety, and depression: a meta-analytic review. *Psychosomatic Medicine, 65*(4), 528–533.

Hofmann, S. G., Asnaani, A., Vonk, I. J., Sawyer, A. T., & Fang, A. (2012). The efficacy of cognitive behavioral therapy: A review of meta-analyses. *Cognitive Therapy and Research, 36*(5), 427–440.

Hofmann, S. G., & Smits, J. A. (2008). Cognitive-behavioral therapy for adult anxiety disorders: A meta-analysis of randomized placebo-controlled trials. *The Journal of Clinical Psychiatry, 69*(4), 621–632.

Hundt, N. E., Bensadon, B. A., Stanley, M. A., Petersen, N. J., Kunik, M. E., Kauth, M. R., et al. (2013). Coping mediates the relationship between disease severity and illness intrusiveness among chronically ill patients. *Journal of Health Psychology* Dec 1.

Hunter, C. L., Goodie, J. L., Dobmeyer, A. C., & Dorrance, K. A. (2014). Tipping points in the department of defense's experience with psychologists in primary care. *American Psychologist, 69*(4), 388–398.

Hyer, L., & Shah, (2009). Integration of psychology, psychiatry, and medication in long-term care. In E. Roswsky, J. M. Casciani, & M. Arnold (Eds.), *Geropsychology amd Long Term Care: A practitioner's guide.* New York: Springer Publishing Co.

Institute of Medicine Board on Health Care Services (2006). *Improving the quality of health care for mental and substance-use conditions: Quality chasm series.* Washington DC: National Academic Press.

Karel, M., Gatz, M., & Smyler, M. (2012). Aging and mental health in the decade ahead: What psychologists need to know. *American Psychologist, 67,* 184–198.

Kaskie, B. (2013). The widespread deployment of integrated models of care. *Public Policy & Aging Report, 3*(1), 3–9 23.

Kathol, R. G., Butler, M., McAlpine, D. D., & Kane, R. L. (2010). Barriers to physical and mental condition integrated service delivery. *Psychosomatic Medicine, 72*(6), 511–518.

Kathol, R. G., deGruy, F., & Rollman, B. L. (2014). Value-based financially sustainable behavioral health components in patient-centered medical homes. *Annals of Family Medicine, 12,* 172–175.

Kaufman, D. W., Kelly, J. P., Rosenberg, L., Anderson, T. E., & Mitchell, A. A. (2002). Recent patterns of medication use in the ambulatory adult population of the United States. *Journal of the American Medical Association, 287*(3), 337–344.

Kerns, R. D., Sellinger, J., & Goodin, B. R. (2011). Psychological treatment of chronic pain. *Annual Review of Clinical Psychology, 7,* 411–434.

Kirsch, I. (2010). *Emperor's new drugs: Exploding the antidepressant myth.* Basic Books.

Klerman, G. L., DiMascio, A., Weissman, M. M., Prusoff, B. A., & Paykel, E. S. (1974). Treatment of depression by drugs and psychotherapy. *Am. J. Psychiat, 131*(2), 186–191.

Klerman, G. L., Weissman, M. M., Rounsaville, B. J., & Chevron, E. S. (1984). *Interpersonal psychotherapy of depression.* New York: Basic Books.

Kohn, L. T., Corrigan, J. M., & Donaldson, M. S. (Eds.), (2000). *To err is human: building a safer health system.* National Academies Press.

Kowal, J., Wilson, K. G., McWilliams, L. A., Péloquin, K., & Duong, D. (2012). Self-perceived burden in chronic pain: Relevance, prevalence, and predictors. *Pain, 153*(8), 1735–1741.

Kuo, W. H., Gallo, J. J., & Eaton, W. W. (2004). Hopelessness, depression, substance disorder, and suicidality – A 13-year community-based study. *Social Psychiatry & Psychiatric Epidemiology, 39*(6), 497–501.

Langer, E. J., & Rodin, J. (1976). The effects of choice and enhanced personal responsibility for the aged: A field experiment in an institutional setting. *Journal of Personality and Social Psychology, 34*(2), 191–198.

Lawton, M. P. (1999, 23 August). Measuring quality of life in nursing homes: The search continues. Invited address, divisions 34, 5, & 20, Annual Meeting of the American Psychological Society, Boston, MA.

Leipzig, R. M., Hall, W. J., & Fried, L. P. (2012). Treating our societal scotoma: The case for investing in geriatrics, our nation's future, and our patients. *Annals of Internal Medicine, 156*(9), 657–659.

Liederman, P. C., & Green, R. (1965). Geriatric outpatient group therapy. *Comprehensive Psychiatry, 6*(1), 51–60.

Lin, W. -C., Zhang, J., Leung, G. Y., & Clark, R. E. (2011). Chronic physical condition in older adults with mental illness and/or substance abuse disorders. *Journal of American Geriatrics Society, 59,* 1913–1921.

Litauska, A. M., Kozikowski, A., Nouryan, C. N., Kline, M., Pekmezaris, R., & Wolf-Klein, G. (2014). Do residents need end-of-life care training? *Palliative & Supportive Care, 12*(3), 195–201.

Luoma, J. B., Martin, C. E., & Pearson, J. L. (2002). Contact with mental health and primary care providers before suicide: A review of the evidence. *The American Journal of Psychiatry, 159*(6), 909–916.

Lysack, C., Leach, C., Russo, T., Paulson, D., & Lichtenberg, P. (2013). DVD training for depression identification and treatment in older adults: A two group randomized waitlist control study. *American Journal of Occupational Therapy, 67*, 1–10. http://dx.doi.org/10.5014/ajot.2013.008060.

Mallet, L., Spinewine, A., & Huang, A. (2007). The challenge of managing drug interactions in elderly people. *The Lancet, 370*(9582), 185–191.

Martin, K. A., Leary, M. R., & Rejeski, W. J. (2000). Self-presentational concerns in older adults: Implications for health and well-being. *Basic and Applied Social Psychology, 22*(3), 169–179.

McClement, S., Chochinov, H. M., Hack, T., Hassard, T., Kristjanson, L. J., & Harlos, M. (2007). Dignity therapy: family member perspectives. *Journal of Palliative Medicine, 10*(5), 1076–1082.

McPherson, C. J., Wilson, K. G., Chyurlia, L., & Leclerc, C. (2010). The balance of give and take in caregiver–partner relationships: An examination of self-perceived burden, relationship equity, and quality of life from the perspective of care recipients following stroke. *Rehabilitation Psychology, 55*(2), 194–203.

McPherson, C. J., Wilson, K. G., & Murray, M. A. (2007). Feeling like a burden to others: A systematic review focusing on the end of life. *Palliative Medicine, 21*(2), 115–128.

Mehta, K. M., Simonsick, E. M., Penninx, B. W., Schulz, R., Rubin, S. M., Satterfield, S., et al. (2003). Prevalence and correlates of anxiety symptoms in well-functioning older adults: Findings from the Health Aging and Body Composition Study. *Journal of the American Geriatrics Society, 51*(4), 499–504.

Meier, D. E., Back, A. L., & Morrison, R. S. (2001). The inner life of physicians and care of the seriously ill. *Journal of the American Medical Association, 286*(23), 3007–3014.

Meier, D. E., & Beresford, L. (2010). Growing the interface between palliative medicine and psychiatry. *Journal of Palliative Medicine, 13*(7), 803–806.

Miller, B. F., Petterson, S., Burke, B. T., Phillips, R. L., Jr., & Green, L. A. (2014). Proximity of providers: Colocating behavioral health and primary care and the prospects for an integrated workforce. *American Psychologist/Special Issue, 69*, 443–451.

Minuchin, S. (1974). *Families and Family Therapy.* Cambridge: Harvard University Press.

Mohlman, J. (2012). A community based survey of older adults' preferences for treatment of anxiety. *Psychology and Aging, 27*(4), 1182.

Monk, A. (1988). Aging, loneliness, and communications. *American Behavioral Scientist, 31*(5), 532–563.

Morin, C. M., Colecchi, C., Stone, J., Sood, R., & Brink, D. (1999). Behavioral and pharmacological therapies for late-life insomnia: A randomized controlled trial. *Journal of the American Medical Association, 281*(11), 991–999.

Morriss, R., Gask, L., Dowrick, C., Dunn, G., Peters, S., Ring, A., et al. (2010). Randomized trial of reattribution on psychosocial talk between doctors and patients with medically unexplained symptoms. *Psychological Medicine, 40*(02), 325–333.

Nemade, R., Reiss, N. S. & Dombeck, M. (2007). Interpersonal therapy for major depression. Available from: <http://www.mentalhelp.net/poc/view_doc.php?type=doc&id=doc&id=13026&cn=5>.

Noel, P. H., Williams, J. W., Unützer, J., Worchel, J., Less, S., Cornell, J., et al. (2004). Depression and comorbid illness in elderly primary care patients: Impact of multiple domains of health status and well-being. *Annals of Family Medicine, 2*, 555–562.

Novack, D. H., Suchman, A. L., Clark, W., Epstein, R. M., Najberg, E., & Kaplan, C. (1997). Calibrating the physician: Personal awareness and effective patient care. *Journal of the American Medical Association, 278*(6), 502–509.

Ogden, J. (2012). *Health psychology: A textbook.* McGraw-Hill International.

Olfson, M., & Marcus, S. C. (2009). National patterns in antidepressant medication treatment. *JAMA Psychiatry, 66*(8), 848–856.

Olfson, M., Marcus, S. C., Druss, B., Elinson, L., Tanielian, T., & Pincus, H. A. (2002). National trends in the outpatient treatment of depression. *Journal of the American Medical Association, 287*(2), 203–209.

Orlander, J. D., Graeme Fincke, B., Hermanns, D., & Johnson, G. A. (2002). Medical residents' first clearly remembered experiences of giving bad news. *Journal of General Internal Medicine, 17*(11), 825–840.

Ormel, J., Kempen, G. I. J. M., Deeg, D. J., Brilman, E. I., Van Sonderen, E., & Relyveld, J. (1998). Functioning, well-being, and health perception in late middle-aged and older people: Comparing the effects of depressive symptoms and chronic medical conditions. *Journal of the American Geriatrics Society, 46*(1), 39–48.

Osgood, N. J., & Thielman, S. (1990). Geriatric suicidal behavior: Assessment and treatment. In S. J. Blumenthal & D. J. Kupfer (Eds.), *Suicide over the Life Cycle: Risk Factors, Assessment, and Treatment of Suicidal Patients* (pp. 341–379).

O'Malley, K. (1998). PACE: Innovative care for the frail older adult Hartman-Stein (Ed.), *Innovative Behavioral Healthcare for Older Adults* (pp. 19–39). San Francisco: Jossey-Bass Publishers.

Owsley, C., Jr., & McGwin, G. (2010). Vision and driving. *Vision Research, 50*(23), 2348–2361.

Pasina, L., Brucato, A. L., Falcone, C., Cucchi, E., Bresciani, A., Sottocorno, M., et al. (2014). Medication non-adherence among elderly patients newly discharged and receiving polypharmacy. *Drugs & Aging, 31*(4), 283–289.

Petrone, K., & Katz, P. (2005). Approaches to appropriate drug prescribing for the older adult. *Primary Care, 32,* 755–775.

Pomerantz, A. S., Shiner, B., Watts, B. V., Detzer, M. J., Kutter, C., Street, B., et al. (2010). The White River model of colocated collaborative care: A platform for mental and behavioral health care in the medical home. *Families, Systems, & Health, 28,* 114–129.

Raue, P. J., Schulberg, H. C., Heo, M., Klimstra, S., & Bruce, M. L. (2009). Patients' depression treatment preferences and initiation, adherence, and outcome: A randomized primary care study. *Psychiatric Services, 60*(3), 337–343.

Rayner, A. V., O'Brien, J. G., & Schoenbachler, B. (2006). Behavior disorders of dementia: Recognition and treatment. *American Family Physicians, 73*(4), 647–652.

Ring, A., Dowrick, C. F., Humphris, G. M., Davies, J., & Salmon, P. (2005). The somatising effect of clinical consultation: What patients and doctors say and do not say when patients present medically unexplained physical symptoms. *Social Science & Medicine, 61*(7), 1505–1515.

Rodin, J., & Langer, E. T. (1977). Long-term effects of control-relevant intervention with the institutionalized aged. *Journal of Personality and Social Psychology, 35,* 897–902.

Rodriguez, S. (2013). Better coordination of care for Medicare beneficiaries with severe mental illness could improve quality of life and lower cost. *Public Policy & Aging Report, 23*(N. 3), 10–15.

Rosowsky, E., Casciani, J. M., & Arnold, M. (2009). *Geropsychology and long term care: A practitioner's guide.* New York: Springer.

Roter, D. L., Hall, J. A., Merisca, R., Nordstrom, B., Cretin, D., & Svarstad, B. (1998). Effectiveness of interventions to improve patient compliance. *Medical Care, 36*(8), 1138–1161.

Roter, D. L., Stewart, M., Putnam, S. M., Lipkin, M., Stiles, W., & Inui, T. S. (1997). Communication patterns of primary care physicians. *Journal of the American Medical Association, 277*(4), 350–356.

Rubak, S., Sandbæk, A., Lauritzen, T., & Christensen, B. (2005). Motivational interviewing: A systematic review and meta-analysis. *British Journal of General Practice, 55*(513), 305–312.

Saul, E. V., & Kass, J. S. (1969). Study of anticipated anxiety in a medical school setting. *Academic Medicine, 44*(6), 526–532.

Schneider, L. S., Dagerman, K. S., & Insel, P. (2005). Risk of death with atypical antipsychotic drug treatment for dementia. *Journal of the American Medical Association, 294*(15), 1934–1943.

Schneider, L. S., Tariot, P. N., Dagerman, K. S., Davis, S. M., Hsiao, J. K., Ismail, M. S., et al. (2006). Effectiveness of atypical antipsychotic drugs in patients with Alzheimer's disease. *New England Journal of Medicine, 355*(15), 1525–1538.

Seyfried, L. S., Kales, H. C., Ignacio, R. V., Conwell, Y., & Valenstein, M. (2011). Predictors of suicide in patients with dementia. *Alzheimers & Dementia, 7*(6), 567–573.

Sink, K. M., Holden, K. F., & Yaffe, K. (2005). Pharmacological treatment of neuropsychiatric symptoms of dementia. *Journal of the American Medical Association, 293*, 596–608.

Stanley, M. A., Beck, J. G., & Glassco, J. D. (1996). Treatment of generalized anxiety in older adults: A preliminary comparison of cognitive-behavioral and supportive approaches. *Behavior Therapy, 27*(4), 565–581.

Steuer, J. L., Mintz, J., Hammen, C. L., Hill, M. A., Jarvik, L. F., McCarley, T., et al. (1984). Cognitive-behavioral and psychodynamic group psychotherapy in treatment of geriatric depression. *Journal of Consulting and Clinical Psychology, 52*(2), 180–189.

Stewart, R. B., & Caranasos, G. J. (1989). Medication compliance in the elderly. *The Medical Clinics of North America., 73*(6), 1551–1563.

Straub, R. O. (2012). *Health psychology*. New York: A Biopsychological Approach. Worth Publishers.

Sullivan, A. D., Hedberg, K., & Hopkins, D. (2001). Legalized physician-assisted suicide in Oregon, 1998–2000. *New England Journal of Medicine, 344*(8), 605–607.

Tannen, D. (2002). *I only say this because I love you: Talking to your parents, partner, sibs, and kids when you're all adults*. Random House LLC.

Taylor, J. E., Alpass, F., Stephens, C., & Towers, A. (2011). Driving anxiety and fear in young older adults in New Zealand. *Age and Ageing, 40*(1), 62–66.

Taylor, J., Deane, F., & Podd, J. (2002). Driving-related fear: A review. *Clinical psychology review, 22*(5), 631–645.

Teri, L., & Gallagher-Thompson, D. G. (1991). Cognitive-behavioral interventions for treatment of depression in Alzheimer's patients. *The Gerontologist, 31*, 413–416.

Teri, L., & Logsdon, R. G. (1991). Identifying pleasant activities for alzheimer's disease patients: The pleasant events schedule-AD. *The Gerontologist, 31*(1), 124–127.

Tsoh, J., Chiu, H. F., Duberstein, P. R., Chan, S. S., Chi, I., Yip, P. S., et al. (2005). Attempted suicide in elderly Chinese persons: A multi-group, controlled study. *The American Journal of Geriatric Psychiatry, 13*(7), 562–571.

Unützer, J., Katon, W., Callahan, C. M., Williams, J. W., Hunkeler, E., Harpole, L., et al. (2003). Depression treatment in a sample of 1,801 depressed older adults in primary care. *Journal of the American Geriatrics Society, 51*(4), 505–514.

Wei, W., Sambamoorthi, U., Olfson, M., Walkup, J. T., & Crystal, S. (2005). Use of psychotherapy for depression in older adults. *American Journal of Psychiatry, 162*(4), 711–717.

Weissman, M. M., Markowitz, J. C., & Klerman, G. L. (2000). *Comprehensive guide to interpersonal psychotherapy*. New York: Basic Books.

Wilson, K. G., Curran, D., & McPherson, C. J. (2005). A burden to others: A common source of distress for the terminally ill. *Cognitive behaviour therapy, 34*(2), 115–123.

Yohannes, A. M., Willgoss, T. G., Baldwin, R. C., & Connolly, M. J. (2010). Depression and anxiety in chronic heart failure and chronic obstructive pulmonary disease: Prevalence, relevance, clinical implications and management principles. *International Journal of Geriatric Psychiatry, 25*(12), 1209–1221.

Zivin, K., Pfeiffer, P. N., Szymanski, B. R., Valenstein, M., Post, E. P., Miller, E. M., et al. (2010). Initiation of primary care mental health integration programs in the VA health system: Association with psychiatric diagnoses in primary care. *Medical Care, 48*(9), 843–851.

7

Managing Safety and Mobility Needs of Older Drivers

Arne Stinchcombe[1], Germaine L. Odenheimer[2], and Michel Bédard[3]

[1]University of Ottawa, Ottawa, Ontario, Canada; [2]University of Oklahoma Health Sciences Center and Oklahoma City VA Medical Center, Oklahoma City, Oklahoma, USA; [3]Lakehead University, Thunder Bay, Ontario, Canada

INTRODUCTION

Driving a motor vehicle is frequently considered synonymous with mobility and independence and is associated with good health and quality of life (Dickerson et al., 2007; Kua, Korner-Bitensky, Desrosiers, Man-Son-Hing, & Marshall, 2007; Oxley, Langford, & Charlton, 2010). Driving is so vital in North America it has been viewed as an Instrumental Activity of Daily Living (IADL) (Ball, Ross, Eby, Molnar, & Meuser, 2013). It facilitates community engagement, access to services, opportunities for social participation, and many employment opportunities. It is also a highly complex behavior. Safe navigation of a motor vehicle simultaneously requires effective functioning of cognitive, motor, sensory, and physical systems (Anstey, Wood, Lord, & Walker, 2005). When any of these is impaired, driving can also lead to costly motor-vehicle collisions and injury.

National collision data show that while older drivers are involved in fewer collisions in comparison to other age groups, they are one of the highest risk groups for collisions resulting in serious injury or death after controlling for distance travelled (Bédard, Guyatt, Stones, & Hirdes, 2002; McGwin, Owsley, & Ball, 1998). Examination of collision statistics by age typically reveals a U-shaped curve, with younger and older drivers at greatest risk (Evans, 2000). The increased risk for serious injury and death among older adults is partly due to collision type (i.e., left-hand turns) and the physical frailty that often accompanies the aging process.

B. Bensadon (Ed): Psychology and Geriatrics.
DOI: http://dx.doi.org/10.1016/B978-0-12-420123-1.00007-1

Several authors report that not all older drivers account for this increased risk, especially those who drive infrequently. In fact, Langford, Methorst, and Hakamies-Blomqvist (2006) reported that after controlling for annual distance driven, most older drivers were safer than all other groups but older drivers traveling less than 3000 km (i.e., 1864 miles) per year were at an elevated risk of collision. This distinction in risk based on annual distance traveled is known as the *low-mileage bias*, and the effect has been reproduced using a number of separate data sets (Fontaine, 2003; Hakamies-Blomqvist, Raitanen, & O'Neill, 2002). Researchers attribute this effect in part to driving location, since low mileage drivers tend to drive in high-density urban environments where complex traffic situations may occur. Moreover, it may be that low mileage drivers reduce their driving in response to changes in their ability to drive safely. Some evidence also suggests that cohort differences account for the variance in older drivers' increased risk and that future generations of older drivers will exhibit lower risk (Evans, 1993; Mullen, Dubois, & Bédard, 2013).

While evidence-based interventions to promote safety and mobility among older drivers are available (e.g., Bédard et al., 2008a; Cassavaugh & Kramer, 2009; Husband, 2010), some older adults may need to cease driving due to aging-associated changes in cognitive, sensory, and physical functions or as a result of medical conditions and medications (Kowalski et al., 2012; Marshall & Man-Son-Hing, 2011). Given the psychological meaning attributed to driving and the independence it affords throughout adulthood, many older adults do not want to modify their driving even when objectively they should. The transition to nondriving status among older adults has been associated with a number of deleterious health outcomes, including rapid declines in overall physical health (Edwards, Lunsman, Perkins, Rebok, & Roth, 2009a), isolation, depression, increased risk of long-term care placement (Freeman, Gange, Munoz, & West, 2006), and even increased mortality (Edwards, Perkins, Ross, & Reynolds, 2009b; Windsor, Anstey, Butterworth, Luszcz, & Andrews, 2007).

To further understand this relationship between driving cessation and increased mortality, O'Connor and colleagues (2013) collected driving status, health, and mortality data from a cohort of community dwelling older adults over a 5-year period. Their results showed that while mortality risk was 1.68 times higher for nondrivers in comparison to drivers, this relationship was mediated by physical performance and health variables. The authors concluded that nondriving status may be indicative of declining health, although the cause and effect have not been fully determined. Clearly, the impact of driving cessation is far reaching, posing significant human and health care costs, not just to retired drivers but also to their caregivers (Taylor & Tripodes, 2001).

As these data illustrate, for many older adults, driving is a critical component of mobility and quality of life, especially when other means of transportation are unavailable (Oxley & Whelan, 2008) as is often the case in rural areas. Public health experts, insurers, advocacy groups, and service delivery professions all have different, at times conflicting, perspectives about older driver safety. Psychologists and physicians who are focused on senior driving strive to support safety, accurately assess driving capacity, and facilitate maintenance of mobility through a smooth transition to nondriving status when an older driver is no longer safe on the road (Dickerson et al., 2007; Eby & Molnar, 2009). Importantly, health care practice and policy aiming to reduce related injury must consider the mobility needs of seniors and how to keep them mobile long after driving ceases (Noland, 2013; Staplin & Freund, 2013).

Psychology and geriatrics play an important role in understanding the challenges facing older drivers in order to help them maintain mobility, positive mental health, and quality of life with or without a driver's license. This chapter describes a number of challenges faced by older drivers, their families, and health care providers, and recommends an integrated approach to optimally address them.

IDENTIFICATION OF UNSAFE OLDER DRIVERS

Neuropsychological Testing

The responsibility for assessing older drivers' fitness to safely operate a motor vehicle depends largely on the jurisdiction in which the driver is licensed and is often held by the licensing authority (i.e., Department of Motor Vehicles), the medical community (e.g., family physicians, neurologists), the private sector, or a combination of these entities. In Canada and the United States (U.S.) provincial jurisdictions or individual states are responsible for granting driver's licenses, and the specific requirements through which older adults are licensed varies significantly between each province/state (Kelly, Nielson, & Snoddon, 2014). But in contrast to the U.S., physicians in most Canadian provinces have a statutory duty to report to licensing authorities any patient they believe to be unfit to operate a motor vehicle (Canadian Medical Association, 2012). In the U.S. all states have policies for the identification of unfit drivers but only six have mandatory reporting laws through which physicians are obliged to report drivers with medical conditions compromising their driving fitness (Berger, Rosner, Kark, & Bennett, 2000). Evidence shows physicians are often uncomfortable assessing driving safety because they lack the appropriate tools and guidelines to do so confidently (Herrmann et al., 2006; Jang et al., 2007; Marshall, 2008; Wernham et al., 2014). To inform medical decisions about fitness to drive, physicians may consult relevant specialists such as occupational therapists who are trained to assess function and neuropsychologists who can assess cognition. After comprehensive evaluation, neuropsychologists provide a formal recommendation to physicians regarding patients' cognitive function related to driving.

Specifically, attention, processing speed, memory and executive function, visuo-spatial processing, and global cognitive functioning have each been associated with driving outcomes among the aged (Anstey et al., 2005; Mathias & Lucas, 2009). Attention is often cited as one of the most critical cognitive determinants of safe driving, especially among older adults. A seminal study by Summala and Mikkola (1994) investigated the primary cause of serious collisions in which one or more vehicle occupants died. The authors found that the proportion of collisions attributed to inattention increased with older age. Attentional deficits among older drivers have been widely researched and there is consensus that attention plays an important role in predicting driving outcomes among older adults (see Trick, Enns, Mills, & Vavrik, 2004) and their younger counterparts, especially given the hazards of texting while driving (e.g., McKnight & McKnight, 2003).

Broadly, the attention process can be described as selective concentration on salient environmental features while ignoring other aspects. According to psychologists Posner and Petersen's (1990) Attentional Network Theory, attention may be subdivided into three attentional systems, each of which is associated with separate neural systems: alerting, orienting, and executive attention. Attention can be measured in a variety of ways, such as pencil and paper tests, computerized and simulator assessments, or through real-time driving tasks.

A growing body of literature has shown strong links between computerized measures of attention and driving outcomes. Among the more well-studied examples used to assess attention among older drivers is the Useful Field of View (UFOV) (Ball & Owsley, 1993), a brief screening tool that can be administered in approximately 15 minutes. The tool consists of three subtests of increasing complexity – processing speed, divided attention, and selective attention. An alternative computerized test based on Posner and Petersen's (1990) theory is the Attentional Network Test, comparable to the UFOV in predicting driving performance in a driving simulator (Weaver, Bédard, McAuliffe, & Parkkari, 2009). The test is available for download without charge and takes approximately 20 minutes to complete.

There are numerous clinically relevant neuropsychological tests to evaluate older adult driving performance. Mathias and Lucas (2009) identified over 30 cognitive tasks found in the literature associated with one or more components of safe driving among healthy older adults. Among them, the authors cite the UFOV, Trail Making Tests, Clock Drawing, Complex Reaction Time, and the Mini-Mental State Exam (MMSE) as promising predictors of driving outcomes. Tests used to assess older drivers usually depend on contextual factors such as computer availability.

Though each measure may be useful, it is advisable not to rely on any single test to determine driving fitness. An analysis of three separate data sets revealed that despite statistically significant associations between commonly used cognitive tests (notably the MMSE, UFOV, and Trails A) and driving performance, prediction of individuals who would have poor driving performance was inconclusive (Bédard, Weaver, Darzins, & Porter, 2008b). This difficulty in accurately identifying poor drivers may be due to the fact that driving is a highly complex task drawing upon a myriad of cognitive, perceptual and physical processes that are difficult to assess with a single test or by examining a single functional domain in isolation. For example, Bédard and colleagues (2008b) describe an at-risk driver with strong cognitive skills but lower extremity dysfunction. Cognitive tests will not adequately capture this person's inability to safely operate the pedals of the vehicle. This logic led an expert panel to formally affirm that a decision about driving "should never be made on the results of one tool in isolation, as there is not enough evidence provided by any one tool to make a decision" (Bédard & Dickerson, 2014). Similar challenges arise in drivers whose health conditions involve symptoms that fluctuate (e.g., multiple sclerosis) or are intermittent (e.g., seizures).

Research has shown that cognitive function is a key determinant of safe driving and that normal cognitive changes associated with aging can lead to decrements in attention, memory and executive functions that threaten driving safety among older adults. However, it is crucial for clinicians to differentiate between changes due to normal cognitive aging and those that indicate pathology, including the effects of medication. As noted elsewhere in this publication, this has historically been a difficult, albeit imperative, distinction.

Neurodegenerative processes, including Alzheimer's disease and related disorders (ADRD), can alter cognitive function, personality, and inevitably result in severe disability and death. The number one known risk factor for ADRD is advancing age (Blennow, de Leon, & Zetterberg, 2006). Some research suggests that healthy older people and those in the early stages of dementia are at comparable risk, especially in the year following a dementia diagnosis. Other findings suggest that individuals with dementia are at a two-fold increase in risk of collisions (Carr & Ott, 2010). Risk increases as the disease progresses (Drachman & Swearer, 1993). Individuals with dementia may lack insight into their decline and inability to safely operate a vehicle, often continuing to drive until they are implicated in one or more collisions (Adler, Rottunda, & Dysken, 2005; Kasziak, Keyl, & Albert, 1991; Meng, Siren, & Teasdale, 2013). Guidelines from both the American Medical Association (AMA) and the Canadian Medical Association (CMA) suggest that while dementia diagnosis is not sufficient to remove a patient's driver's license, in situations where fitness to drive is uncertain, a road test is recommended (American Medical Association, 2003; Canadian Medical Association, 2012).

In their practice guidelines, the American Academy of Neurology (AAN) advises using the Clinical Dementia Rating scale (CDR) to determine driving risk among individuals with dementia. The CDR encompasses determination of cognitive functions as well as basic activities of daily living (ADL) and more complex IADL mentioned earlier. Based on this information the stage of dementia ranges from 0 to 3, where 0 indicates no dementia and 3 indicates severe or late stage dementia (Iverson et al., 2010). Evidence suggests that a CDR score of 1 (mild or early stage dementia) or greater significantly increases the risk of unsafe driving. Unfortunately though, this recommendation is not clinically practical since the CDR has largely been used in clinical research and is not widely used or familiar to general practitioners. Both AMA & CMA guidelines, however, indicate that no test has high enough sensitivity and specificity to be relied upon as a determinant of driving ability. Instead, abnormalities on the MMSE, clock drawing, and Trail Making Test (B) should lead to more in-depth assessment of driving ability (American Medical Association, 2003; Canadian Medical Association, 2012).

Clinically, while a dementia diagnosis alone may not immediately necessitate driving cessation, it does alert the practitioner that the patient will likely progress and eventually have to stop driving. Thus, if a driver's license is retained after dementia is diagnosed, it is imperative that the clinician closely monitor the cognitive and functional status of the patient for decline that may increase crash risk, notably inattention, visuo-spatial skills, and executive function. The CMA recommends the patient with mild dementia who retains a driver's license be reevaluated every 6 to 12 months (Canadian Medical Association, 2012).

Cognitive Interventions to Support Safe Driving

Assessment of at-risk drivers addresses larger public safety concerns but often fails to consider the continued mobility needs of the older adults themselves. Research has shown that driver retraining for older drivers without dementia can improve driver and public safety. These interventions typically include a combination of education, on-road feedback, physical training, and cognitive training methods (Korner-Bitensky, Kua, von Zweck, & Van Benthem, 2009).

Education-based driver retraining programs are often conducted in a classroom setting and focus on road rules and the impact of the aging process on driving. One example, the 55-Alive older driver refresher program, provides a curriculum designed to increase knowledge and awareness and ultimately reduce risk among older drivers (Joanisse, Stinchcombe, & Yamin, 2010). Though helpful in principle, evidence of benefit of classroom education alone is mixed (e.g., Janke, 1994). Bédard and colleagues (2008a) combined the 55-Alive refresher program with two 30- to 40-minute on-road training sessions with a certified instructor and found better performance on a standard road assessment among healthy older drivers who participated in the intervention compared to those who did not (Bédard et al., 2008a).

Cognitive training for older adults is a growing field and researchers have investigated whether computerized cognitive training can improve safety. Edwards, Delahunt, & Mahncke (2009c) found that healthy community dwellers randomly assigned to receive speed of processing training were less likely to cease driving in comparison to individuals assigned to a control condition. Moreover, research shows that in cognitively normal individuals such training using the UFOV may improve processing speed, reduce crash risk, and have a positive impact on health and functional well-being (Edwards et al., 2009c; Wood & Owsley, 2014). Though promising, the precise mechanisms responsible for positive driving outcomes as a result of such intervention remain unclear (Bédard & Weaver, 2011). A better understanding as well as replication of cognitive training studies are therefore necessary to determine their clinical relevance and potential impact on safety, especially among cognitively impaired drivers.

Some older drivers compensate for age-related changes by engaging in self-regulatory behaviors (Horswill, Anstey, Hatherly, Wood, & Pachana, 2011; Molnar et al., 2014). In an effort to increase safety, drivers who perceive themselves as "at risk" limit exposure by driving less and avoiding complex driving situations such as left-hand turns, peak traffic times or bad weather. Research generally shows an inverse relationship between drivers' confidence and self-regulation such that less confident drivers tend to avoid difficult driving situations and drive less frequently (Baldock, Mathias, McLean, & Berndt, 2006; Horswill, Sullivan, Lurie-Beck, & Smith, 2013; Ross, Dodson, Edwards, Ackerman, & Ball, 2012).

However, not all drivers have insight into their driving ability, and the majority of older drivers rate their skill level as better than average (Gosselin, Gagnon, Stinchcombe, & Joanisse, 2010; Horswill et al., 2013). Classroom-based interventions targeting older drivers may be a means to improve the accuracy of drivers' self-assessments and promote self-regulatory behaviors. For example, Owsley, McGwin, Phillips, McNeal, and Stalvey (2004) found that visually impaired older drivers who received a 3-hour education-based intervention on safe driving strategies were more likely to avoid challenging driving situations in comparison to controls.

PSYCHOLOGY OF DRIVING

While physicians in some jurisdictions/states have a responsibility to report medically unfit older drivers to the appropriate licensing authority, psychologists have a unique, complimentary role to play in identifying and counseling older drivers likely to be unsafe. Driving is a multifactorial behavior, and physicians often have access to multiple sources of information when determining fitness to drive. These include medical diagnoses, physical fitness (e.g., balance, dexterity), sensory function (e.g., vision), brain imaging results, neuropsychological test results, and the results of functional assessments. But access to information does not automatically translate into comfort. In fact, even with this clinical information at their disposal, physicians are still uncomfortable making a determination about fitness to drive and feel they lack the tools to adequately do so (Jang et al., 2007; Marshall, Demmings, Woolnough, Salim, & Man-Son-Hing, 2012). But why?

Multiple psychological factors affect physicians' comfort in assessing and determining driving fitness, including concern about damaging the patient-physician relationship, lack of familiarity with guidelines, and fear of personal or corporate liability (Moorhouse, Hamilton, Fisher, & Rockwood, 2011). Indeed, discussions with patients about driving cessation can be extremely delicate, anxiety provoking, and emotionally intense. Driving is often closely linked with patients' identity and may be synonymous with independence and freedom. Without psychological adjustment to the concept of driving retirement and awareness of available alternatives to support and maintain mobility, patients (and their physicians) may fearfully perceive these discussions as significant threats to their identity and lifestyle. By triangulating sources of information and by engaging in a dialogue with psychologists, family members, and patients, physicians' confidence in their ability to determine fitness to drive can be vastly improved. Collaboration would enable discussion to occur in a palatable fashion, drawing on the integration of evidence from multiple sources. Physicians and psychologists together represent a comprehensive, biopsychosocial approach to identifying and managing at-risk older drivers (Ball et al., 2006; Bédard et al., 2008a).

When physicians have trouble identifying the precise cause of an older adult's driving difficulty, the CMA's *Determining Medical Fitness to Drive: A Guide for Physicians* recommends using the CANDRIVE Fitness-to-Drive Assessment Mnemonic to focus inquiry. The mnemonic focuses on the domains of Cognition, Acute or fluctuating illness, Neuromusculoskeletal disease or neurological effects, Drugs, (driving) Record, In-car Experiences, Vision, and Ethanol use.

Once the evidence points to driving difficulties, physicians may choose to engage in a dialogue with their patients about driving safety and potential cessation. Such discussion can be emotionally stressful for all involved – clinician, patient, and family (Persson, 1993; Ralston et al., 2001). This likely explains why generally, physicians are late in initiating discussions about driving safety. When initiated, these conversations may be suboptimal due, in part, to time constraints (Betz, Jones, Petroff, & Schwartz, 2013).

Advance Driving Directives (ADD), which enable the driver to identify a professional, family member, or trusted friend who can help make a decision about driving cessation (Oxley & Whelan, 2008), can facilitate conversations between drivers and health professionals and aid in planning for driving cessation (Betz et al., 2013; Betz, Schwartz, Valley, & Lowenstein, 2012). Other tools, such as the Assessment of Readiness for Mobility Transition (ARMT) developed by psychologist Tom Meuser, can be used to assess emotional and attitudinal precursors to adaptive coping in response to a significant mobility change, such as driving cessation (Meuser, Berg-Weger, Chibnall, Harmon, & Stowe, 2013).

Patients' reactions to driving fitness-related feedback vary and can be influenced by the cohort to which they belong, their gender, and who is actually providing it. Some older drivers, for example, report that the decision to stop driving is theirs alone to make, while others indicate that they would expect feedback from their physician and family members. In a qualitative study by Rudman, Friedland, Chipman, and Sciortino (2006), pre-seniors (aged 55–64) reported they would accept feedback from their spouses while seniors reported a role for children in providing feedback related to driving safety. These discussions can have profound impacts on family dynamics, as evidenced by the following comment: "Some family members have had such difficulty taking Dad's car keys away. ... It's just created such heartbreak in the whole family situation." (Rudman et al., 2006). While older drivers report a preference for physicians to monitor driving safety, they also believe that physicians may avoid these conversations and allow older drivers to continue driving even in cases where it is no longer safe for them to do so (Persson, 1993; Rudman et al., 2006).

As discussed, in current practice, official determination of medical fitness to drive is typically a physician's responsibility. However, managing the concomitant psychological distress and threats to identity are better addressed by clinical geropsychologists. Brief, targeted family psychotherapy can focus on challenges such as overcoming perceived loss, related mood disturbance (e.g., anxiety and depression), lifestyle adjustment, and promoting behavior change. Ideally, supportive behavioral interventions can help mitigate the negative impact of driving cessation and alleviate tensions between physicians and patients that arise from these highly sensitive conversations. Psychologists must support and empower both patients and physician colleagues during this process. This could enhance patients' ability to recognize potential personal safety risks and facilitate insight into what driving reduction or cessation signifies for them and how their lives might change after driving cessation. Additionally, it might enable physicians to modulate their own guilt and associated discomfort with being the one responsible for terminating a patient's driving privilege.

Remedial programs or policies in place might facilitate healthy transitions to nondriving status, such as restricted licensing or financial supports for alternative transportation. However, physicians cannot be expected to maintain expertise on policies, programs and services that support mobility as they are often jurisdiction-specific and can change regularly. The emergence of family health teams within clinical care settings could ensure that seniors and families are informed of available programs.

TRANSITIONING TO NONDRIVING STATUS

Negative Health Effects

Driving is the primary means of transportation in many parts of the world and research shows that older adults use personal vehicles for almost 90% of their daily travel, serving as the driver approximately 75% of the time (Collia, Sharp, & Giesbrecht, 2003). Not surprisingly, research has documented several negative psychological and physical outcomes following the decision to retire from driving. Older adults describe a void in their lives after driving retirement. This void has been associated with loss of freedom, independence, role, and occupation (Ralston et al., 2001). Several longitudinal studies have found that driving cessation is associated with an increase in depressive symptoms, even after adjusting for variables such as sociodemographics, cognition, and physical health (Marottoli et al., 1997; Ragland, Satariano, & MacLeod, 2005; Windsor et al., 2007).

In a series of studies, Johnson (1995, 1998, 1999) found that former drivers often reported isolation as a consequence of driving cessation, which subsequently led to feelings of severe loneliness in both urban and rural settings. Indeed, evidence points to a reduction in the range of out-of-home activities, frequency of travel, and distance travelled following driving cessation (Bonnel, 1999; Corn & Rosenblum, 2002; Marottoli et al., 2000; Taylor & Tripodes, 2001). Older adults who no longer drive rely heavily on family and friends for their transportation needs (Rosenblum and Corn, 2002). Some suggest, due to gender norms, it is more acceptable for women than men to rely on informal networks for mobility (e.g., Adler & Rottunda, 2006). Family members who are responsible for providing this transportation often report a sense of obligation, burden, and added responsibility (Ralston et al., 2001). Depression, perceptions of burden, and loss are also experienced by both those who no longer drive and those who relied on the older driver when he or she did drive (Bonnel, 1999; Peel, Westmoreland, & Steinberg, 2002).

Individual responses to driving cessation can be moderated by demographic and personality variables, the degree to which the decision was voluntary or involuntary, and whether the process was gradual or abrupt (Bauer, Rottunda, & Adler, 2003; Corn & Rosenblum, 2002; Davey, 2007; Windsor et al., 2007). By engaging earlier in a dialogue with physicians about possible driving cessation and by planning appropriately, driving cessation can be a voluntary decision that takes place gradually, leading to more successful outcomes (Bauer et al., 2003). Conversely, involuntary license removal is a deeply traumatic experience characterized by loss of independence and identity (Whitehead, Howie, & Lovell, 2006).

Evidence-based interventions to support a healthy transition to nondriving show promise (Windsor & Anstey, 2006). In particular, the UQDRIVE program aims to promote community engagement and mobility and prevent depression and isolation for older adults facing driving cessation (Liddle, McKenna, & Bartlett, 2007). The program is facilitated by a former driver who successfully transitioned and takes place over six separate sessions, each lasting between 3 and 4 hours. Intervention activities include information sharing, group discussion, speakers, practical exercises, and outings. Results demonstrated that older drivers without dementia who received the UQDRIVE used public transportation and walked more frequently, had greater self-efficacy related to community mobility, and higher satisfaction with transportation in comparison to individuals who did not receive the intervention (Liddle et al., 2014).

There is clear evidence that driving cessation is often accompanied by poor mental and physical health among older adults, whether it is a cause, effect, or a combination of both. In cases where an older adult can no longer drive safely and driving cessation is required, it is essential that physicians and psychologists work together to support a healthy and humane transition to nondriver status. Through psychotherapeutic approaches, psychologists can facilitate patients' insight into the need to modify their driving behavior, and help them develop coping strategies for subsequent mobility changes (for a case study, see Bahro, Silber, Box, & Sunderland, 1995). Similarly, psychologists may support the former driver in regaining a sense of control that may have been lost along with driving privileges, and help maintain social networks in the absence of a driver's license. If former drivers experience feelings of worthlessness that stem from a loss of identity associated with driving cessation, psychologists can help them redefine themselves and shift focus to other meaningful areas of their lives, including their social networks, family, employment, and volunteerism.

Retained Mobility after Driving

Of course, driving is not the only means through which satisfactory community mobility can be achieved. In some urban areas, a range of transportation options are available, such as public and paratransit services, specialized transit services, and senior transport services (Dickerson et al., 2007). Evidence suggests, however, that former drivers prefer depending on their family and friends for meeting their transportation needs (Azad, Byszewski, Molnar, & Amos, 2003; Davey, 2007; DeCarlo, Scilley, Wells, & Owsley, 2003; Rosenbloom, 2001). This is understandable, given that family and friends are more flexible than public transportation schedules and more easily trusted (Bonnel, 1999).

Maintaining mobility after driving cessation may require a multipronged approach that involves: a) residing in an accessible neighborhood within walking distance to critical services, b) use of public or private forms of transportation for regularly scheduled appointments or events, and c) reliance on informal transportation from friends and family to reach destinations that are difficult to access through other means. Relocation to a residence within close proximity to essential services may seem like a practical approach to countering mobility losses associated with driving cessation. In practice, however, older adults are reluctant to relocate and prefer to stay in their family homes despite evidence to support making a move.

Initiatives that seek to improve alternative transportation options could be an enormous benefit to nondriving seniors. The Independent Transportation Network America (ITNAmerica) is a prime example. ITNAmerica is a national nonprofit transportation system with the goal of supporting sustainable, community-based transportation services for older adults. Through annual memberships, ITNAmerica matches seniors with drivers at a rate that costs less than a taxi. A different approach is the World Health Organization's Age Friendly Cities (AFC) concept where the physical and social environments within a community are tailored to older adults' needs. Menec and Nowicki (2014) measured the age friendliness of 29 communities located in the province of Manitoba (Canada) and collected data from 593 younger and older residents. They found that age friendliness, including transportation options, was significantly associated with life satisfaction among older adults. It follows that features of an older adult's community can moderate seniors' success in transitioning to nondriver status.

Though driving cessation research is generally skewed toward negative health-related impact, it is reasonable to speculate that as long as mobility is maintained, driving cessation may also have positive impacts on the older individual's health and well-being. Driving a motor vehicle without recent practice or while managing cognitive decline can be a highly stressful experience (Hakamies-Blomqvist & Wahlstrom, 1998). Driving cessation may represent gains in the form of financial benefits (i.e., lack of vehicle maintenance or insurance costs), improved physical activity through walking, and social contact associated with being a passenger in a vehicle. King and colleagues (2011) found that older adults who lived in more walkable neighborhoods vs. those living in less walkable neighborhoods had greater "transport activity" (self-reported walking or bicycling for errands) and greater moderate-to-vigorous physical activity as well as lower body mass. While the successful transition to nondriving for older adults may result in unintended positive benefits, research has generally not studied this possibility of successful transitions.

INTERPROFESSIONAL APPROACHES

At its core, driving is an emotionally laden human *behavior* (i.e., psychological in nature) embedded within community safety, health service delivery, and public policy contexts. It impacts families, communities, and the health and well-being of older adults themselves. This chapter has outlined a number of research findings related to older drivers, and has identified opportunities for geriatrics and psychology professionals to support them by facilitating smooth transitions and coping strategies for improved safety and continued mobility. Clinicians should collaboratively leverage their respective skills and expertise.

Psychologists are trained to function in a number of health care environments, be they community-based, private practice, or hospitals. Too often though, psychologists and physicians practice in separate clinical settings. Psychologists spend longer periods of time with patients and discuss their complex emotional experiences and behavioral patterns in greater depth. Thus, while physicians are often required to make a formal determination regarding medical fitness to drive, informing this decision should be insights gleaned by clinical geropsychologists about patients' and families' respective goals, concerns, and fears related to driving. Similarly, consultation with neuropsychologists can help in determining recommendations for older drivers' cognitive capacity to safely and independently operate a motor vehicle. Physicians may refer older adults to psychologists to help plan for driving retirement and develop an ADD. Psychologists can facilitate support groups aimed at easing the transition to nondriving status, engaging families and friends of older drivers, and developing educational resources about alternative transportation options. They can also guide older adults through the emotional discomfort inherent in identity changes and related anxiety, depression, and grief that can accompany the driving cessation process. Moreover, psychologists can support caregivers who must adjust to new roles and manage perceptions of related burden.

While physicians are well-positioned to treat medical conditions affecting mobility, psychologists can target the emotional impact of such changes as well as motivation to engage in health maintenance and mobility-preserving behaviors that may serve as a lifeline in the absence of driving privileges. Patients stand to benefit from having a biopsychosocial approach to the myriad factors associated with aging, driving, and related decision-making. Physicians, themselves, may benefit from support in managing their own concerns or feelings of guilt that may contribute to their reluctance to ask related questions, let alone suggest that their patients stop driving. When physicians do make this recommendation, and patients do lose their driving privileges, the emotional impact on both can be even more intense.

Traditionally, in the absence of psychology-geriatrics integration, psychologists have not been called upon by the medical community to assist in the management of impaired older drivers. Given the major psychological relevance and symbolism of driving, age-associated challenges to mobility, and life-altering impact of driving cessation, it is apparent that psychologists are significantly underutilized in the area of clinical medicine where they can greatly facilitate positive outcomes.

References

Adler, G., & Rottunda, S. (2006). Older adults' perspectives on driving cessation. *Journal of Aging Studies, 20*(3), 227–235.

Adler, G., Rottunda, S., & Dysken, M. (2005). The older driver with dementia: An updated literature review. *Journal of Safety Research, 36*(4), 399–407.

American Medical Association (2003). *Physician's guide to assessing and counseling older drivers.* Chicago, IL: American Medical Association.

Anstey, K. J., Wood, J., Lord, S., & Walker, J. G. (2005). Cognitive, sensory and physical factors enabling driving safety in older adults. *Clinical Psychology Review, 25*(1), 45–65.

Azad, N., Byszewski, A., Molnar, F. J., & Amos, S. (2003). A survey of the impact of driving cessation on older drivers. *Geriatrics Today, 5*(4), 170–174.

Bahro, M., Silber, E., Box, P., & Sunderland, T. (1995). Giving up driving in Alzheimer's disease – An integrative therapeutic approach. *International Journal of Geriatric Psychiatry, 10*(10), 871–874.

Baldock, M. R., Mathias, J. L., McLean, A. J., & Berndt, A. (2006). Self-regulation of driving and its relationship to driving ability among older adults. *Accident Analysis and Prevention, 38*(5), 1038–1045.

Ball, K., & Owsley, C. (1993). The useful field of view test: A new technique for evaluating age-related declines in visual function. *American Optometric Association Journal, 64*(1), 71–79.

Ball, K., Ross, L. A., Eby, D. W., Molnar, L. J., & Meuser, T. M. (2013). Emerging issues in safe and sustainable mobility for older persons. *Accident Analysis and Prevention, 61*, 138–140.

Ball, K. K., Roenker, D. L., Wadley, V. G., Edwards, J. D., Roth, D. L., McGwin, G., Jr., et al. (2006). Can high-risk older drivers be identified through performance-based measures in a department of motor vehicles setting? *Journal of the American Geriatrics Society, 54*(1), 77–84.

Bauer, M. J., Rottunda, S., & Adler, G. (2003). Older women and driving cessation. *Qualitative Social Work, 2*(3), 309–325.

Bédard, M., & Dickerson, A. E. (2014). Consensus statements for screening and assessment tools. *Occupational Therapy in Health Care, 28*(2), 127–131.

Bédard, M., Guyatt, G. H., Stones, M. J., & Hirdes, J. P. (2002). The independent contribution of driver, crash, and vehicle characteristics to driver fatalities. *Accident Analysis and Prevention, 34*, 717–727.

Bédard, M., Porter, M. M., Marshall, S., Isherwood, I., Riendeau, J., Weaver, B., et al. (2008a). The combination of two training approaches to improve older adults' driving safety. *Traffic Injury Prevention, 9*(1), 70–76.

Bédard, M., & Weaver, B. (2011). Commentary on: Cognitive training for older drivers can reduce the frequency of involvement in motor vehicle collisions. *Evidence-Based Mental Health, 14*(2), 52.

Bédard, M., Weaver, B., Darzins, P., & Porter, M. (2008b). Predicting driver performance in older adults: We are not there yet! *Annual Conference of the Association for the Advancement of Automotive Medicine.* San Diego, CA.

Berger, J. T., Rosner, F., Kark, P., & Bennett, A. J. (2000). Reporting by physicians of impaired drivers and potentially impaired drivers. The committee on bioethical issues of the medical society of the State of New York. *Journal of General Internal Medicine, 15*(9), 667–672.

Betz, M. E., Jones, J., Petroff, E., & Schwartz, R. (2013). "I wish we could normalize driving health": A qualitative study of clinician discussions with older drivers. *Journal of General Internal Medicine, 28*(12), 1573–1580.

Betz, M. E., Schwartz, R., Valley, M., & Lowenstein, S. R. (2012). Older adult opinions about driving cessation: A role for advanced driving directives. *Journal of Primary Care & Community Health, 3*(3), 150–154.

Blennow, K., de Leon, M. J., & Zetterberg, H. (2006). Alzheimer's disease. *Lancet, 368*(9533), 387–403.

Bonnel, W. B. (1999). Giving up the car: Older women's losses and experiences. *Journal of Psychosocial Nursing and Mental Health Service, 37*(5), 10–15.

Canadian Medical Association, (2012). *CMA driver's guide: Determining medical fitness to operate motor vehicles* (8th ed.). Ottawa, ON: Canadian Medical Association.

Carr, D. B., & Ott, B. R. (2010). The older adult driver with cognitive impairment: "It's a very frustrating life". *JAMA, 303*(16), 1632–1641.

Cassavaugh, N. D., & Kramer, A. F. (2009). Transfer of computer-based training to simulated driving in older adults. *Applied Ergonomics, 40*(5), 943–952.

Collia, D. V., Sharp, J., & Giesbrecht, L. (2003). The 2001 national household travel survey: A look into the travel patterns of older Americans. *Journal of Safety Research, 34*(4), 461–470.

Corn, A. L., & Rosenblum, L. P. (2002). Experiences of older adults who stopped driving because of their visual impairments: Part 2. *Journal of Visual Impairment and Blindness, 96*, 485–500.

Davey, J. A. (2007). Older people and transport: Coping without a car. *Ageing & Society, 27*(1), 49–66.

DeCarlo, D. K., Scilley, K., Wells, J., & Owsley, C. (2003). Driving habits and health-related quality of life in patients with age-related maculopathy. *Optometry & Vision Science, 80*(3), 207–213.

Dickerson, A. E., Molnar, L. J., Eby, D. W., Adler, G., Bédard, M., Berg-Weger, M., et al. (2007). Transportation and aging: A research agenda for advancing safe mobility. *The Gerontologist, 47*(5), 578–590. (0016–9013).

Drachman, D., & Swearer, J. M. (1993). Driving and Alzheimer's disease: The risk of crashes. *Neurology, 43*, 2448–2456.

Eby, D. W., & Molnar, L. J. (2009). Older adult safety and mobility: Issues and research needs. *Public Works Management & Policy, 13*(4), 288–300.

Edwards, J. D., Delahunt, P. B., & Mahncke, H. W. (2009c). Cognitive speed of processing training delays driving cessation. *The Journals of Gerontology. Series A, Biological Sciences and Medical Sciences, 64*(12), 1262–1267.

Edwards, J. D., Lunsman, M., Perkins, M., Rebok, G. W., & Roth, D. L. (2009a). Driving cessation and health trajectories in older adults. *The Journals of Gerontology. Series A, Biological Sciences and Medical Sciences, 64*(12), 1290–1295.

Edwards, J. D., Perkins, M., Ross, L. A., & Reynolds, S. L. (2009b). Driving status and three-year mortality among community-dwelling older adults. *The Journals of Gerontology. Series A, Biological Sciences and Medical Sciences, 64*(2), 300–305.

Evans, L. (1993). How safe were today's older drivers when they were younger? *American Journal of Epidemiology, 137*, 769–775.

Evans, L. (2000). Risks older drivers face themselves and threats they pose to other road users. *International Journal of Epidemiology, 29*(2), 315–322. (0300-5771).

Fontaine, H. (2003). Âge des conducteurs de voiture et accidents de la route: Quel risque pour les seniors? *Recherche – Transports – Sécurité, 79–80*(0), 107–120.

Freeman, E. E., Gange, S. J., Munoz, B., & West, S. K. (2006). Driving status and risk of entry into long-term care in older adults. *American Journal of Public Health, 96*(7), 1254–1259.

Gosselin, D., Gagnon, S., Stinchcombe, A., & Joanisse, M. (2010). Comparative optimism among drivers: An intergenerational portrait. *Accident Analysis and Prevention, 42*(2), 734–740.

Hakamies-Blomqvist, L., Raitanen, T., & O'Neill, D. (2002). Driver ageing does not cause higher accident rates per km. *Transportation Research Part F: Traffic Psychology and Behaviour, 5*(4), 271–274.

Hakamies-Blomqvist, L., & Wahlstrom, B. (1998). Why do older drivers give up driving? *Accident Analysis and Prevention, 30*(3), 305–312.

Herrmann, N., Rapoport, M. J., Sambrook, R., Hébert, R., McCracken, P., & Robillard, A. (2006). Predictors of driving cessation in mild-to-moderate dementia. *Canadian Medical Association Journal, 175*(6), 591–595.

Horswill, M. S., Anstey, K. J., Hatherly, C., Wood, J. M., & Pachana, N. A. (2011). Older drivers' insight into their hazard perception ability. *Accident Analysis and Prevention, 43*(6), 2121–2127.

Horswill, M. S., Sullivan, K., Lurie-Beck, J. K., & Smith, S. (2013). How realistic are older drivers' ratings of their driving ability? *Accident Analysis and Prevention, 50*, 130–137.

Husband, P. (2010). A literature review of older driver training interventions: Implications for the delivery programmes by Devon County Council and Devon Road Casualty Reduction Partnership. Retrieved from: <www.devon.gov.uk/fullreport.pdf>.

Iverson, D. J., Gronseth, G. S., Reger, M. A., Classen, S., Dubinsky, R. M., & Rizzo, M. (2010). Practice parameter update: Evaluation and management of driving risk in dementia. Report of the quality standards subcommittee of the American Academy of Neurology. *Neurology, 74*(16), 1316–1324.

Jang, R. W., Man-Son-Hing, M., Molnar, F. J., Hogan, D. B., Marshall, S. C., Auger, J., et al. (2007). Family physicians' attitudes and practices regarding assessments of medical fitness to drive in older persons. *Journal of General Internal Medicine, 22*(4), 531–543.

Janke, M. K. (1994). Mature driver improvement program in California. *Transportation Research Record, 1438*, 77–83.

Joanisse, M., Stinchcombe, A., & Yamin, S. (2010). Evaluability assessment of a national driver retraining program: Are we evaluating in the right lane? *Canadian Journal of Program Evaluation, 1*, 27–50.

Johnson, J. E. (1995). Rural elders and the decision to stop driving. *Journal of Community Health Nursing, 12*(3), 131–138.

Johnson, J. E. (1998). Older rural adults and the decision to stop driving: The influence of family and friends. *Journal of Community Health Nursing, 15*(4), 205–216.

Johnson, J. E. (1999). Urban older adults and the forfeiture of a driver's license. *Journal of Gerontological Nursing, 25*(12), 12–18.

Kasziak, A. W., Keyl, P. M., & Albert, M. S. (1991). Dementia and the older driver. *Human Factors, 33*, 527–537.

Kelly, M., Nielson, N., & Snoddon, T. (2014). Aging population and driver licensing: A policy perspective. *Canadian Public Policy, 40*(1), 31–44.

King, A. C., Sallis, J. F., Frank, L. D., Saelens, B. E., Cain, K., Conway, T. L., et al. (2011). Aging in neighborhoods differing in walkability and income: Associations with physical activity and obesity in older adults. *Social Science & Medicine, 73*(10), 1525–1533. (1982).

Korner-Bitensky, N., Kua, A., von Zweck, C., & Van Benthem, K. (2009). Older driver retraining: An updated systematic review of evidence of effectiveness. *Journal of Safety Research, 40*(2), 105–111.

Kowalski, K., Love, J., Tuokko, H., MacDonald, S., Hultsch, D., & Strauss, E. (2012). The influence of cognitive impairment with no dementia on driving restriction and cessation in older adults. *Accident Analysis and Prevention, 49*(0), 308–315.

Kua, A., Korner-Bitensky, N., Desrosiers, J., Man-Son-Hing, M., & Marshall, S. (2007). Older driver retraining: A systematic review of evidence of effectiveness. *Journal of Safety Research, 38*(1), 81–90.

Langford, J., Methorst, R., & Hakamies-Blomqvist, L. (2006). Older drivers do not have a high crash risk – A replication of low mileage bias. *Accident Analysis and Prevention, 38*(3), 574–578.

Liddle, J., Haynes, M., Pachana, N. A., Mitchell, G., McKenna, K., & Gustafsson, L. (2014). Effect of a group intervention to promote older adults' adjustment to driving cessation on community mobility: A randomized controlled trial. *The Gerontologist, 54*(3), 409–422.

Liddle, J., McKenna, K., & Bartlett, H. (2007). Improving outcomes for older retired drivers: The QUDrive program. *Australian Occupational Therapy Journal, 54*, 303–306.

Marottoli, R. A., Mendes de Leon, C. F., Glass, T. A., Williams, C. S., Cooney, L. M. J., Berkman, L. F., et al. (1997). Driving cessation and increased depressive symptoms: Prospective evidence from the New Haven EPESE. *Journal of the American Geriatrics Society, 45*, 202–206.

Marottoli, R. A., Mendes de Leon, C. F., Glass, T. A., Williams, C. S., Cooney, L. M. J., & Berkman, L. F. (2000). Consequences of driving cessation: Decreased out-of-home activity levels. *Journal of Gerontology: Social Sciences, 55B*(6), S334–S340.

Marshall, S., Demmings, E. M., Woolnough, A., Salim, D., & Man-Son-Hing, M. (2012). Determining fitness to drive in older persons: A survey of medical and surgical specialists. *Canadian Geriatrics Journal, 15*(4), 101–119.

Marshall, S. C. (2008). The role of reduced fitness to drive due to medical impairments in explaining crashes involving older drivers. *Traffic Injury Prevention, 9*(4), 291–298.

Marshall, S. C., & Man-Son-Hing, M. (2011). Multiple chronic medical conditions and associated driving risk: A systematic review. *Traffic Injury Prevention, 12*(2), 142–148.

Mathias, J. L., & Lucas, L. K. (2009). Cognitive predictors of unsafe driving in older drivers: A meta-analysis. *International Psychogeriatrics/IPA, 21*(4), 637–653.

McGwin, G. J., Owsley, C., & Ball, K. (1998). Identifying crash involvement among older drivers: Agreement between self-report and state records. *Accident Analysis and Prevention, 30*(6), 781–791.

McKnight, A. J., & McKnight, A. S. (2003). Young novice drivers: Careless or clueless? *Accident Analysis and Prevention, 35*(6), 921–925.

Menec, V. H., & Nowicki, S. (2014). Examining the relationship between communities' "age-friendliness" and life satisfaction and self-perceived health in rural Manitoba, Canada. *Rural and Remote Health, 14*, 2594.

Meng, A., Siren, A., & Teasdale, T. W. (2013). Older drivers with cognitive impairment: Perceived changes in driving skills, driving-related discomfort and self-regulation of driving. *European Geriatric Medicine, 4*(3), 154–160.

Meuser, T. M., Berg-Weger, M., Chibnall, J. T., Harmon, A. C., & Stowe, J. D. (2013). Assessment of readiness for mobility transition (ARMT): A tool for mobility transition counseling with older adults. *Journal of Applied Gerontology, 32*(4), 484–507.

Molnar, L. J., Charlton, J. L., Eby, D. W., Langford, J., Koppel, S., Kolenic, G. E., et al. (2014). Factors affecting self-regulatory driving practices among older adults. *Traffic Injury Prevention, 15*(3), 262–272.

Moorhouse, P., Hamilton, L., Fisher, T., & Rockwood, K. (2011). Barriers to assessing fitness to drive in dementia in Nova Scotia: Informing strategies for knowledge translation. *Canadian Geriatrics Journal, 14*(3), 61–65.

Mullen, N., Dubois, S., & Bédard, M. (2013). Fatality trends and projections for drivers and passengers: Differences between observed and expected fatality rates with a focus on older adults. *Safety Science, 59*(0), 106–115.

Noland, R. B. (2013). From theory to practice in road safety policy: Understanding risk versus mobility. *Research in Transportation Economics, 43*(1), 71–84.

O'Connor, M. L., Edwards, J. D., Waters, M. P., Hudak, E. M., & Valdes, E. G. (2013). Mediators of the association between driving cessation and mortality among older adults. *Journal of Aging and Health, 25*(Suppl. 8), 249S–269SS. http://dx.doi.org/10.1177/0898264313497796

Owsley, C. O., McGwin, G., Phillips, J. M., McNeal, S. F., & Stalvey, B. T. (2004). Impact of an educational program on the safety of high-risk, visually impaired, older drivers. *American Journal of Preventive Medicine, 26*(3), 222–229.

Oxley, J., Langford, J., & Charlton, J. (2010). The safe mobility of older drivers: A challenge for urban road designers. *Journal of Transport Geography, 18*(5), 642–648.

Oxley, J., & Whelan, M. (2008). It cannot be all about safety: The benefits of prolonged mobility. *Traffic Injury Prevention, 9*(4), 367–378.

Peel, N., Westmoreland, J., & Steinberg, M. (2002). Transport safety for older people: A study of their experiences, perceptions and management needs. *Injury Control & Safety Promotion, 9*(1), 19–24.

Persson, D. (1993). The elderly driver: Deciding when to stop. *The Gerontologist, 33*(1), 88–91.

Posner, M. I., & Petersen, S. E. (1990). The attention system of the human brain. *Annual Review of Neuroscience, 13*, 25–42.

Ragland, D. R., Satariano, W. A., & MacLeod, K. E. (2005). Driving cessation and increased depressive symptoms. *Journals of Gerontology Series A: Biological Sciences and Medical Sciences, 60A*(3), 399.

Ralston, L. S., Bell, S. L., Mote, J. K., Rainey, T. B., Brayman, S., & Shotwell, M. (2001). Giving up the car keys: Perceptions of well elders and families. *Physical & Occupational Therapy in Geriatrics, 19*(4), 59–70.

Rosenbloom, S. (2001). Driving cessation among older people: When does it happen and what impact does it have? *Transportation Research Record, 1779*, 93–99.

Rosenblum, L. P, & Corn, A. L (2002). Experiences of older adults who stopped driving because of their visual impairments: Part 1. *Journal of Visual Impairment and Blindness, 96*(6), 389–398.

Ross, L. A., Dodson, J. E., Edwards, J. D., Ackerman, M. L., & Ball, K. (2012). Self-rated driving and driving safety in older adults. *Accident Analysis and Prevention, 48*, 523–527.

Rudman, D. L., Friedland, J., Chipman, M., & Sciortino, P. (2006). Holding on and letting go: The perspectives of pre-seniors and seniors on driving self-regulation in later life. *Canadian Journal on Aging/La Revue Canadienne Du Vieillissement, 25*(1), 65–76.

Staplin, L., & Freund, K. (2013). Policy prescriptions to preserve mobility for seniors – A dose of realism. *Accident Analysis and Prevention, 61*, 212–221.

Summala, H., & Mikkola, T. (1994). Fatal accidents among car and truck drivers: Effects of fatigue, age, and alcohol consumption. *Human Factors, 36*(2), 315–326.

Taylor, B. D., & Tripodes, S. (2001). The effects of driving cessation on the elderly with dementia and their caregivers. *Accident Analysis and Prevention, 33*(4), 519–528.

Trick, L. M., Enns, J. T., Mills, J., & Vavrik, J. (2004). Paying attention behind the wheel: A framework for studying the role of attention in driving. *Theoretical Issues in Ergonomics Science, 5*(5), 385–424.

Weaver, B., Bédard, M., McAuliffe, J., & Parkkari, M. (2009). Using the attention network test to predict driving test scores. *Accident Analysis and Prevention, 41*(1), 76–83.

Wernham, M., Jarrett, P. G., Stewart, C., MacDonald, E., MacNeil, D., & Hobbs, C. (2014). Comparison of the SIMARD MD to clinical impression in assessing fitness to drive in patients with cognitive impairment. *Canadian Geriatrics Journal, 17*(2), 63–69.

Whitehead, B. J., Howie, L., & Lovell, R. K. (2006). Older people's experience of driver licence cancellation: A phenomenological study. *Australian Occupational Therapy Journal, 53*(3), 173–180.

Windsor, T. D., & Anstey, K. J. (2006). Interventions to reduce the adverse psychosocial impact of driving cessation on older adults. *Clinical Interventions in Aging, 1*(3), 205–211.

Windsor, T. D., Anstey, K. J., Butterworth, P., Luszcz, M. A., & Andrews, G. R. (2007). The role of perceived control in explaining depressive symptoms associated with driving cessation in a longitudinal study. *The Gerontologist, 47*(2), 215–223.

Wood, J. M., & Owsley, C. (2014). Useful field of view test. *Gerontology, 60*(4), 315–318.

8

Person-Centered Suicide Prevention

Paul R. Duberstein, and Marsha N. Wittink

University of Rochester Medical Center, Rochester, New York, USA

"Do everything for the patient while doing as little as possible to the patient."

—Bernard Lown

"It is more important to know what type of person has the disease than to know what type of disease the person has."

—William Osler

INTRODUCTION

Aging brings change. Chronic diseases develop, physical functioning deteriorates, and cognitive function declines. Occupational roles disappear with retirement, family roles change or erode as children and grandchildren grow up, and ageism is encountered. Some friends and family members die; others need round-the-clock assistance. Aging brings positive change as well, such as increases in wisdom (Baltes, 1997) and improvements in the capacity to regulate emotions (Carstensen, Isaacowitz, & Charles, 1999). Nonetheless, as nature takes its course and death approaches, changes-for-the-worse often outweigh changes-for-the-better (Baltes, 1997). A goal of geriatric care is to enable older adults to bear life changes with dignity and equanimity. This goal remains elusive. For too many individuals, the seemingly unrelenting accretion of changes-for-the-worse leads to unbearable suffering, defined by Cassell (1982, p. 639) as a "specific state of severe distress induced by the loss of integrity, intactness, cohesiveness, or wholeness of person, or by a threat that the person believes will result in the dissolution of his or her integrity." As Gerstorf and colleagues (2010) put it, "something is seriously wrong

B. Bensadon (Ed): Psychology and Geriatrics.
DOI: http://dx.doi.org/10.1016/B978-0-12-420123-1.00008-3

at the end of life." One of the clearest indicators of that "something" is the suicide rate, which increases with age in most Western countries, including the United States (U.S.) (Duberstein, Heisel, & Conwell, 2011).

Over the past 50 years, suicide prevention efforts worldwide have largely been informed by a biomedical paradigm (Clarke, Mamo, Fosket, Fishman, & Shim, 2009). The medicalization of suicide (Kushner, 1991) has deflected attention away from nonbiomedical risk factors and interventions (e.g., social isolation and aging services) while motivating scientists and clinicians to concentrate on medically framed risk factors (e.g., symptoms of mental illness) and interventions (e.g., psychotropic medication, psychotherapy). Given that older adults are more likely to see a primary care provider than a mental health specialist in the weeks prior to suicide (Ahmedani et al., 2014; Luoma, Martin, & Pearson, 2002), primary care providers (PCPs) have a key role to play in suicide prevention among older adults.

Advantages of the biomedicalization of suicide are numerous. There is now more open discussion about suicide in scientific journals and in the media. More advocacy groups for suicide prevention exist, and more support groups have been created for people who have lost a family member, partner, or friend to suicide. More money from industry, government, and nongovernmental organizations has been directed at suicide research and prevention. Other secular shifts might account for these changes, but biomedicalization has arguably played a leading role. Yet the more we learn about suicide, the more it seems that automatic, unfettered reliance on the biomedical model – what may be termed exuberant biomedicalism (Duberstein & Jerant, 2014) – is unwise at best and harmful at worst.

Consider the opportunity costs. Allocation of disproportionately more resources (time, effort, money) to biomedicalism has led to the underdevelopment of care models for older adults who are suffering despite receiving standard biomedical care (e.g., Angell, 1997; Foley, 1997). Noting the arbitrary distinction in the U.S. between institutions devoted to health as opposed to social services, Joanne Lynn (2013) has suggested that the financial waste caused by biomedicalization (Berwick & Hackbarth, 2012) could be harvested and reallocated to our flagging aging and social services infrastructure. Shoring up that frail infrastructure will mitigate if not eliminate the types of suffering (e.g., loneliness, financial strain, loss of function) that precipitate suicide and assisted suicide.

Biomedicalism's harm in the care of suffering older adults is not confined to opportunity costs. For example, the physical harm engendered by psychotropic medications (Coupland et al., 2011; Hampton, Daubresse, Chang, Alexander, & Budnitz, 2014) does not appear to be outweighed by the benefits (Erlangsen, Agerbo, Hawton, & Conwell, 2009). Moreover, the medicalization of suffering can rob patients of their identity and cause other psychological harms (Drought & Koenig, 2002; Entwistle,

Carter, Cribb, & McCaffery, 2010; Frank, 1997; Kaufman, 1998; Solomon & Lawlor, 2011). Given that older patients frequently have nonbiomedical explanations for their suffering, PCPs risk alienating patients when they try to convince them of a biomedical explanation and treatment (Wittink, Givens, Knott, Coyne, & Barg, 2011). Moreover, the standard approach to suicide prevention in primary care involves mental health screening and referral to mental health treat (Bruce et al., 2004; Duberstein & Heisel, 2014; Duberstein et al., 2011), an approach that can lead to fragmentation of care rather than engagement in care (Pincus, 2003; Wittink, Duberstein, & Lyness, 2013). Finally, unfettered biomedicalism in the form of over-treatment wastes financial resources, estimated at roughly $200 billion annually in the U.S. alone (Berwick & Hackbarth, 2012).

Over the past few decades, the prevailing biomedicalism has shaped the societal conversation about suicide prevention. By focusing more on suffering persons and less on diagnosing and treating disease, this chapter aims to realign the conversation to be more consistent with the public's native understanding of suffering and suicide (Epstein et al., 2010; Gask et al., 2012; Hjelmeland, Dieserud, Dyregrov, Knizek, & Leenaars, 2012; Kjolseth, Ekeberg, & Steihaug, 2010). Drawing from research on suicide in older adults, our *main premise* is that age-related increases in suicide rates are tied more to suffering and anticipated suffering than to the presence of mental disorders alone. Acknowledging that disease-centered care can, in some instances, be person-centered[1], we argue that person-centered interventions are needed to decrease suicide risk, reduce the harm associated with unfettered biomedicalism, and improve other patient outcomes.

Care of older adults ought to be more person-centered[1] and less disease-centered. This is not a new idea. Some of medicine's great thinkers have counseled clinicians to avoid confusing the treatment of disease with the treatment of persons. This chapter's epigraphs represent a sampling of that collective wisdom. Before George Engel (1980, 1992) launched his salvo on biomedical hegemony, Adolph Meyer (Rutter, 1986) had launched his own. Why, despite the counsel of Osler, Meyer, Engel, Lown,

---

[1] Notwithstanding the popularity of the term patient-centered, we and others (Starfield, 2011) prefer the term person-centered. First, in order to be effective, suicide prevention initiatives must reach well beyond those who self-define as "a patient" and show up in medical clinics or facilities for intervention. Second, many patients are accompanied by caregivers when visiting the PCP, and PCPs' interactions with these third parties can influence patient outcomes. Third, interventions targeting patients in health care settings will not reach their full potential unless they account for the needs of nonpatients, namely, health care providers and other personnel in the health care system. In other words, patients will receive person-centered care only insofar as the needs of the persons involved in care provision (e.g., PCPs, administrative personnel) are accommodated.

and countless other individuals (Brown, 1998; Eisenberg, 1988; Epstein et al., 2005; Sullivan, 2003), not to mention the Institute of Medicine (2001), has a disease focus remained so entrenched? To the best of our knowledge, this question has received little, if any, scholarly attention. This lack of curiosity is striking when one considers the accumulated costs of wisdom ignored: wasted societal resources, psychological harms, lives lost. Given the passage of the Patient Protection and Affordable Care Act (PPACA), with its numerous incentives for patient-centered provisions (e.g., medical homes), it is timely to consider why it has been so difficult to heed the calls for person-centeredness. Our *secondary premise* is that these calls (and incentives) will remain hollow until we understand why disease-centeredness remains a reflex-like default.

Chapter Organization

This chapter is divided into three main sections. In the first, "Biomedicalism Misdirected," we explain why unfettered biomedicalism is poorly suited both for suicide prevention and for the practice of primary care medicine. Unsurprisingly, biomedically oriented interventions have not been shown to reduce suicide mortality in older adults (Duberstein & Heisel, 2014). Not only have these interventions generated opportunity costs, they have also led to unintended psychological harm that, we theorize, are largely byproducts of two cognitive heuristics (or problem-solving strategies) inherent in biomedicalism, essentialism (Gelman, 2003) and focalism (Kahneman, 2011). In the second section, "Biomedicalism Retained," we offer a hypothesis that seeks to explain why person-centered care has not gained traction in medicine. We suggest that economic arguments, while compelling (e.g., Relman, 1994), have limited explanatory power. Moreover, economic theories of unfettered biomedicalism seem to presume, incorrectly, that clinicians (or their employers) are motivated primarily or exclusively by money. By integrating two psychological theories, terror management theory (TMT) (Greenberg, Pyszczynski, & Solomon, 1986) and self-determination theory (SDT) (Ryan & Deci, 2000), we offer a hypothesis that is premised on a more nuanced view of human motivation. Moreover, unlike economic theories, our hypothesis can explain the implications of essentialism and focalism for the clinician's cognitive activity. In the third section, "Humanism Reimagined," we discuss how developments in information technology can improve person-centered suicide prevention (Duberstein & Heisel, 2014). Whereas the prevailing biomedicalism prioritizes the treatment of mental disorders, humanistic person-centeredness prioritizes the relief of patient suffering by mitigating precisely those cognitive heuristics, essentialism and focalism, that we theorize make it difficult for clinicians to bear and respond to patient suffering.

Two caveats delimit our discussion. First, this chapter focuses principally on suicide mortality, not attempted suicide or suicide ideation. As argued elsewhere (Duberstein & Heisel, 2014; Useda et al., 2007), the desire to draw conclusions about suicide mortality from clinical experience with "suicidal" patients or from research on attempted suicide or suicide ideation must be resisted. Second, this chapter is not intended to serve as a review of risk markers for suicide or as a practical guide to risk management or suicide prevention. These topics are covered elsewhere (Duberstein et al., 2011; Heisel & Duberstein, 2005).

BIOMEDICALISM MISDIRECTED

Part 1: Suicide is not a Biomedical Problem

As one of several approaches to solving clinical or public health problems, biomedicalism has many strengths and can claim many victories (Le Fanu, 2012). Childhood leukemia, incurable decades ago, is now curable. In many parts of the globe, diphtheria, smallpox, and polio are faint memories. Yet there is also a history of failure in biomedicalism: People succumb to diseases that are purportedly treatable. Their family members are harmed in the process, and societal resources are laid to waste. Some of these failures result from misdirecting biomedicalism to problems that it simply cannot solve. Philosophers call this type of misdirection a category error. The biomedical paradigm is well-suited to the treatment of diseases that obey mechanistic laws of nature but is poorly suited to many other phenomena that are thought to warrant clinical attention.

Compare what is known about suicide with what is known about an exemplar biomedical condition, influenza. Whereas the pathogenic effects of influenza are largely independent of the social, cultural, or historic context, suicide risk is *contingent upon* social, cultural, economic, and historical contextual considerations (Neeleman, 2002), such as the gross domestic product, employment rate, and media coverage of suicide. Research over the past few decades, much of it at considerable taxpayer expense, has uncovered "information" about suicide but has yet to show, even tentatively, that suicide obeys mechanistic laws. Humans – scientists included – conflate information with mechanistic knowledge (Tuomi, 1999). As Keil (2012, p. 329) put it, "… people of all ages have strikingly impoverished mechanistic understandings – often far worse than they assume."

A considerable body of research suggests that suicide risk in older adulthood is tied to suffering and anticipated suffering stemming from sentinel events (widowhood, the recent diagnosis of terminal illness or dementia) or ongoing strains (financial hardship, functional impairment, social isolation, burden of caring for a loved one). This conclusion is strengthened by the diversity of methodological approaches employed, ranging from large-sample epidemiological studies (Fang et al., 2012; Turvey et al., 2002) to smaller-sample psychological autopsy research (Conwell et al., 2010; Duberstein, Conwell, Conner, Eberly, & Caine, 2004b; Duberstein et al., 2004a; Harwood, Hawton, Hope, & Jacoby, 2006a; Harwood, Hawton, Hope, Harriss, & Jacoby, 2006b; Rubenowitz, Waern, Wilhelmson, & Allebeck, 2001; Waern et al., 2002) and qualitative research (Kjolseth et al., 2010). For example, in a prospective study of more than 6 million Swedes (Fang et al., 2012), those who had recently been diagnosed with cancer had an increased risk of suicide during the week (RR = 12.6) (95% Confidence Interval (CI), 8.6 to 17.8) and year (RR = 3.1) (95% CI, 2.7, 3.5) following diagnosis. Among the nearly 800 terminally ill people who have died by suicide in Oregon under the auspices of the Death with Dignity Act (Oregon Public Health Division, 2014), loss of autonomy is the number one reason endorsed, offered by more than 90% of respondents. Other reasons include inability to engage in pleasant activities (89%), loss of dignity (81%), loss of control of bodily functions (50.3%), burden on caregivers (40%) and inadequate pain control (24%).

Many of the themes documented in Oregon have been identified in studies of suicide mortality. For example, the theme of "losing oneself" emerged in a qualitative study of 23 suicides in Norway (Kjolseth et al., 2010). Loss was experienced not just in bodily and sensory domains but in the broader sense of identity. One respondent reported that her father had said, "Now I just don't exist anymore." Another "felt as if he was just disappearing" and a third felt "robbed of his identity."

Given that thinking can be distorted in suicidal people (Szanto et al., 2012), feelings of identity loss, perceived burdensomeness, or profound social isolation might be byproducts of a treatable mood disorder. When confronted with a patient who appears to be suffering existentially, the biomedical paradigm encourages providers to adopt specific cognitive heuristics (Table 8.1) that, in effect, empower them to consider patients' suffering in terms of specific categorical diseases (e.g., major depression) and causal mechanisms of action (e.g., serotonergic dysregulation). These heuristics encourage providers to offer a biomedical solution for suffering (Brickman et al., 1982). While helpful for some patients and in some circumstances, the deployment of these heuristics could generate psychological harms (Cunningham, Sirey, & Bruce, 2007; Dar-Nimrod & Heine, 2011; Kvaale, Gottdiener, & Haslam, 2013a; Kvaale, Haslam, & Gottdiener, 2013b) and lead to overdiagnosis and overtreatment (Brownlee, 2007; Dowrick & Frances, 2013; Mojtabai, 2013). Older individuals who have begun to feel robbed of their identity, autonomy, or sense of control are subjected to interventions that could exacerbate psychological suffering while also conferring physical harms.

TABLE 8.1 Cognitive Biases in Suicidology

Cognitive bias	Definition	Manifestation in suicidology
Biomedical Essentialism	Codified view that people could be categorized on the basis of their intrinsically different genetics, physiology or anatomy.	Propagation of belief that a particular physical essence distinguishes suicidal and nonsuicidal people. For decades the search for that essence has focused on serotonin, 5-HIAA, and cortisol levels in cerebrospinal fluid, and more recently on genetic biomarkers. It has yet to yield laboratory tests suggestive of imminent or longer-term suicide risk.
Focalism	Tendency to rely on one attribute or criterion when making decisions, even when there is reason to believe that no single attribute or criterion should be disproportionately weighted.	Disproportionate emphasis placed on depression and other putative manifestations of serotonergic dysfunction when making decisions about suicide risk and when allocating resources for suicide research and suicide prevention.

Biomedicalism's heuristics tacitly give the clinician permission to avoid the painful work (Larson & Yao, 2005) of exploring patient suffering. Not surprisingly, research on interactions between suicidal patients and their physicians revealed that physician response to patient suffering quickly became adversarial or surprisingly superficial (Vannoy, Tai-Seale, Duberstein, Eaton, & Cook, 2011). Watching these tapes, one of us could not help but feel the genuineness of the physicians' desire to help, but they seemed bereft, as if their training had left them unprepared for these exchanges. As Meier (2014, p. 897) wrote, physicians "care deeply about their patients" and "express … care exactly as they were taught to express it." Merely imploring physicians to change their habits or behave in a person-centered manner is insufficient.

The biomedical model offers two types of interventions for individuals at risk for suicide: psychotropic medication and psychotherapy. But, as the following example illustrates, there are other ways of intervening. After receiving the diagnosis of motor neuron disease 4 years earlier, a 67-year-old retired accountant was 90% sure that he would eventually take his own life, but he now pegs his chances of suicide at only 10% (Chamberlain, 2014, p. 1). He observed, "I have accepted more personal care than I thought I would want because of the professionalism of my main carer." In this case, a simple nonbiomedical intervention involving the provision of home care appears to have modified his affective forecasting bias (Hoerger, Chapman, Epstein, & Duberstein, 2012) and decreased suicide risk.

Part 2: Primary vs Specialty Care

Differences in the ways PCPs and specialty providers interact with patients, think about their professional roles, and provide clinical care (Lampe et al., 2013) must be acknowledged to improve the conceptualization of suicide prevention in primary care. Patients often present to PCPs with unfiltered stories – multiple, vague symptoms. Whereas the top 6 diagnostic clusters account for up to 90% of patient visits to specialists, the top 20 diagnostic clusters account for roughly half of patient visits to PCPs (Stange et al., 1998). In specialty care, the patient's story has been filtered (Marino, Gallo, Ford, & Anthony, 1995), leaving distilled biomedical facts (lab values, imaging results) that authorize the physician to initiate a discussion about whether, and which, intervention is warranted. In contrast, PCPs wade through more material and, in the words of Julian Tudor Hart (1971, p. 411), occasionally "dig beneath the presenting symptom, and encourage a return when something appears to have been left unsaid."

If specialist-biomedicalists fix their attention on distilled (if misleading) facts, the PCP-humanist must solicit and attend to patients' stories. Primary care interventions can be offered in the context of an ongoing relationship that enhances continuity of care, as well as the capacity to monitor the change and impact of symptoms over time. Thus, even though suicide rates are elevated among patients seen by oncologists and neurologists, it is hardly surprising that suicide prevention initiatives have been mounted in primary care, not in those specialty settings.

Prior Studies of Suicide Prevention in Primary Care

A clinician-directed initiative was launched in 1983 and 1984 on the Swedish island of Gotland (population 58,000). All 18 primary care physicians on that Baltic island were trained to detect and treat depression (Rutz, 2001). Two years into the study, the number of suicides had decreased by 60%. The suicide rate declined in women, but was unchanged in men and rose following program discontinuation.

The Prevention of Suicide in Primary Care Elderly-Collaborative Trial (Bruce et al., 2004) was designed to determine whether *collaborative care*, involving the colocalization of specialty mental health providers in primary care, reduced depression and suicide ideation among patients ≥ 60 years old. Indeed, those exposed to collaborative care showed a greater decrease in prevalence of suicide ideation (Bruce et al., 2004; similar findings were reported by Unützer et al., 2006). Follow-up analyses showed that depressed patients exposed to collaborative care experienced a greater decline in suicide ideation and depressive symptoms at 2-year follow-up (Alexopoulos et al., 2009) and had lower rates of all-cause mortality (Gallo et al., 2013). Effects on suicide mortality have not been demonstrated.

Australian researchers (Almeida et al., 2012) opted to conduct a cluster randomized trial of practice audit, not collaborative care (for reasons discussed below). PCPs (n = 373) and their patients ≥60 years old (n = 21,762) were assigned to intervention or control. The intervention consisted mainly of practice audit with the provision of detailed, personalized feedback along with printed educational material about the assessment and management of depression in later life. PCPs in the control condition received a practice audit but were given pooled, not personalized, feedback. Control PCPs were given no education about screening, depression, or suicide but they did receive monthly newsletters about study progress. Patients were followed for 24 months.

The results were intriguing. Even though patients of intervention PCPs were not more likely to have received antidepressants or mental health care, they had lower rates of self-harm and scored lower on a composite outcome made up of clinically significant depression and self-harm. Noting that their findings were consistent with another educational intervention (Gask et al., 2004), the authors hypothesized that educational interventions might improve PCP empathy and willingness to discuss patients' emotional concerns, an interpretation that is consistent with a meta-analysis of patient–clinician interventions (Kelley, Kraft-Todd, Schapira, Kossowsky, & Riess, 2014) and with psychotherapy research (Crits-Christoph, Gibbons, Hamilton, Ring-Kurtz, & Gallop, 2011; Flueckiger, Del Re, Wampold, Symonds, & Horvath, 2012; Horvath, Del Re, Flueckiger, & Symonds, 2011). Teaching physicians to give patients the space to voice and explore their symptoms could have a direct therapeutic effect independent of the effects of specialty referrals (Bertakis & Azari, 2011).

Collaborative care might intuitively seem more potent than a clinician-directed informational intervention, but Almeida et al. (2012) argued that the effects of collaborative care in prior studies were modest, and they also questioned its expense and sustainability. They are not the only ones to critique collaborative care (Wittink et al., 2013). For example, some have complained about the increased strain on their workload generated by the addition of a mental health specialist to the team and others have argued that collaborative care reinforces the idea that depression is a separate component of health, the treatment of which should be outsourced to a specialist (Wittink et al., 2013). This could signal to patients that PCPs will selectively focus on their (physical) health issues (Henke et al., 2008), potentially undermining the provision of person-centered care (Wittink et al, 2013). In the third section, we describe an approach that addresses these important critiques, but first we will consider why, even amidst compelling calls for person-centeredness, unfettered disease-centered biomedicalism abides in most health care settings.

BIOMEDICALISM RETAINED: INSTITUTIONAL AND PROVIDER CONSIDERATIONS

Without theory, proposed solutions for reining in exuberant biomedicalism will remain piecemeal, *ad hoc*, or merely exhortatory. Drawing on TMT (Greenberg et al., 1986) and SDT (Ryan & Deci, 2000), we offer a two-pronged argument, focusing on institutional norms and individual motivations. We argue that calls for person-centeredness represent a threat both to a) the *identities of institutions* with a vested (and not solely financial) interest in biomedicalism, and to b) the *self-determination of providers*.

Institutional Considerations

Thomas Kuhn (1970) said that "paradigms gain status to the extent that they are successful in solving problems, and they lose status as paradoxes multiply." If a measure of biomedicalism's favorable status in suicidology is the number or importance of problems solved, then a measure of its unfavorable status is the number or importance of problems unsolved or generated. The biomedicalization of suicide has not led to lowered suicide rates in older adulthood. No specific treatment has been shown to decrease risk of suicide mortality in primary care patients, and the United States Preventive Services Task Force (LeFevre & US Preventive Services Task Force, 2014) has concluded that there are insufficient data to recommend screening for suicide risk in primary care.

In the face of this evidence, it might be wise to identify an alternative to the disease-centered paradigm. An established but somewhat marginalized tradition of humanistic scholarship in suicidology (Jobes, 1995; Shneidman, 1993) could readily displace the biomedical approach to suicide prevention in primary care. That has not happened. When paradigms begin to lose explanatory power or generate paradoxes, status quo bias motivates paradigm-refinement, not paradigm-replacement. That is what has happened in the pharmacological treatment of suicide risk, though the recent repurposing of ketamine is a potential conceptual advance (Griffiths, Zarate, & Rasimas, 2014). In general, pharmacological interventions in medicine have been characterized more by methodological refinement than by conceptual advances (Angell & Relman, 2002). In the psychosocial realm, resources have been devoted to treatment-engagement interventions (e.g., motivational interviewing) to increase the uptake of treatments that themselves are unlikely to have a demonstrable influence on suicide mortality. Paradoxes have multiplied, but the biomedical paradigm retains its status.

Why do paradigms abide in the face of countervailing evidence? One explanation holds that institutions, because they are vulnerable to the *sunk-cost fallacy* (Kahneman, 2011), are reluctant to abandon objects or ideas in which considerable resources have been invested. This fallacy leads to *status-quo bias* (sticking with the same approach even when it has not proven helpful and alternatives have been proposed) and the paradox of throwing good money after bad. The *sunk-cost fallacy* and *status quo bias* are descriptive labels, not theoretical explanations, however. Yet theoretical explanations for why unfettered biomedicalism abides are needed. Without an understanding of the human motives sustaining unfettered biomedicalism, proposed solutions will be ineffective. Any attempt to modify human behavior does so in the face of deep resistance (Graham & Martin, 2012) among stakeholder institutions and individuals (patients, providers, administrators). Two broad classes of theoretical explanations can be invoked to explain this resistance economic and psychosocial.

Economic Explanations: Financial Incentives

Much has been written about the adverse influence of money in health care and the need for economic incentives to improve health care. For example, Arnold Relman repeatedly urged physicians to change their behavior, once scolding his colleagues for acting like "competing businessmen" rather than "trustworthy advocates for patients" (1994, p. 24). Products developed and marketed by the pharmaceutical and medical device industries are, understandably, designed to improve disease-centered care more than person-centered care. But when direct-to-consumer advertising leads clinicians to prescribe medications for diseases that patients do not have (Kravitz et al., 2005), money is wasted and person-centeredness suffers.

Clinicians and their employers can justifiably say that, historically, they have not been paid to behave in a person-centered manner. But what if physicians were paid to provide person-centered care? No direct data are available, but some indirect evidence (Doran et al., 2011; Jha, Joynt, Orav, & Epstein, 2012) suggests that paying providers to enact person-centeredness is unlikely to confer long-term benefit, to individuals or to society. Economic explanations of human behavior in health care, education, and other moral endeavors are not as powerful as policymakers would like to believe. With few notable exceptions (e.g., Petry, Andrade, Barry, & Byrne, 2013), economic incentives have rarely generated the expected, desired effects. Moreover, experimental evidence suggests that extrinsic (monetary) rewards might, in some instances, sap intrinsic motivation (Deci, Koestner, & Ryan, 1999).

Psychosocial Explanations: Social Norms

When Medicare became law more than 50 years ago, one of its aims was to reduce the widespread geographic variability in the practice of disease-centered health care. Scholars are now painfully aware that the legislation has had little, if any, impact on geographic variability, and they have begun searching for explanations. Even economists and health services researchers, who by virtue of their training and professional socialization might be favorably inclined toward economic explanations, have offered psychosocial explanations focused on *individual* attitudes and beliefs or *social* norms (Barnato et al., 2014; Cutler, Skinner, Stern, & Wennberg, 2013). Given that the provision of health care is a ritualized group activity, the most compelling of these explanations concern norms.

Social norms are established early in clinical training, but the process of identifying suitable candidates for medical school itself probably prioritizes the selection of individuals who are more likely to abide by a particular norm (Charlton, 2009). Like all individuals in the workforce, clinicians come of age in institutions that establish the rules and norms for proper behavior, implement messaging strategies to reinforce these rules and norms among the membership, and strive to convey a particular public image (Good & DelVecchio-Good, 1993). For most, this socialization process occurs in their mid- to late 20s, a time in life when personality traits are beginning to cohere (McCrae & Costa, 1990). Institutions confer a sense of identity for their members (Douglas, 1986), offer opportunities to create lifelong bonds with like-minded people, guidance in times of uncertainty, and sanctuary in times of adversity. As death, dying, and suffering are encountered like never before, the young medical professional is exposed to institutional norms that are frankly inimical to introspection, self-reflection, and compassionate vulnerability (Coulehan, 2009). Norms such as depersonalization of patients ("the pancreas in room 5B"), detached concern, and denial of feeling have evolved to prevent the development of overwhelming anguish (Menzies, 1960; Mount, 1986). Individuals who value conformity will conform to the social norm. Doing otherwise exacts psychological costs, including diminished well-being (Fulmer et al., 2010) and the potential for humiliation (Marques, Abrams, Paez, & Martinez-Taboada, 1998). Not only are people motivated to behave in a manner than increases their psychological similarity to the in-group (Fulmer et al., 2010) but they will also derogate group members who threaten to disrupt group norms (Marques et al., 1998).

Why is the biomedical social norm so resistant to change? One reason is that the medical profession has historically been self-regulating (Freidson, 1970), limiting the extent to which outside forces can disrupt the norm. But to say "the profession has historically been self-regulating" is to relabel the problem without explaining it. Drawing from TMT (Greenberg et al., 1986), we hypothesize that the need to abide by fixed as opposed to flexible social norms is particularly strong in work settings where exposure to death (dying people, dead people, suicidal people) is so common that it becomes routinized, no longer jarring. Most medical settings, particularly those serving older individuals, would meet that criterion. Inspired by the work of cultural anthropologist Ernest Becker (1973), TMT's driving ideas are that people experience death anxiety when exposed to a reminder of death. To defend against death anxiety, TMT presumes, humans created social institutions (e.g., religions, professions), replete with identity-conferring ideologies and *social norms* ("the pancreas in 5B"). Although the theory's fundamental premise about the historic origins of social institutions is untestable, and some of its main tenets have been disputed (Proulx & Heine, 2006), well-controlled experiments have supported many of its predictions (Burke, Martens, & Faucher, 2010; Landau et al., 2004; Martens, Burke, Schimel, & Faucher, 2011; Niemiec et al., 2010; Renkema, Stapel, & Van Yperen, 2008; Simon et al., 1997).

Of greatest relevance are studies showing that exposure to reminders of death motivates conformity behaviors (Renkema et al., 2008) as well as habitual patterns of information processing that sustain conformity (Landau et al., 2004). Specifically, exposure to reminders of death has been shown to motivate yielding to in-group opinion, defense of group norms, derogation of out-group opinion as well as the tendency to "freeze" on and prefer initial (vs. subsequent), stereotypical (vs. statistical), or unambiguous (vs. ambiguous) information (Landau et al., 2004). Clinicians, like nonclinicians, are vulnerable to a host of social cognitive biases. In the clinical setting these biases could insidiously influence patient care, outside the clinician's conscious awareness (Solomon & Lawlor, 2011).

From this perspective, disease-centered biomedicalism abides not because it is lucrative (Relman, 1994) or because it is a behavior that can be modified by manipulating a policy lever or by changing personnel management strategies (Berwick & Hackbarth, 2012), but because it is the product of a shared cognitive mindset (a norm) that seizes on unambiguous, readily tractable problems that are thought to be solvable by authorities who have historically discouraged, and even derogated, challenges to their codified views. The authority's most powerful weapon is the capacity to define a problem (biomedical, in my purview, not yours); arrogance is his most powerful ammunition.

Writing about his physician-father, Berwick (2009, p. 129) recalled:

> With his great responsibility came great authority. Sometimes arrogance came, too. I was 11 years old. At dinnertime, the telephone rang. A patient was calling. I watched my father listen, and then scowl. "I'm the doctor," he seethed. "You're not. You'll get penicillin when I say, and not a moment sooner." He slammed the phone handset down so violently that its plastic cradle shattered, sending shards into my beef stew.

Some people are more arrogant than others, but TMT suggests that the arrogance that sustains unfettered biomedicalism is, partly, a product of social norms that were created to contain anxiety. To meet their needs for care, patients have historically paid the price of absorbing that arrogance ("I'm the doctor. You're not.").

Derogation of patient identity (Drought & Koenig, 2002; Entwistle et al., 2010; Kaufman, 1998) is part of another problem: derogation of humanism in medicine more broadly. Humanism is derogated in many ways. It is derogated by the hidden curriculum, which places enormous pressure on young people to conform, appear tough, and adopt a narrow view of science (Eisenberg, 1988). It is derogated when lawmakers are unwilling to fight for policies that would have incentivized providers to have meaningful conversations about anticipated suffering and end-of-life care (Tinetti, 2012). It is derogated by the salary structure in American medicine, which handsomely rewards proceduralists at the expense of clinicians who believe, along with Bernard Lown (1999), that words are their most powerful tools. It is derogated when it is assumed that the skill, knowledge, labor, and expertise required to perform a pancreoduodenectomy is somehow "greater" or of greater societal value than the skill, knowledge, labor, and expertise required to empathize and bear another's suffering.

A century after William Osler offered the counsel appearing in this chapter's epigraph, Edwin Shneidman (1992, p. 890) offered this advice about suicide prevention: "A focus on mental illness is often misleading. Physicians and other health professionals need the courage and wisdom to work on a person's suffering at the phenomenological level." The word *courage* was carefully chosen. TMT suggests that courage is needed not only to countenance death anxiety but also to resist the desire to conform to social norms that discount "work on a person's suffering at the phenomenological level."

Provider Considerations

There's a joke about an older man who went to see his doctor because he was suffering from a bad cold. His doctor prescribed some pills, to no avail. On his next visit, the doctor gave the man an injection, but that didn't do any good, either. On his third visit, the doctor told the man to go home and take a hot bath. Then, as soon as he gets out of the bath, he must open all the windows and stand in the draft. "But doctor," protested the man, "I'll get pneumonia." "I know," said his doctor, "I can cure pneumonia."

Of course, providers do not intentionally make their patients sick in an effort to give themselves a problem they can solve. However, providers, like all humans, have fundamental psychological needs that influence the way they interpret ambiguous data. What are those fundamental needs? SDT (Ryan & Deci, 2000) points to three: autonomy, competence, and relatedness. Clinicians want to interact with patients who present with problems they can solve competently and with some degree of autonomy.

The influence of fundamental psychological motives is perhaps most evident when clinicians and scientists are faced with ambiguities, either in clinical care, in scientific data, or in the scientific literature. Consider, for example, research suggesting that a nontrivial proportion of people who die by suicide have no identifiable mental disorder (Ahmedani et al., 2014; Ernst et al., 2004; Harwood et al., 2006a; Owens, Booth, Briscoe, Lawrence, & Lloyd, 2003). On the one hand, these findings can be taken at face value, as evidence that suicide occurs in the absence of a diagnosable disorder (Owens et al., 2003). On the other hand, these findings can be viewed as inaccurate, because they are based on flawed diagnostic procedures (Ahmedani et al., 2014; Ernst et al., 2004). We believe the latter interpretation is an example of a form of *confirmation bias*, one motivated by the need to view one's profession as possessing relevant competencies. Mental health professionals who define their competencies mainly or exclusively in terms of treating patients with mental illness are more motivated to diagnose mental illness when it is not unambiguously present than those who define their competencies differently.

In oncologist Balfour Mount's (1986, p. 1128) moving reflection on futility when caring for incurable patients, he observed that "the psychodynamic cost of ... irrelevance is great since so much of the caregiver's professional identity is tied in his own perception and in the view of his colleagues, to his perceived skills as diagnostician and therapist." Irrelevance confers "a sense of impotence, since from the traditional perspective of diagnosis and fighting disease, there is indeed nothing more to be done." Balfour Mount transformed that feeling of irrelevance into a societal good. He is a pioneer in palliative care.

What is a mental health clinician to do when confronted with a patient with multiple chronic conditions (diabetes, arthritis, heart disease) who is suffering existentially, expresses a desire to die, but does not spontaneously report other symptoms of depression? This situation is not anomalous. A study of community-dwelling 97-year-olds revealed that most participants who reported suicide ideation (77%) met criteria for neither major nor minor depression (Fassberg, Ostling, Borjesson-Hanson, Skoog, & Waern, 2013). Clinicians can search long and hard for evidence of depression but no gold-standard diagnostic tool exists, the available tools are largely dependent on patient self-report, and many questionnaire items are themselves symptoms of chronic diseases. Although the impact of clinicians' psychological propensities or biases on patient safety has received scant attention (Meier, Back, & Morrison, 2001), the psychology of the health care provider cannot be separated from the psychology of the patient, perhaps especially in matters of life and death (Conwell, 1994; Miles, 1994). A psychiatrist and internist steeped in nosologic research confessed that the diagnostic process "often boils down to subtle perceptions, distinctions, and judgments. Such decisions are almost always made subjectively and with some degree of uncertainty, and are therefore easily swayed by the physician's own biases" (Koenig, 1993, p. 176). Clinicians are biased because they are humans, not machines. However, machines can help clinicians provide more humane care.

HUMANISM RE-IMAGINED

In the prior section, we suggested that calls for person-centeredness represent a threat both to the *identities of institutions* and the *self-determination of providers*. One way of responding to these dual threats is to derogate humanism. In this section, we argue that humanism has been a target of derision because it has been perceived, inaccurately, as an unscientific approach that could foster clinical pessimism and abandonment if not nihilism. Although humanism is not inherently unscientific, it does pose significant challenges to clinicians (who wish to experience feelings of competence and autonomy) and to health systems (that have historically not been expected to provide person-centered care). Fortunately, recent developments in information technology (IT) can enable clinicians and health systems to overcome these challenges by improving individual and organizational decision-making. We hypothesize that IT-interventions deployed in patients' homes or at the point-of-care can enhance the provision of person-centered care and thereby mitigate suicide risk and improve other health outcomes.

The Old Humanism

With titles like *On Being a Person* (Rogers, 1961) and *Love and Will* (May, 1969), humanistic writings could be inspirational and provocative. They have had little measurable impact on the delivery of health care services outside mental health services, however. Even in psychiatry and clinical psychology, humanism's appeal has waned since the 1970s. The ever-increasing number of psychiatric diagnoses, the growing market for psychotropic medications, and unrelenting efforts to confirm genetic hypotheses that spawn more essentialist biases than scientific insights reflect both biomedicalism's swagger and, to some extent, humanism's effete fecklessness.

Contrarian (Breggin, 1991; Szasz, 1974) and nondirective (Rogers, 1951, 1961) themes in the humanistic oeuvre could be readily misinterpreted as fostering therapeutic nihilism or abandonment. Moreover, while some forms of biomedicalism can be justifiably criticized for adopting a blinkered view of science (Eisenberg, 1988), some forms of humanism can be criticized as inherently unscientific (Habermas, 1991). Humanism is not inherently unscientific or nihilistic, however. For example, one humanistic theory, SDT (Ryan & Deci, 2000), has been empirically scrutinized and helpfully applied to diverse areas of human endeavor, including health care (Ng et al., 2012) and public policy (Moller, Ryan, & Deci, 2006).

Challenges of the New Humanism

Drawing on SDT (Ryan & Deci, 2000), Duberstein and Heisel (2014) theorize that person-centered approaches to suicide prevention in primary care will succeed to the extent that they enhance autonomous decision-making and self-determination on the part of all stakeholders, including at-risk individuals, their family members, clinicians and staff. Unlike biomedical approaches to patient-centeredness, which typically emphasize *genetic* processes (Hamburg & Collins, 2010), the humanistic approach to person-centeredness emphasizes the modification of individual and organizational *decision-making* processes (Duberstein & Heisel, 2014). Whereas biomedicalism's optimism is rooted mainly in its faith in technological progress, humanism's optimism derives from the conjoining of technological progress (e.g., biomedical, information, assistive) and social change (e.g., changing social norms). Technological advances without social progress and community buy-in invites exploitation (Tebes, Thai, & Matlin, 2014).

Although the legitimization (Douglas, 1986) of patients as decision-makers with expertise in their own circumstances is a sign of social progress (Coulter & Collins, 2011), implementation challenges face any clinician or health system that desires to provide "the care patients want and no more." Most suicidal patients want relief of suffering, but medicine's historic emphasis on diagnosis and treatment, and its key heuristics (essentialism, focalism), leave little room for PCPs to genuinely elicit patients' wants or explore their suffering.

For their part, patients have not been socialized to disclose the everyday worries and day-to-day circumstances that fuel their thoughts of suicide (disability, finances, caregiving, their living conditions, loneliness, anticipation of suffering), and they have not been empowered or reinforced for doing so. Keenly aware of the attention and reassurance they receive for reporting symptoms such as chest pain or breathing difficulties (Wittink, Barg, & Gallo, 2006), they know that discussions of the worries that lead them to have thoughts of self-harm are rarely reinforced in the same manner. It is not difficult to understand why. Patients' everyday circumstances and worries about suffering and dying have historically received disproportionately less attention in the medical curriculum than "hard sciences." The narrowness of the curriculum is reflected in care settings, which have historically not been outfitted to enable patients to access an array of social and aging services (Wittink et al., 2013). Even when patients and clinicians both agree that a patient is suicidal, the physician's "biomedical" explanation will seem "off" to patients who are inclined to think about suicide in spiritual (Wittink, Joo, Lewis, & Barg, 2009), existential, or other terms. Reflecting their biomedical training and professional socialization, clinicians will occasionally unwittingly choose the "wrong" explanatory model for many patients, potentially undermining patient care and motivation (Brickman et al., 1982).

Engineering Humanism

Care delivery systems can be engineered to enable primary care providers to exercise professional judgment and offer personalized solutions to their patients' presenting problems, including the everyday worries that fuel thoughts of suicide. Although some primary care practices already may be designed to enable clinicians to do this in a manner that makes clinicians feel good about themselves and their jobs, the prevailing unfettered biomedicalism has prepared few clinicians and practices in the United States for that task.

But there is reason for optimism. Whereas early IT interventions involved merely administering questionnaires by computer, perhaps with the assistance of computerized adaptive testing (Boudreaux & Horowitz, 2014), a new generation of IT interventions is on the horizon. Deployed on-line or at the point-of-care (i.e., in primary care waiting rooms), these interventions can be used to educate patients, elicit patients' wants, and assess their psychosocial circumstances along with their health beliefs – all while gently encouraging patients to broach stigmatized or taboo topics (such as suicide) with their clinicians (Duberstein & Heisel, 2014; Duberstein & Jerant, 2014; Duberstein, Wittink, & Pigeon, in press; Wittink et al., 2013). A primary care practice's use of computer-generated personalized assessments (CPAs) would signal to patients that the provision of high-quality personalized health care is more than ordering laboratory tests or prescribing guideline-concordant treatments for the correct diagnosis. It is also about being open to the patient's perspective, reducing the power asymmetries that have historically characterized the patient-PCP encounter, and enhancing the motivation of patients to take care of themselves. In theory, CPAs could improve decision-making processes (individual, dyadic, organizational), enhance the provision of person-centered care, increase PCP and patient self-determination (autonomy, competence, relatedness), and decrease suicide risk. Table 8.2 compares this person-centered approach with the more standard approach to collaborative care.

One recent study, designed to motivate patients with at least mild depression symptoms to discuss symptoms of depression and encourage openness to PCP treatment offers (Kravitz et al., 2013), reported surprisingly promising findings regarding suicide (Shah et al., 2014). Patients

TABLE 8.2 Comparison of Disease-Centered Collaborative Care and Person-Centered Care

	Disease-centered collaborative care	Person-centered care
Importance of patient–PCP communication	No assumptions made	Quality of patient–PCP communication is an important driver of health outcomes (Epstein et al., 2005; Street, Makoul, Arora & Epstein 2009)
Who frames the problem	PCP and mental health (MH) specialists	Patients and family caregivers (if applicable)
Tools used to frame problem	Screening tests, diagnostic interviews, lab tests	Information technology, Computerized personalized assessments
Involvement of MH specialists	Paid to provide a structured manualized treatment	No assumptions made
Patient expertise	No assumptions made	Patients have expertise that should be brought to bear in the clinical encounter
PCP attitudes toward involvement of specialist MH providers	No assumptions made	Ambivalent about specialist involvement in MH care; concerned about autonomy erosion
Patient attitudes toward involvement of specialist MH providers	No assumptions made	Ambivalent; many want to receive care from PCP
Resources required	Colocalized space, psychiatrists, other MH providers	Information technology

Table adapted from Wittink et al. (2013).

completed a CPA while waiting to see their doctor (median use time 5 minutes). The CPA provided text, audio, and video messages tailored to patient presentation (symptom level, visit agenda), causal explanations of depression, and views about mental health treatment. Despite little suicide-specific content, the CPA led to increased clinician inquiry about suicidal thoughts, without disturbing workflow. One likely advantage of the CPA over screening or assessment is less vulnerability to focalism and essentialism biases. Moreover, CPAs might be more acceptable to PCPs and primary care practices than off-the-shelf questionnaires. Questionnaires typically include a prespecified number of items administered in the same way to all patients. Yet if each patient is different, is it useful to ask all patients the same questions, in the same order, using exactly the same words? Experienced clinicians do not behave that way when interviewing patients, but when we employ screening questionnaires or assessment instruments, that is precisely what we do. In theory, individual practices and PCPs could develop their own CPAs, and ask only the questions they want, worded however they wish. Doing so would address reservations that clinicians and patients harbor about questionnaires (Dowrick et al., 2009; Ganzini et al., 2013).

Properly deployed, CPAs could be used to persuade older adults to talk with their health care providers about their thoughts of suicide. CPAs can help jumpstart difficult conversations and increase patient openness to interventions that are tailored to their particular circumstances. Whereas the options typically available in biomedically informed care are relatively limited (medication, psychotherapy, medication plus psychotherapy), person-centered humanism demands personalizing treatment and exploding the option set beyond mere combinations and permutations of medications and psychotherapies (Wittink et al., 2013). Other interventions must be considered, including bibliotherapy, supportive phone calls (Vaiva et al., 2006) and postcards (Carter, Clover, Whyte, Dawson, & D'Este, 2013) in conjunction with social and aging services (e.g., caregiver respite). Suicide has many causes, and many potential solutions.

CONCLUSION

Over the past few decades, the prevailing biomedicalism has profoundly influenced thinking about suicide prevention and the societal conversation about health and disease more broadly. Although much has been written about the influence of financial incentives on unfettered biomedicalism, our conceptual analysis highlights other influences: the complicated psychology of terror-management that affects the professional socialization and acculturation of health care personnel, their need for self-determination, the power asymmetries that stoke essentialism and focalism, confirmation biases, conformity, and other social and organizational processes that have the net effect of biomedicalizing the societal conversation about suicide while stifling discussion of alternatives.

Unbearable suffering – that is why older adults have the highest suicide rates in virtually all countries worldwide. A goal of geriatric care is to relieve suffering and enable older adults to bear life changes with dignity and equanimity. Biomedicalism has won many victories but it is not victorious at the end of life. Too many people suffer for too long. Too many people end that suffering by taking matters into their own hands. Even as more biomedical resources have been directed at suicide, suffering remains.

Care needs to be more humane and less biomedical, more person-centered and less disease-centered. Timeless calls for person-centered care will not gain traction until unfettered biomedicalism's inherent appeal is properly understood and counterbalanced. Our analysis suggests that unfettered biomedicalism is not merely an economic problem (Relman, 1994) that could be fixed with an economic overhaul (although financing changes would be helpful). It is not merely a behavior problem (Berwick & Hackbarth, 2012) that could be fixed by incentivizing or exhorting clinicians to change their habits[2] (although behavior change would be desirable). It is not an educational problem (Eisenberg, 1988) that could be fixed by adding coursework in psychology and social sciences to the curriculum (although curricular changes aimed at modifying the culture of care delivery would help). Nor is it a human resources problem that could be fixed, as some have suggested, by modifying the criteria used to select medical students. As he lay dying, Franz Ingelfinger (1980), former editor of the *New England Journal of Medicine*, wrote an essay on arrogance that was published posthumously. In it, he mused, "One might suggest ... that only those who have been hospitalized during their adolescent or adult years be admitted to medical school. Such a practice would ... increase the number of empathic doctors." Ingelfinger understood that empathy is in short supply in medicine but he seemed to believe that empathy is a fixed, static entity, and it is not (Schumann, Zaki, & Dweck, 2014).

Our analysis suggests that unfettered biomedicalism is, above all, a social norm problem that affects how patients and providers alike think about themselves and their roles. All norms, even those with deep historical roots (Clarke et al., 2009) involving the expression of care and empathy, are modifiable. By re-engineering encounters between patients and clinicians at the point-of-care, and offering far more options for care than are currently available (Wittink et al., 2013), we hypothesize that patients will be more likely to get the care they need and no more, and the care they want and no less. As a result, suffering, and suicide risk, will be mitigated.

Suicidologists have long known that large samples are needed to demonstrate that any intervention has a real, robust, and sustained effect on the suicide rate. Enterprising scholars interested in suicide may wish to spend more of their precious time exploring the effects of laws, regulations, or policy changes than studying specific treatments in small samples

---

[2] In a speech on December 3, 2013 at the Lown Conference *From Avoidable Care to Right Care*, Don Berwick said professionals must "unlearn disciplinary habits of excellence... not venal ones....It's going to take a very deep breath to drop back and begin to ask the question 'what do I do that heals, and what do I do that does not?'" A video of the speech is available here: http://www.youtube.com/watch?v=TkV5tnNulP4.

(Lewis, Hawton, & Jones, 1997). The PPACA includes many provisions, such as patient-centered medical homes and IT innovations, that could improve person-centeredness. Time will tell whether implementation of the PPACA decreases suffering and suicide risk in older adults.

References

Ahmedani, B. K., Simon, G. E., Stewart, C., Beck, A., Waitzfelder, B. E., Rossom, R., et al. (2014). Health care contacts in the year before suicide death. *Journal of General Internal Medicine, 29*(6), 870–877.

Alexopoulos, G. S., Reynolds, C. F., III, et al., Bruce, M. L., Katz, I. R., Raue, P. J., Mulsant, B. H., et al. (2009). Reducing suicidal ideation and depression in older primary care patients: 24-month outcomes of the PROSPECT study. *The American Journal of Psychiatry, 166*(8), 882–890.

Almeida, O. P., Pirkis, J., Kerse, N., Sim, M., Flicker, L., Snowdon, J., et al. (2012). A randomized trial to reduce the prevalence of depression and self-harm behavior in older primary care patients. *Annals of Family Medicine, 10*(4), 347–356.

Angell, M. (1997). The Supreme Court and physician-assisted suicide – The ultimate right. *The New England Journal of Medicine, 336*(1), 50–53.

Angell, M., & Relman, A. (2002). Patients, profits, and American medicine: Conflicts of interest in the testing and marketing of new drugs. *Daedalus, 131*(2), 102–111.

Baltes, P. B. (1997). On the incomplete architecture of human ontogeny: Selection, optimization, and compensation as foundation of developmental theory. *American Psychologist, 52*(4), 366–380.

Barnato, A. E., Mohan, D., Lane, R. K., Huang, Y. M., Angus, D. C., Farris, C., et al. (2014). Advance care planning norms may contribute to hospital variation in end-of-life ICU use: A simulation study. *Medical Decision Making, 34*(4), 473–484.

Becker, E. (1973). *The denial of death.* New York, NY: Free Press.

Bertakis, K. D., & Azari, R. (2011). Patient-centered care is associated with decreased health care utilization. *Journal of the American Board of Family Medicine, 24*(3), 229–239.

Berwick, D. M. (2009). The epitaph of profession. *The British Journal of General Practice, 59*(559), 128–131.

Berwick, D. M., & Hackbarth, A. D. (2012). Eliminating waste in US health care. *Journal of the American Medical Association, 307*(14), 1513–1516.

Boudreaux, E. D., & Horowitz, L. (2014). Suicide risk screening and assessment: Designing instruments with dissemination in mind. American Journal of Preventive Medicine, 47(3S2), S163–S169.

Breggin, P. R. (1991). *Toxic psychiatry: Why therapy, empathy, and love must replace the drugs, electroshock, and biochemical theories of the "new psychiatry".* New York, NY: St Martin's Press.

Brickman, P., Rabinowitz, V. C., Karuza, J., Coates, D., Cohn, E., & Kidder, L. (1982). Models of helping and coping. *American Psychologist, 37*(4), 368–384.

Brown, T. M. (1998). George Canby Robinson and the "patient as a person". In C. Lawrence & G. Weisz (Eds.), *Greater than the parts: Holism in biomedicine 1920–1950* (pp. 136–160). New York, NY: Oxford University Press.

Brownlee, S. (2007). *Overtreated: Why too much medicine is making us sicker and poorer.* New York, NY: Bloomsbury.

Bruce, M. L., Ten Have, T. R., Reynolds, C. F., III, et al., Katz, I. I., Schulberg, H. C., Mulsant, B. H., et al. (2004). Reducing suicidal ideation and depressive symptoms in depressed older primary care patients: A randomized controlled trial. *Journal of the American Medical Association, 291*(9), 1081–1091.

Burke, B. L., Martens, A., & Faucher, E. H. (2010). Two decades of terror management theory: A meta-analysis of mortality salience research. *Personality and Social Psychology Review*, 14(2), 155–195.

Carstensen, L. L., Isaacowitz, D. M., & Charles, S. T. (1999). Taking time seriously. A theory of socioemotional selectivity. *The American Psychologist*, 54(3), 165–181.

Carter, G. L., Clover, K., Whyte, I. M., Dawson, A. H., & D'Este, C. (2013). Postcards from the EDge: 5-year outcomes of a randomised controlled trial for hospital-treated self-poisoning. *British Journal of Psychiatry*, 202(5), 372–380.

Cassel, E. J. (1982). The nature of suffering and the goals of medicine. *The New England Journal of Medicine*, 306(11), 639–645.

Chamberlain, P. I. (2014). An assisted dying law might save me from a lingering and unpleasant death. *BMJ (Clinical Research Ed.)*, 349, g4784.

Charlton, B. G. (2009). Why are modern scientists so dull? how science selects for perseverance and sociability at the expense of intelligence and creativity. *Medical Hypotheses*, 72(3), 237–243.

Clarke, A. E., Mamo, L., Fosket, J. R., Fishman, J. R., & Shim, J. K. (Eds.), (2009). *Biomedicalization: Technoscience, health, and illness in the US*. Durham, NC: Duke University Press.

Conwell, Y. (1994). Physician-assisted suicide: A mental health perspective. *Suicide & Life-Threatening Behavior*, 24(4), 326–333.

Conwell, Y., Duberstein, P. R., Hirsch, J. K., Conner, K. R., Eberly, S., & Caine, E. D. (2010). Health status and suicide in the second half of life. *International Journal of Geriatric Psychiatry*, 25(4), 371–379.

Coulehan, J. (2009). Compassionate solidarity: Suffering, poetry, and medicine. *Perspectives in Biology and Medicine*, 52(4), 585–603.

Coulter, A., & Collins, A. (2011). *Making shared decision-making a reality: No decision about me, without me*. London, UK: The King's Fund.

Coupland, C., Dhiman, P., Morriss, R., Arthur, A., Barton, G., & Hippisley-Cox, J. (2011). Antidepressant use and risk of adverse outcomes in older people: Population based cohort study. *BMJ (Clinical Research Ed.)*, 343, d4551.

Crits-Christoph, P., Gibbons, M. B. C., Hamilton, J., Ring-Kurtz, S., & Gallop, R. (2011). The dependability of alliance assessments: The alliance-outcome correlation is larger than you might think. *Journal of Consulting and Clinical Psychology*, 79(3), 267–278.

Cunningham, J., Sirey, J. A., & Bruce, M. L. (2007). Matching services to patients' beliefs about depression in Dublin, Ireland. *Psychiatric Services*, 58(5), 696–699.

Cutler, D., Skinner, J., Stern, A. D., & Wennberg, D. (2013). *Physician beliefs and patient preferences: A new look at regional variation in health care spending. (NBER Working Paper No. 19320)*. Cambridge, MA: National Bureau of Economic Research.

Dar-Nimrod, I., & Heine, S. J. (2011). Genetic essentialism: On the deceptive determinism of DNA. *Psychological Bulletin*, 137(5), 800–818.

Deci, E. L., Koestner, R., & Ryan, R. M. (1999). A meta-analytic review of experiments examining the effects of extrinsic rewards on intrinsic motivation. *Psychological Bulletin*, 125(6), 627–668. (discussion 692–700).

Doran, T., Kontopantelis, E., Valderas, J. M., Campbell, S., Roland, M., Salisbury, C., et al. (2011). Effect of financial incentives on incentivised and non-incentivised clinical activities: Longitudinal analysis of data from the UK quality and outcomes framework. *BMJ (Clinical Research Ed.)*, 342, d3590.

Douglas, M. (1986). *How institutions think*. Syracuse, NY: Syracuse University Press.

Dowrick, C., & Frances, A. (2013). Medicalising unhappiness: New classification of depression risks more patients being put on drug treatment from which they will not benefit. *BMJ (Clinical Research Ed.)*, 347, f7140.

Dowrick, C., Leydon, G. M., McBride, A., Howe, A., Burgess, H., Clarke, P., et al. (2009). Patients' and doctors' views on depression severity questionnaires incentivised in UK quality and outcomes framework: Qualitative study. *BMJ (Clinical Research Ed.)*, 338, 1–6.

Drought, T. S., & Koenig, B. A. (2002). "Choice" in end-of-life decision making: Researching fact or fiction? *The Gerontologist, 42*(Spec No 3), 114–128.

Duberstein, P. R., Conwell, Y., Conner, K. R., Eberly, S., & Caine, E. D. (2004b). Suicide at 50 years of age and older: Perceived physical illness, family discord and financial strain. *Psychological Medicine, 34*(1), 137–146.

Duberstein, P. R., Conwell, Y., Conner, K. R., Eberly, S., Evinger, J. S., & Caine, E. D. (2004a). Poor social integration and suicide: Fact or artifact? A case–control study. *Psychological Medicine, 34*(7), 1331–1337.

Duberstein, P. R., & Heisel, M. J. (2014). Person-centered prevention of suicide among older adults. In M. Nock (Ed.), *Oxford handbook of suicide and self-injury* (pp. 113–132). New York, NY: Oxford University Press.

Duberstein, P. R., Heisel, M. J., & Conwell, Y. (2011). Suicide in older adults. In M. E. Agronin & G. J. Maletta (Eds.), *Principles and practice of geriatric psychiatry* (pp. 451–463) (2nd ed.). Philadelphia, PA: Walters Kluwer Health/LWW.

Duberstein, P. R., & Jerant, A. F. (2014). Suicide prevention in primary care: Optimistic humanism imagined and engineered. *Journal of General Internal Medicine.*

Duberstein, P. R., Wittink, M., & Pigeon, W. (in press). Person-centered suicide prevention in primary care. In G. R. Sullivan, L. James, & B. Bongar (Eds.), *Handbook of suicide in veterans and military populations.* New York: Oxford University Press.

Eisenberg, L. (1988). Science in medicine: Too much or too little and too limited in scope? *The American Journal of Medicine, 84*(3 Pt 1), 483–491.

Engel, G. (1992). How much longer must medicine's science be bound by a 17th-century world-view? *Psychotherapy and Psychosomatics, 57*(1–2), 3–16.

Engel, G. L. (1980). The clinical application of the biopsychosocial model. *American Journal of Psychiatry, 137*(5), 535–544.

Entwistle, V. A., Carter, S. M., Cribb, A., & McCaffery, K. (2010). Supporting patient autonomy: The importance of clinician–patient relationships. *Journal of General Internal Medicine, 25*(7), 741–745.

Epstein, R. M., Duberstein, P. R., Feldman, M. D., Rochlen, A. B., Bell, R. A., Kravitz, R. L., et al. (2010). "I didn't know what was wrong:" How people with undiagnosed depression recognize, name and explain their distress. *Journal of General Internal Medicine, 25*(9), 954–961.

Epstein, R. M., Franks, P., Fiscella, K., Shields, G. C., Meldrum, S. C., Kravitz, R. L., et al. (2005). Measuring patient-centered communication in patient-physician consultations: Theoretical and practical issues. *Social Science & Medicine, 61*(7), 1516–1528.

Erlangsen, A., Agerbo, E., Hawton, K., & Conwell, Y. (2009). Early discontinuation of antidepressant treatment and suicide risk among persons aged 50 and over: A population-based register study. *Journal of Affective Disorders, 119*(1–3), 194–199.

Ernst, C., Lalovic, A., Lesage, A., Seguin, M., Tousignant, M., & Turecki, G. (2004). Suicide and no axis I psychopathology. *BMC Psychiatry, 4*, 7.

Fang, F., Fall, K., Mittleman, M. A., Sparen, P., Ye, W., Adami, H., et al. (2012). Suicide and cardiovascular death after a cancer diagnosis. *New England Journal of Medicine, 366*(14), 1310–1318.

Fassberg, M. M., Ostling, S., Borjesson-Hanson, A., Skoog, I., & Waern, M. (2013). Suicidal feelings in the twilight of life: A cross-sectional population-based study of 97-year-olds. *BMJ Open, 3*(2), 10.

Flueckiger, C., Del Re, A. C., Wampold, B. E., Symonds, D., & Horvath, A. O. (2012). How central is the alliance in psychotherapy? A multilevel longitudinal meta-analysis. *Journal of Counseling Psychology, 59*(1), 10–17.

Foley, K. M. (1997). Competent care for the dying instead of physician-assisted suicide. *The New England Journal of Medicine, 336*(1), 54–58.

Frank, A. W. (1997). Illness as moral occasion: Restoring agency to ill people. *Health, 1*(2), 131–148.

Freidson, E. (1970). *Professional dominance: The social structure of medical care*. New York, NY: Atherton Press.

Fulmer, C. A., Gelfand, M. J., Kruglanski, A. W., Kim-Prieto, C., Diener, E., Pierro, A., et al. (2010). On "feeling right" in cultural contexts: How person-culture match affects self-esteem and subjective well-being. *Psychological Science, 21*(11), 1563–1569.

Gallo, J. J., Morales, K. H., Bogner, H. R., Raue, P. J., Zee, J., Bruce, M. L., et al. (2013). Long term effect of depression care management on mortality in older adults: Follow-up of cluster randomized clinical trial in primary care. *BMJ (Clinical Research Ed.), 346*, f2570.

Ganzini, L., Denneson, L. M., Press, N., Bair, M. J., Helmer, D. A., Poat, J., et al. (2013). Trust is the basis for effective suicide risk screening and assessment in veterans. *Journal of General Internal Medicine, 28*(9), 1215–1221.

Gask, L., Bower, P., Lamb, J., Burroughs, H., Chew-Graham, C., Edwards, S., AMP Research Group, (2012). Improving access to psychosocial interventions for common mental health problems in the United Kingdom: Narrative review and development of a conceptual model for complex interventions. *BMC Health Services Research, 12*, 249. 6963-12-249.

Gask, L., Dowrick, C., Dixon, C., Sutton, C., Perry, R., Torgerson, D., et al. (2004). A pragmatic cluster randomized controlled trial of an educational intervention for GPs in the assessment and management of depression. *Psychological Medicine, 34*(1), 63–72.

Gelman, S. A. (2003). *The essential child: Origins of essentialism in everyday thought*. New York, NY: Oxford University Press.

Gerstorf, D., Ram, N., Mayraz, G., Hidajat, M., Lindenberger, U., Wagner, G. G., et al. (2010). Late-life decline in well-being across adulthood in Germany, the United Kingdom, and the United States: Something is seriously wrong at the end of life. *Psychology and Aging, 25*(2), 477–485.

Good, B. J., & DelVecchio-Good, M. J. (1993). "Learning medicine": The construction of medical knowledge at Harvard Medical School. In S. Lindenbaum & M. M. Lock (Eds.), *Knowledge, power, and practice: The anthropology of medicine and everyday life* (pp. 81–107). Berkeley, CA: University of California Press.

Graham, R. G., & Martin, G. I. (2012). Health behavior: A Darwinian reconceptualization. *American Journal of Preventive Medicine, 43*(4), 451–455.

Greenberg, J., Pyszczynski, T., & Solomon, S. (1986). The causes and consequences of a need for self-esteem: A terror management theory. In R. F. Baumeister (Ed.), *Public self and private self* (pp. 189–212). New York, NY: Springer-Verlag.

Griffiths, J. J., Zarate, C. A., Jr., & Rasimas, J. J. (2014). Existing and novel biological therapeutics in suicide prevention. *American Journal of Preventive Medicine, 47*(3 Suppl. 2), S195–S203.

Habermas, J. (1991). *On the logic of the social sciences* (S. W. Nicholsen, J. A. Stark, Trans.). Cambridge, MA: MIT Press.

Hamburg, M. A., & Collins, F. S. (2010). The path to personalized medicine. *The New England Journal of Medicine, 363*(4), 301–304.

Hampton, L. M., Daubresse, M., Chang, H. Y., Alexander, G. C., & Budnitz, D. S. (2014). Emergency department visits by adults for psychiatric medication adverse events. *JAMA Psychiatry, 71*(9), 1006–1014.

Hart, J. T. (1971). Inverse care law. *Lancet, 1*(7696), 405–412.

Harwood, D., Hawton, K., Hope, T., & Jacoby, R. (2006a). Suicide in older people without psychiatric disorder. *International Journal of Geriatric Psychiatry, 21*(4), 363–367.

Harwood, D. M., Hawton, K., Hope, T., Harriss, L., & Jacoby, R. (2006b). Life problems and physical illness as risk factors for suicide in older people: A descriptive and case–control study. *Psychological Medicine, 36*(9), 1265–1274.

Heisel, M. J., & Duberstein, P. R. (2005). Suicide prevention in older adults. *Clinical Psychology: Science and Practice, 12*(3), 242–259.

Henke, R. M., McGuire, T. G., Zaslavsky, A. M., Ford, D. E., Meredith, L. S., & Arbelaez, J. J. (2008). Clinician- and organization-level factors in the adoption of evidence-based care for depression in primary care. *Health Care Management Review*, *33*(4), 289–299.

Hjelmeland, H., Dieserud, G., Dyregrov, K., Knizek, B. L., & Leenaars, A. A. (2012). Psychological autopsy studies as diagnostic tools: Are they methodologically flawed? *Death Studies*, *36*(7), 605–626.

Hoerger, M., Chapman, B. P., Epstein, R. M., & Duberstein, P. R. (2012). Emotional intelligence: A theoretical framework for individual differences in affective forecasting. *Emotion*, *12*(4), 716–725.

Horvath, A. O., Del Re, A. C., Flueckiger, C., & Symonds, D. (2011). Alliance in individual psychotherapy. *Psychotherapy*, *48*(1), 9–16.

Ingelfinger, F. J. (1980). Arrogance. *The New England Journal of Medicine*, *303*(26), 1507–1511.

Institute of Medicine, (2001). *Crossing the quality chasm: A new health system for the 21st century*. Washington, DC: National Academies Press.

Jha, A. K., Joynt, K. E., Orav, E. J., & Epstein, A. M. (2012). The long-term effect of premier pay for performance on patient outcomes. *The New England Journal of Medicine*, *366*(17), 1606–1615.

Jobes, D. A. (1995). The challenge and the promise of clinical suicidology. *Suicide & Life-Threatening Behavior*, *25*(4), 437–449.

Kahneman, D. (2011). *Thinking, fast and slow*. New York, NY: Farrar Straus & Giroux.

Kaufman, S. R. (1998). Intensive care, old age, and the problem of death in America. *The Gerontologist*, *38*(6), 715–725.

Keil, F. C. (2012). Running on empty? How folk science gets by with less. *Current Directions in Psychological Science*, *21*(5), 329–334.

Kelley, J. M., Kraft-Todd, G., Schapira, L., Kossowsky, J., & Riess, H. (2014). The influence of the patient-clinician relationship on healthcare outcomes: A systematic review and meta-analysis of randomized controlled trials. *PloS One*, *9*(4), e94207.

Kjolseth, I., Ekeberg, O., & Steihaug, S. (2010). Why suicide? Elderly people who committed suicide and their experience of life in the period before their death. *International Psychogeriatrics*, *22*(2), 209–218.

Koenig, H. G. (1993). Legalizing physician-assisted suicide: Some thoughts and concerns. *The Journal of Family Practice*, *37*(2), 171–179.

Kravitz, R. L., Epstein, R. M., Feldman, M. D., Franz, C. E., Azari, R., Wilkes, M. S., et al. (2005). Influence of patients' requests for direct-to-consumer advertised antidepressants: A randomized controlled trial. *Journal of the American Medical Association*, *293*(16), 1995–2002.

Kravitz, R. L., Franks, P., Feldman, M. D., Tancredi, D. J., Slee, C. A., Epstein, R. M., et al. (2013). Patient engagement programs for recognition and initial treatment of depression in primary care: A randomized trial. *Journal of the American Medical Association*, *310*(17), 1818–1828.

Kuhn, T. S. (1970). *The structure of scientific revolutions* (2nd ed.). Chicago, IL: University of Chicago Press.

Kushner, H. I. (1991). *American suicide: A psychocultural exploration*. New Brunswick, NJ: Rutgers University Press.

Kvaale, E. P., Gottdiener, W. H., & Haslam, N. (2013a). Biogenetic explanations and stigma: A meta-analytic review of associations among laypeople. *Social Science & Medicine*, *96*, 95–103. (1982).

Kvaale, E. P., Haslam, N., & Gottdiener, W. H. (2013b). The "side effects" of medicalization: A meta-analytic review of how biogenetic explanations affect stigma. *Clinical Psychology Review*, *33*(6), 782–794.

Lampe, L., Fritz, K., Boyce, P., Starcevic, V., Brakoulias, V., Walter, G., et al. (2013). Psychiatrists and GPs: Diagnostic decision making, personality profiles and attitudes toward depression and anxiety. *Australasian Psychiatry*, *21*(3), 231–237.

Landau, M. J., Johns, M., Greenberg, J., Pyszczynski, T., Martens, A., Goldenberg, J. L., et al. (2004). A function of form: Terror management and structuring the social world. *Journal of Personality and Social Psychology, 87*(2), 190–210.

Larson, E. B., & Yao, X. (2005). Clinical empathy as emotional labor in the patient-physician relationship. *The Journal of the American Medical Association, 293*(9), 1100–1106.

Le Fanu, J. (2012). *The rise and fall of modern medicine* (2nd ed.). New York, NY: Basic Books.

LeFevre, M. L., & US Preventive Services Task Force, (2014). Screening for suicide risk in adolescents, adults, and older adults in primary care: U.S. preventive services task force recommendation statement. *Annals of Internal Medicine, 160*(10), 719–726.

Lewis, G., Hawton, K., & Jones, P. (1997). Strategies for preventing suicide. *The British Journal of Psychiatry, 171*, 351–354.

Lown, B. (1999). *The lost art of healing: Practicing compassion in medicine.* New York, NY: Ballantine Books/Random House.

Luoma, J. B., Martin, C. E., & Pearson, J. L. (2002). Contact with mental health and primary care providers before suicide: A review of the evidence. *The American Journal of Psychiatry, 159*(6), 909–916.

Lynn, J. (2013). Reliable and sustainable comprehensive care for frail elderly people. *Journal of the American Medical Association, 310*(18), 1935–1936.

Marino, S., Gallo, J. J., Ford, D., & Anthony, J. C. (1995). Filters on the pathway to mental-health-care. 1. incident mental-disorders. *Psychological Medicine, 25*(6), 1135–1148.

Marques, J. M., Abrams, D., Paez, D., & Martinez-Taboada, C. (1998). The role of categorization and in-group norms in judgments of groups and their members. *Journal of Personality and Social Psychology, 75*(4), 976–988.

Martens, A., Burke, B. L., Schimel, J., & Faucher, E. H. (2011). Same but different: Meta-analytically examining the uniqueness of mortality salience effects. *European Journal of Social Psychology, 41*, 6–10.

May, R. (1969). *Love and will.* New York, NY: Norton.

McCrae, R. R., & Costa, P. T., Jr. (1990). *Personality in adulthood.* New York, NY: Guilford Press.

Meier, D. E. (2014). "I don't want Jenny to think I'm abandoning her": Views on overtreatment. *Health Affairs (Project Hope), 33*(5), 895–898.

Meier, D. E., Back, A. L., & Morrison, R. S. (2001). The inner life of physicians and care of the seriously ill. *The Journal of the American Medical Association, 286*(23), 3007–3014.

Menzies, I. (1960). A case study in the functioning of social systems as a defense against anxiety. *Human Relations, 13*, 95–121.

Miles, S. H. (1994). Physicians and their patient's suicides. *Journal of the American Medical Association, 271*(22), 1786–1788.

Mojtabai, R. (2013). Clinician-identified depression in community settings: Concordance with structured-interview diagnoses. *Psychotherapy and Psychosomatics, 82*(3), 161–169.

Moller, A. C., Ryan, R. M., & Deci, E. L. (2006). Self-determination theory and public policy: Improving the quality of consumer decisions without using coercion. *Journal of Public Policy & Marketing, 25*(1), 104–116.

Mount, B. (1986). Dealing with our losses. *Journal of Clinical Oncology, 4*(7), 1127–1134.

Neeleman, J. (2002). Beyond risk theory: Suicidal behavior in its social and epidemiological context. *Crisis, 23*(3), 114–120.

Ng, J. Y. Y., Ntoumanis, N., Thogersen-Ntoumani, C., Deci, E. L., Ryan, R. M., Duda, J. L., et al. (2012). Self-determination theory applied to health contexts: A meta-analysis. *Perspectives on Psychological Science, 7*(4), 325–340.

Niemiec, C. P., Brown, K. W., Kashdan, T. B., Cozzolino, P. J., Breen, W. E., Levesque-Bristol, C., et al. (2010). Being present in the face of existential threat: The role of trait mindfulness in reducing defensive responses to mortality salience. *Journal of Personality and Social Psychology, 99*(2), 344–365.

Oregon Public Health Division (2014). *2013 Death with dignity act report*. Available at: <http://public.health.oregon.gov/ProviderPartnerResources/EvaluationResearch/DeathwithDignityAct/Documents/year16.pdf>.

Owens, C., Booth, N., Briscoe, M., Lawrence, C., & Lloyd, K. (2003). Suicide outside the care of mental health services: A case-controlled psychological autopsy study. *Crisis, 24*, 113–121.

Petry, N. M., Andrade, L. F., Barry, D., & Byrne, S. (2013). A randomized study of reinforcing ambulatory exercise in older adults. *Psychology and Aging, 28*(4), 1164–1173.

Pincus, H. A. (2003). The future of behavioral health and primary care: Drowning in the mainstream or left on the bank? *Psychosomatics, 44*(1), 1–11.

Proulx, T., & Heine, S. J. (2006). Death and black diamonds: Meaning, mortality, and the meaning maintenance model. *Psychological Inquiry, 17*(4), 309–318.

Relman, A. S. (1994). The impact of market forces on the physician-patient relationship. *Journal of the Royal Society of Medicine, 87*(Suppl. 22), 22–24. (discussion 24–25).

Renkema, L. J., Stapel, D. A., & Van Yperen, N. W. (2008). Go with the flow: Conforming to others in the face of existential threat. *European Journal of Social Psychology, 38*(4), 747–756.

Rogers, C. R. (1951). *Client-centered therapy: Its current practice, implications and theory*. London, UK: Constable.

Rogers, C. R. (1961). *On becoming a person; A therapist's view of psychotherapy*. Boston, MA: Houghton Mifflin.

Rubenowitz, E., Waern, M., Wilhelmson, K., & Allebeck, P. (2001). Life events and psychosocial factors in elderly suicides – A case-control study. *Psychological Medicine, 31*(7), 1193–1202.

Rutter, M. J. (1986). Meyerian psychobiology. personality development, and the role of life experiences. *American Journal of Psychiatry, 143*, 1077–1087.

Rutz, W. (2001). Preventing suicide and premature death by education and treatment. *Journal of Affective Disorders, 62*(1–2), 123–129.

Ryan, R. M., & Deci, E. L. (2000). Self-determination theory and the facilitation of intrinsic motivation, social development, and well-being. *American Psychologist, 55*(1), 68–78.

Schumann, K., Zaki, J., & Dweck, C. S. (2014). Addressing the empathy deficit: Beliefs about the malleability of empathy predict effortful responses when empathy is challenging. *Journal of Personality and Social Psychology, 107*(3), 475–493.

Shah, R., Franks, P., Jerant, A., Feldman, M., Duberstein, P., Fernandez y Garcia, E., et al. (2014). The effect of targeted and tailored patient depression engagement interventions on clinician inquiry about suicidal thoughts: A randomized control trial. *Journal of General Internal Medicine, 29*, 1148–1154.

Shneidman, E. S. (1992). Rational suicide and psychiatric disorders. *The New England Journal of Medicine, 326*(13), 889–890. (author reply 890–891).

Shneidman, E. S. (1993). Suicide as psychache. *The Journal of Nervous and Mental Disease, 181*(3), 145–147.

Simon, L., Greenberg, J., Arndt, J., Pyszczynski, T., Clement, R., & Solomon, S. (1997). Perceived consensus, uniqueness, and terror management: Compensatory responses to threats to inclusion and distinctiveness following mortality salience. *Personality and Social Psychology Bulletin, 23*(10), 1055–1065.

Solomon, S., & Lawlor, K. (2011). Death anxiety: The challenge and the promise of whole person care. In T. A. Hutchinson (Ed.), *Whole person care: A new paradigm for the 21st century* (pp. 97–107). New York, NY: Springer Science + Business Media.

Stange, K., Zyzanski, S., Jaen, C., Callahan, E., Kelly, R., Gillanders, W., et al. (1998). Illuminating the "black box" – A description of 4454 patient visits to 138 family physicians. *Journal of Family Practice, 46*(5), 377–389.

Starfield, B. (2011). Is patient-centered care the same as person-focused care? *Permanente Journal, 15*(2), 63–69.

Street, R. L. J., Makoul, G., Arora, N. K., & Epstein, R. M. (2009). How does communication heal? Pathways linking clinician-patient communication to health outcomes. *Patient Education and Counseling, 74*(3), 295–301.

Sullivan, M. (2003). The new subjective medicine: Taking the patient's point of view on health care and health. *Social Science & Medicine, 56*(7), 1595–1604.

Szanto, K., Dombrovski, A. Y., Sahakian, B. J., Mulsant, B. H., Houck, P. R., Reynolds, C. F., et al. (2012). Social emotion recognition, social functioning, and attempted suicide in late-life depression. *The American Journal of Geriatric Psychiatry, 20*(3), 257–265.

Szasz, T. (1974). *The myth of mental illness (rev. ed.)*. New York: Harper & Row.

Tebes, J. K., Thai, N. D., & Matlin, S. L. (2014). Twenty-first century science as a relational process: From Eureka! to team science and a place for community psychology. *American Journal of Community Psychology, 53*(3–4), 475–490.

Tinetti, M. E. (2012). The retreat from advanced care planning. *Journal of the American Medical Association, 307*(9), 915–916.

Tuomi, I. (1999). Data is more than knowledge: Implications of the reversed knowledge hierarchy for knowledge management and organizational memory. *Systems Sciences, 1999. HICSS-32. Proceedings of the 32nd annual Hawaii international conference on system sciences.*

Turvey, C. L., Conwell, Y., Jones, M. P., Phillips, C., Simonsick, E., Pearson, J. L., et al. (2002). Risk factors for late-life suicide: A prospective, community-based study. *The American Journal of Geriatric Psychiatry, 10*(4), 398–406.

Unützer, J., Tang, L., Oishi, S., Katon, W., Williams, J. W., Jr., et al., Hunkeler, E., et al. (2006). Reducing suicidal ideation in depressed older primary care patients. *Journal of the American Geriatrics Society, 54*(10), 1550–1556.

Useda, J. D., Duberstein, P. R., Conner, K. R., Beckman, A., Franus, N., Tu, X., et al. (2007). Personality differences in attempted suicide versus suicide in adults 50 years of age or older. *Journal of Consulting and Clinical Psychology, 75*(1), 126–133.

Vaiva, G., Vaiva, G., Ducrocq, F., Meyer, P., Mathieu, D., Philippe, A., et al. (2006). Effect of telephone contact on further suicide attempts in patients discharged from an emergency department: Randomised controlled study. *BMJ (Clinical Research Ed.), 332*(7552), 1241–1245.

Vannoy, S. D., Tai-Seale, M., Duberstein, P., Eaton, L. J., & Cook, M. A. (2011). Now what should I do? Primary care physicians' responses to older adults expressing thoughts of suicide. *Journal of General Internal Medicine, 26*(9), 1005–1011.

Waern, M., Rubenowitz, E., Runeson, B., Skoog, I., Wilhelmson, K., & Allebeck, P. (2002). Burden of illness and suicide in elderly people: Case-control study. *BMJ (Clinical Research Ed.), 324*(7350), 1355.

Wittink, M. N., Barg, F. K., & Gallo, J. J. (2006). Unwritten rules of talking to doctors about depression: Integrating qualitative and quantitative methods. *The Annals of Family Medicine, 4*(4), 302–309.

Wittink, M. N., Duberstein, P., & Lyness, J. (2013). Late life depression in the primary care setting: Building the case for customized care. In H. Lavretsky, M. Sajatovic, & C. Reynolds (Eds.), *Late life mood disorders* (pp. 500–515). New York, NY: Oxford University Press.

Wittink, M. N., Givens, J. L., Knott, K. A., Coyne, J. C., & Barg, F. K. (2011). Negotiating depression treatment with older adults: Primary care providers' perspectives. *Journal of Mental Health, 20*(5), 429–437.

Wittink, M. N., Joo, J. H., Lewis, L. M., & Barg, F. K. (2009). Losing faith and using faith: Older African Americans discuss spirituality, religious activities, and depression. *Journal of General Internal Medicine, 24*(3), 402–407.

9

End-of-Life Care

Elizabeth C. Gundersen

Florida Atlantic University, Boca Raton, Florida, USA

INTRODUCTION

"If you come into this hospital, we're not going to let you die."

There are multiple ways to interpret these famous words uttered by UCLA Medical Center CEO Dr. David T. Feinberg. While the intent may have been reassurance that patients were top priority, this seemingly admirable mission to save lives encapsulates what has become a highly controversial, emotionally laden debate throughout the nation. As life expectancy in the United States continues to grow, so does the perception among many Americans, conscious or not, that death is "optional."

Physicians and other health care providers are generally trained to restore or preserve health and fight illness. Comparatively little time is spent learning how to treat, manage, and communicate with patients at the end of life (Bickel-Swenson, 2007). In part this should not be surprising given the significant existential challenge and psychological discomfort death represents for patients, families, and clinicians alike. Yet while most people are intellectually aware that death is a biological certainty, very few are equipped to prepare for it emotionally. This is best reflected in the nation's current health care system in which inadequate end-of-life care leads to increased conflict, stress, and depression among patients, families, and the health care team (Detering, Hancock, Reade, & Sylvester, 2010).

This chapter addresses multiple factors compromising the ability of the nation's health care system to deliver quality end-of-life care. Consistent with the prevailing themes of this publication, the relevance of beliefs and behavior is emphasized, as are current gaps in end-of-life care that clinical geropsychologists are most qualified to fill.

B. Bensadon (Ed): *Psychology and Geriatrics.*
DOI: http://dx.doi.org/10.1016/B978-0-12-420123-1.00009-5

THE CURRENT STATE OF END-OF-LIFE CARE

What is end-of-life care? While many may immediately think of the last days or hours of a person's life, this may not be entirely accurate. End-of-life care refers to the services provided to terminally ill patients whose incurable disease has advanced to a stage near death. Such care may span weeks, months, or even years and applies to multiple disease states. In the United States, most people aged 65 and over die from chronic conditions such as heart disease, cerebrovascular disease, chronic obstructive pulmonary disease, and dementia, while only about 22% of deaths are from cancer (Hogan et al., 2000). This distinction is especially important since it is more difficult to predict the timing of death from chronic diseases other than cancer, and this difficulty often translates into increased vulnerability of these patients and their families.

Generally, chronic disease is characterized by steadily declining health and periodic exacerbations of illness resulting in multiple hospitalizations (Lynn, 2001; Lynn, Schall, Milne, Nolan, & Kabcenell, 2000). During these episodes, patients may come quite close to dying but, through medical intervention, are stabilized enough to be discharged from the hospital. Underlying disease is not cured and the patient and family may not be told that the disease is terminal. Further, although the course of chronic disease usually includes future bouts of "critical" illness, the patient's personal preferences for care are all too often not elicited, leading to repeated health crises for which patients and their families are unprepared (Frost, Cook, Heyland, & Fowler, 2011). But why?

COMMUNICATION

End-of-life communication is vital. Effective clinical communication establishes trust, increases patient and family satisfaction, and prevents stress and conflict at the end of life. But when suboptimal, treatments, conditions, prognoses, and decision-making are extremely confusing (Baker et al., 2000; Danis, 1998; Hanson, Danis, & Garrett, 1997a; Lynn et al., 2000; Steinhauser et al., 2000; Teno et al., 2000; Teno, Stevens, Spernak, & Lynn, 1998). This is compounded when conversations regarding treatment options have not occurred with patients before they become incapacitated and unable to speak for themselves. When this occurs, family members or health care surrogates must determine the patient's wishes.

Trainees and junior physicians tend to learn the manner of communication that is modeled for them. Unfortunately, surveys suggest this training has been inadequate (Maguire, 1999). Often, trainees see few or poor examples of how to conduct sensitive conversations such as breaking bad news, facilitating a family meeting, or discussing advance directives. But when they do observe them, they are often appreciative. As a hospitalist, I recall telling a patient he had cancer in front of a resident physician in her final year of training. This was her first experience and she thanked me profusely.

The dearth of formal modeling makes it unsurprising to find so many physicians uncomfortable having these conversations. Physicians' own awareness of this lack of training and low perceived self-efficacy can put them at greater risk of burnout (Ramirez, Graham, Richards, Cull, & Gregory, 1996). Inadequate training and poor communication is a vicious (but resolvable) cycle.

Many patients assume physicians will broach these topics when the time is appropriate, but physicians often assume (or hope) patients will introduce them if they want to. Whether an understandable assumption or perhaps wishful thinking, there are two crucial points to remember:

1. patients, by definition, are the vulnerable party
2. the discomfort on both sides when facing end-of-life care often results in neither initiating the conversation.

Again, psychological discomfort and related reluctance likely explain some of the discrepancy between what patients want, in *theory*, and what they actually receive, in *practice*.

LANGUAGE MATTERS

Particularly revealing is the vocabulary used by physicians who are not adequately trained (DeBakey, 1966). In an attempt to be patient-centered when talking with families about diagnoses, some may ask, "How much would you like to know?" Families will not necessarily understand this question, so a better alternative would be "Is there anything you do not want to know about your diagnosis or condition?" Similarly, when discussing care preferences, families are often asked "Do you want us to do everything possible?" But it is only natural for most families to want "everything done" for their loved ones. Without accurate understanding of the available options and implications of each, anything less could be perceived as incomplete care.

In terms of treatment and management, families often hear "There's nothing more we can do." Again, while physicians may feel they are merely being honest and not sugarcoating the truth, this phrase may instill in patients and families a sense of hopelessness and even emotional abandonment, the implication being patients and families must now face the end of life alone. What's more, especially if clinical psychologists are part of the care, the phrase may simply be inaccurate. In such cases, there may be nothing more to do *medically*, but there is likely more that can be done *psychosocially*, such as holding a hand (Bensadon & Odenheimer, 2014), admitting limitations (Gawande, 2014), or delivering a final in-person goodbye (Meier, 2014). Language also affects clinical decision-making. How physicians inquire about cardiopulmonary resuscitation (CPR) influences whether patients and families choose that option. If asked whether the team should "allow natural death" as opposed to "resuscitate," more families will decide against CPR (Barnato & Arnold, 2013).

ADVANCE CARE PLANNING

Theoretically, advance care planning can solve some of these problems. Through this process patients make decisions about their health care ahead of time and share their wishes with others, for instance by documenting them in an advance directive. Advance directives include the patient's preferences for treatment options such as CPR, artificial nutrition and hydration, and other potentially life-prolonging treatments. The creation of advance directives has been promoted by the Patient Self Determination Act (PSDA), passed by Congress in 1991. This occurred in the wake of the emotionally charged Nancy Cruzan case that focused national attention on whether families have the right to withdraw artificial nutrition and other medical treatments from an incapacitated loved one.

The PSDA mandates that individuals receiving medical care be given written information about their rights to make decisions about their care. These include 1) the right to facilitate their own health care decisions; 2) the right to accept or refuse medical treatment, and 3) the right to establish an advance health care directive. Under the PSDA, all health care agencies must, by law, ask patients whether they have an advance directive and must recognize living wills and durable powers of attorney for health care.

Advance directives are often associated with many positive outcomes. Decades of data suggest patients who have talked to their physicians or families about their preferences for end-of-life care feel less anxious, more comfortable and empowered, and that their physicians better understand their treatment wishes (Smucker et al., 1993). Similarly, decision-makers who have discussed advance directives with a patient report increased confidence in predicting the patient's preferences as compared with decision-makers for patients without advance directives (Ditto et al., 2001). Yet, as shown by psychologist Angela Fagerlin and colleagues, while benefits of such discussion are clear theoretically, in practice they rarely occur (Fagerlin & Schneider, 2004; Fagerlin, Ditto, Hawkins, Schneider, & Smucker, 2002). In fact, a national survey revealed that while more than 90% of people think it's important to talk with their loved ones about their end-of-life care wishes, less than 30% have actually discussed what they or their family would want (The Conversation Project, 2013). Similar data were revealed by an earlier survey that showed 80% of people would want to talk to their physician about end-of-life care if they were seriously ill, yet only 7% have actually done so (California Health Care Foundation, 2012). These discrepancies between what people want to do and actually do persist, even though chronically ill patients often have repeated contact with the health care system as their conditions worsen and, thus, multiple opportunities to broach the topic with clinicians and vice versa. So what stands in the way of such discussion?

CONFLICT

Conflict is a common element of end-of-life care. Even though they can be beneficial, advance directives alone cannot prevent stress, which, when unrecognized and poorly managed, can lead to or exacerbate conflict, particularly when patients have not discussed their preferences with their families or surrogates. Interestingly, the advent of advance directives and the PSDA have not had much impact on resuscitation events (Baker, Einstadter, Husak, & Cebul, 2003; Connors Jr. et al., 1995; Danis et al., 1991; Ditto et al., 2001; Hanson, Tulsky, & Danis, 1997b; Molloy et al., 2000; Teno et al., 1997; Yates & Glick, 1997). In part this is due to the difficult and hypothetical nature of predicting one's choice in advance of the actual situation. At the same time, attempts to allow flexibility result in advance directives that are often too vague to be helpful and are not communicated effectively (Tulsky, Fischer, Rose, & Arnold, 1998). Family members may disagree with patients' preferences, and even if patient and family communicate well with each other about such directives, health care providers may be uncomfortable following them (Connors Jr. et al., 1995). In the current United States (U.S.) health care system, there is no identified expert on the team responsible for (or perhaps capable of) recognizing and addressing this discomfort. As a patient's condition changes, it may be difficult to interpret the advance directive or determine whether it should be applied. In short, advance directives can be considered critical but insufficient to ensure the delivery of quality end-of-life care.

A study of intensive care units (ICU) determined conflict was present in nearly a third of cases involving patients with longer than average stays (Studdert et al., 2003). Typically such conflicts are not between patients and clinicians but rather families and clinicians or even among the members of the health care team themselves. Many physicians and nurses may view conflict as negative and something to be avoided. Because of related psychological discomfort, clinicians may avoid communicating with patients and families or do it poorly, leading to feelings of distrust. Conversely, when conflict is managed well at the end of life, it can lead to better relationships, clearer decision-making, and ultimately higher satisfaction among all involved (Back & Arnold, 2005). Consistent with themes throughout this publication, the emotional challenge of effective communication and conflict resolution between patients, family, and clinicians is clear, but the available health care team members and resources identified to buffer and manage it are not.

HOSPICE

Intertwined with end-of-life care are hospice and palliative care. Hospice was inspired by English nursing student Dame Cicely Saunders during World War II. She described three needs individuals required at the end of life:

- relief from physical pain and suffering
- preservation of dignity
- help with the spiritual and psychological pain of death.

In order to meet these needs, Saunders opened the first hospice in London in 1967. The first U.S. hospice opened 7 years later. Access to hospice care was expanded in 1982 with the passage of the Medicare Hospice Benefit, through which hospices receive federal funding for the care they provide eligible patients. By definition, these patients must have an anticipated prognosis of 6 months or less as certified by two physicians. Although hospice is often envisioned as a specific place, the majority of care takes place in patients' homes, though it can occur in other settings, such as skilled nursing facilities, hospitals, and freestanding hospice centers.

By definition, hospice care attempts to address the needs of both patients and families. All Medicare-certified hospice programs are required to provide interdisciplinary care teams to address physical, psychosocial, and spiritual suffering. Specifically, these teams must consist of physicians, registered nurses, social workers, and counselors (usually chaplains). Surprisingly, psychologists, the best-trained and experienced health care professionals to manage psychosocial needs, are not generally part of this team. But other therapies, such as dietary counseling, physical therapy, and respiratory therapy, may be provided as appropriate.

Hospice is an emotionally laden term. Although 70% of people say they prefer to die at home – a choice which can be facilitated by enrolling in hospice services – 70% of people die in hospitals, nursing homes, or long-term care facilities (Centers for Disease Control and Prevention, 2005). Family members of deceased persons are more likely to report a favorable dying experience for the patient when hospice or palliative care is chosen as compared with being in the hospital (Dawson, 1991; Hanson et al., 1997a; Nolen-Hoeksema, Larson & Bishop 2000; Teno et al., 2004). Considering that clinical psychologists are not standard providers of hospice care, it is interesting to note the most common unmet needs identified by dissatisfied family members (besides adequate treatment of physical symptoms) are psychological. Generally, these relate to perceptions of communication, respect, and emotional support (Connor, Teno, Spence, & Smith, 2005).

Nationally, perceived benefit among those who utilize hospice appears strong. Stronger still, however, is the resistance to using it. The number of Medicare beneficiaries enrolled in hospice at the time of death is increasing while the number of deaths in acute care hospitals is decreasing. However, in terms of benefit, enrollment is not as meaningful as timing. Time spent on ICU during the final month of life continues to increase as does the incidence of health care transitions during the last 3 days of life (Teno et al., 2013). The potential iatrogenic impact of such transfers is well-described (Ouslander et al., 2010).

Experts suggest a hospice stay of at least 3 months is required to adequately address patient and family needs, yet the average length of stay is less than 60 days (Christakis & Iwashyna, 2000). In 2007, only 30% of Medicare beneficiaries were enrolled in hospice for at least 3 days prior to their death. Perhaps most telling, however, is that studies in 2004 and 2006 revealed 10% of hospice patients were enrolled in the last 24 hours of their life (National Hospice and Palliative Care Organization, 2004; 2006; 2012).

These data demonstrate a major disconnect between what patients want and what they receive during life's last phase. It is not uncommon to hear patients themselves voice fears of pain more than of death itself. This is particularly perplexing since surveys of physicians' own end-of-life preferences reveal the same concerns. They do not want, and may fear, the same aggressive, invasive treatments that they themselves are nonetheless administering to their patients at the end of life (Periyakoil, Neri, Fong, & Kraemer, 2014).

PALLIATIVE CARE

All hospice is palliative care, but not all palliative care is hospice. Palliative care is specialized medical care targeting quality of life, physical pain and symptom relief along with matching the treatment plan to patients' goals of care. Many may share the perception that palliative care is reserved for the end of life, or that it is essentially "giving up" on the patient. Actually, palliative care can be provided at any stage of illness and can occur alongside curative treatments. As with hospice, in theory, palliative care is administered by an interprofessional team in order to comprehensively address a patient's biopsychosocial needs. In practice, however, palliative care is still a relatively young specialty within the health care system and it is often delivered by a single practitioner. Although there are growing numbers of outpatient and home-based services, the current (and increasing) trend is for much of palliative care to take place in the inpatient hospital setting. In 2000, less than one-fourth of hospitals with 50 or more beds offered palliative care, while in 2011, more than two-thirds of these hospitals had a palliative care program (Center to Advance Palliative Care, 2013).

Some data suggest multiple benefits to hospital-based palliative care. This includes physical and psychological symptom management, improved caregiver well-being and family satisfaction, and lower costs of care and ICU utilization (Bendaly, Groves, Juliar, & Gramelspacher, 2008; Ciemens, Blum, Nunley, Lasher, & Newman, 2007; Gade et al., 2008; Morrison et al., 2008; Penrod et al., 2010; Ravakkah, Chideme-Munodawafa, & Nakagawa, 2010). In one landmark study, patients with newly diagnosed lung cancer who received palliative care in addition to standard care had a better quality of life and longer survival rates than patients receiving standard care alone (Temel et al., 2010).

Taken together, it appears the national system of end-of-life care is riddled with inconsistencies between what patients would want for themselves and the care they ultimately receive. Similarly inconsistent is (aggressive) care physicians provide, and comfort measures physicians choose to receive for their own end of life (Gallo et al., 2003; Gramelspacher, Zhou, Hanna, & Tierney, 1997; Hillier, Patterson, Hodges, & Rosenberg, 1995). But what is consistent is the strong (often inadequately addressed) psychological toll that manifests as stress, conflict, anxiety, anger, and dissatisfaction at the end of life.

PHYSICIAN PERSPECTIVES

Death is inevitable. But so, it seems, is denial and the avoidance of discussing or acknowledging it. Decades ago psychologist Rollo May addressed death and related anxiety when introducing the concept of existential psychology (1961) and of course decades earlier neurologist Sigmund Freud, and later his daughter Anna, provided a comprehensive account of human defense mechanisms, including denial (Freud, 1936).

It is hard not to see this at play as a physician providing end-of-life care. Rather than address the topic, most people live their life avoiding it. In the face of rapid medical and technological advances during the latter part of the 20th century, medical practice has shifted from management to cure, and fighting disease at all costs is seen and marketed as the ideal, while death is increasingly seen and marketed as failure. Whether such beliefs are tacit or explicit, they nonetheless shape clinicians' practice and the expectations patients and families have of their health care.

The failure of physicians to engage patients and families in the treatment plan is not necessarily a conscious one. Though medical training programs vary, physicians are generally taught to cure disease, fight illness, and restore or at least preserve health. Little time is dedicated to specific training in end-of-life care (Rabow, Hardie, Fair, & McPhee, 2000; Ury, Berkman, Weber, Pignotti, & Leipzig, 2003). As a result, we have difficulty breaking bad news, accurately prognosticating in the face of serious illness, and talking to patients and families about their wishes at the end of life. When faced with gravely ill patients, physicians more often than not move from one aggressive therapy to another, often without pausing to discuss prognosis or reassess patient and family goals of care.

Only after years of practice and reflection have I recognized a tendency to resort to "auto-pilot" mode, convinced I should do everything possible to cure patients, regardless of their quality of life. Though I discussed the plan with patients and families, I seldom asked them what their goals of care were or whether the treatment fit those goals. When patients' illness neared the point of death, I would talk more about do not resuscitate orders or hospice, but in retrospect I wish I had those conversations much earlier, when the patient still had months or even years to live. By no means was I attempting to ignore the patients' wishes. I just never thought to ask, "Is this what you or your loved one wants?" or to let them know of other care options that focused on comfort rather than cure. This lack of awareness might be rectified by psychologist team members since their clinical training largely centers on methods of increasing and measuring mindfulness (Brown & Ryan, 2003).

Training

As noted earlier, medical training traditionally focuses on curing disease and fighting illness, with little time dedicated to preparing patients, families, and of course, oneself, for the end of life. At the same time, evidence of patient and family benefit from physicians' interpersonal skill (e.g., empathy and compassion) has been documented for more than half a century (Beecher, 1955), as have the complaints and lack of satisfaction generally due to suboptimal communication (Korsch, Gozzi, & Francis, 1968). Physician personality and empathic insight may vary, but techniques and strategies to optimize communication are teachable and learnable (Haskard et al., 2008; Rao, Anderson, Inui, & Frankel, 2007). Recent recognition of this fact has led medical curricula across the nation to slowly but steadily incorporate related training that includes student experiences with both actual and standardized patients. Palliative care competencies, including communication skills, have also been developed (e.g., Schaefer et al., 2014).

While promising, the culture of academic medicine continues to prioritize knowledge of basic sciences above relationship-building, and when disease processes are taught, prognostication, symptom control, and recognition of end-stage illness may not be included. As a result, instead of talking with patients and families about their values and goals of care, the focus is too often on what the next test or procedure will be. Because physicians are trained to cure, they default to curing. Because physicians are reimbursed for procedures, they default to procedures. But physicians are also vulnerable to being human. Physicians engaged in long-term relationships with patients are particularly prone to overestimating prognosis (Christakis & Lamont, 2000). Understandably, they do not want to see their patients die; however, not conveying a realistic picture of a patient's illness and not discussing a patient's goals of care does the patient and family a disservice. It deprives patients and their loved ones of the ability to make informed choices and live the end of their lives in a way that is personally meaningful *to them*.

Unlike psychologists, physicians are not taught to identify, understand, and effectively respond to emotions – of patients, families, or their own. In hospice, it is not uncommon to hear family members arrive to visit their loved ones with the question, "Why didn't anyone tell us it was this bad?" There are certainly times when patients and families may not fully register the gravity of "bad" news delivered to them by a skilled physician. There are also many cases of poor or even avoided communication as well. But with appropriately trained clinicians, this can and must be recognized and rectified. There is urgent need to train clinicians to prognosticate, communicate, and empathically respond to patients' emotional needs.

As demonstrated elsewhere in this publication, while medical training may never include the same depth of communication skills as clinical psychology training, better integration allows clinical psychologists to model for physicians-in-training how to build rapport, identify and respond to emotion with empathy, and communicate transparently without fear. In addition, integration can *show rather than tell* future physicians what psychologists do and familiarize them with an often subtle skill set that has proven challenging to articulate persuasively. It stands to reason that holistic, biopsychosocial end-of-life care can only be optimized when psychologists and physicians collaborate on the same care team.

FEAR AND GUILT

Intense emotion influences more than just patient and family coping ability. Fear, whether recognized or not, is a major driver of behavior within the health care team. Many physicians fear taking away patients' hope. Though a valid concern, unfortunately, attempts to manage and control this emotion result in avoidance of discussing prognosis. As described extensively throughout this publication, while such concerns are important and valid, there is currently no formal mechanism or professional in place to gauge how much of these fears or concerns are rooted in physicians, patients, or both. Multiple studies have shown that prognosis does not increase depression or reduce *patients'* hope (Smith et al., 2010; Smith et al., 2011; Wright et al., 2008). Rather, what patients depend on is a sense that their physician will partner with them throughout their illness. When fear leads to avoidance of discussing terminal conditions, physicians prevent their patients from expressing their own goals and priorities.

For decades psychologists and trainees have discussed the potential therapeutic benefit of personal self-disclosure (Knox, Petersen, & Hill, 1997). In medicine, however, this is less clear. Studies examining whether physicians should express uncertainty have revealed mixed data (Ogden et al., 2002) and some physician educators have recently recommended formal training to increase physicians' tolerance for ambiguity (Luther & Crandall, 2011). Clearly, managing such situations is emotionally complex. But tragically, when physicians direct a care plan in contrast to patient wishes, and the patient feels unable to share this view due to the physician's discomfort, the roles become reversed. Patients end up taking care of physicians.

Again, some of these emotions may be rooted in a sense of benevolence for patients; others may stem from physicians' inability to put their own personal beliefs aside. Regardless of etiology, both can contribute to avoidance of end-of-life care discussion, and influence patient decisions in one direction or another.

Physicians also fear failure. Because medical training focuses so much on fighting disease, death and failure are often conflated. Many physicians feel guilty or powerless managing patients at the end of life. On one hand, they are frustrated with patients and families who request care they see as futile. On the other hand, physicians are often uncomfortable when patients do not wish to be resuscitated. A colleague about to change a patient's code status from full code (do everything) to DNR (do not resuscitate) once quipped, "I'll be the bad guy." But to the patient (and me), he was actually "the good guy." He was merely giving the patient, afflicted with progressive, incurable and painful metastatic cancer, the care he wanted. This exemplified the perceived guilt, even unconsciously, that physicians often feel at the thought of their patients perishing. On one hand, we care enough to not want patients to die, but on the other hand we have trouble convincing ourselves that caring, by definition, must include talking about and abiding by patients' wishes. Reconciling this dichotomy remains difficult, though psychologist integration would help.

DON'T SHOOT THE MESSENGER

There is also the fear of the potentially overwhelming emotional response patients and families will have to end-of-life discussions. Even once patients are enrolled in hospice, their families may be particularly skeptical about services provided. Some have instructed me to avoid pain medication since they believe that is what is killing their loved one. Medically knowledgeable clinicians are often taken aback and must fight the urge to become defensive and blame families for trying to "dictate" care. In standard (nonhospice) medicine, suffering patients are often treated with pain medications and family members do not seem bothered. But there is something psychologically different once people are enrolled in hospice. Terminal illness means inevitable decline. It is not a matter of if but when, and what it will look like. By definition this requires close and frequent attention by care providers so they may adequately manage symptoms and optimize comfort. While at times it can feel like a thankless position, the families are often emotionally desperate. The harsh reality of their loved one dying is so painful or surprising that families strive for control and lash out. Health care workers may feel like the target, even though it is more likely the situation. Nonetheless, without this crucial insight (i.e., *is it me or the situation?*) clinicians may take things personally and respond with emotion of their own, which can adversely affect their interaction with the patient and family, and their own well-being (Zinn, 1988; Friedman, 1990; Novack, Suchman, Clark, Epstein, Najberg, & Kaplan, 1997; Meier, Back, & Morrison, 2001).

Although such situations are never easy, recognizing the source of the powerful emotions patients and families direct toward the health care team can be helpful in working through the situation. A physical therapist once described to me the father of a dying 12-year-old boy: "the father was so angry, punching holes in the wall, and refusing to do anything the hospice team suggested." But instead of criticizing or attempting to correct or control the father's behavior, the therapist empathically acknowledged the father's commitment to his son. This *understanding rather than blame* caught the father off guard. He then enthusiastically described the special foods he was preparing for his son. Clinical empathy provided validation and permission for the father to lead the conversation to a positive place where he and the therapist could work together and helped extinguish the conflict.

TRUST

Underpinning many of these challenges may be damaged trust. Hebert and colleagues (2008) interviewed bereaved caregivers to determine what questions they wanted to discuss in order to prepare for the death of a loved one. A variety of elicited responses were classified as medical, practical, psychosocial, and spiritual. These were further divided into whether the questions were actually discussed or whether they went unasked. Not surprisingly, most prevalent in the asked category were medical questions, with many caregivers wanting to know about prognosis or clinical course. Practical concerns included how to reach the physician, make insurance payments, and finances. Within the psychosocial realm, caregivers needed guidance about what to tell children, or how to manage disagreements within the family about the patient's care.

Several types of questions were *not* discussed with the health care team. Of the medical questions, the most common were what death "looked like" – that is, what signs or symptoms could be expected. Also common and not discussed were concerns about poor clinical care. These stemmed from caregivers who perceived communication from the medical team to be poor overall, leading them to fear that the health care providers were "hiding something." Most caregivers asked their psychosocial questions, but some wished for help when there was a family conflict. One caregiver recalled wishing she had been asked about family conflict due to her mother's illness. Spiritual questions tended to be particularly agonizing, leading caregivers to feel conflicted and guilty for questioning God when they weren't supposed to.

Unfortunately for caregivers, when questions are not raised and therefore remain unanswered, the resulting uncertainty can be traumatic. Grieving families often replay the course of their loved ones' illnesses in their minds, amplifying any nagging unexpressed concerns and causing further pain. According to one caregiver struggling 5 months after a loved one's death, "Dr. X just disappeared into thin air … it was a completely mystifying experience … I still can't sleep at night just thinking, who missed what? … I still have thousands of questions in my mind" (Hebert et al., 2008; p. 480). Evidently the families in such cases simply do not trust that the medical team cares about their loved ones. Conversely, adequately inviting and addressing questions and reassuring doubts can bring them immense relief, peace, and a sense of closure.

It seems reasonable to expect and encourage patients to advocate for themselves. So why don't caregivers speak their minds? Many patients and families feel ill-equipped to navigate the course of their illnesses and the fragmented system in which they receive care. They may simply be overwhelmed to the point of not knowing what to ask. As discussed earlier, many patients and families are totally unprepared for death, making it difficult to think clearly about the issues at hand. Even when they have specific questions, they may shy away from asking them due to fear of appearing ignorant. Patients and family members often admit to poor understanding of medical terminology and may simply nod their head in approval of physician-determined plans to avoid revealing their lack of understanding. Geriatric patients in particular often possess low health literacy and perceive physicians as authority figures not to be questioned. Patients and families are also reluctant to communicate openly with members of the health care team when they do not trust them.

Trust is aided by time and continuity, both increasingly scarce. In fact, the proportion of chronically ill Medicare beneficiaries seeing 10 or more specialists in their last 6 months of life continues to grow (Goodman, Esty, Fisher, & Chang, 2011). Establishing rapport in an often stressful, emotionally charged, chaotic end-of-life care context can be challenging and when the health care team is not skilled at relationship-building, a lack of trust can all too easily ensue (Tulsky, 2005). To garner trust, health care professionals must make every effort to anticipate and elicit the concerns and needs of the patients and families they are treating.

ADVERSARIES

Many clinicians feel ill-equipped to manage end-of-life situations and a combination of discomfort and lack of training often lead to disastrous outcomes, culminating in an adversarial dynamic between patients, families, and the health care team and system. This can often harm the quality of care delivery (e.g., Friedman, 1990; Zinn, 1988). Unfortunately, as U.S. health care is currently structured, potential buffers such as standard inclusion of clinical psychologist team members rarely exist. Acute stress is endured on a routine basis without formal mechanisms for patients, families, and their care providers to process and address them. Many involved remain unaware as adversarial dynamics (i.e., *us vs. them*) develop. Clinical psychologists could fill a niche by working supportively with both the family and the health care team to better understand each other, arrive at mutually acceptable solutions, and ease moral distress.

One situation which tends to be laden with conflict is when patients, families, and caregivers have different viewpoints as to what constitutes "futile" care. While it is widely accepted that patients have the right to refuse life-sustaining treatments, some health care workers have contrary beliefs. They believe in sustaining life at all costs. When physician decisions are disproportionately influenced by their own personal beliefs and values, conflict can arise with patients, families, and colleagues. For example, after a patient's daughter stated her father would not want to be kept alive on a ventilator, a physician colleague responded, "You might as well put a pillow on your father's face and suffocate him." The physician refused to honor the patient's wishes. Needless to say, the daughter felt intimidated and unclear how to manage the situation.

Cumulatively, these conflicts, combined with patient, family, and clinician misconceptions of palliative care, can paradoxically result in a hostile "care" environment. Surveys have shown that more than half of hospice and palliative physicians have received derogatory comments from health care professionals or from patients and families implying that they are committing murder (Goldstein et al., 2012).

SYSTEMS BARRIERS

Beyond clinician and patient factors, systemic obstacles impede quality end-of-life care. While hospitals or skilled nursing facilities are legally required to ask patients about advance directives, this is often framed and delivered in a rote yes/no fashion about whether a patient wants to be resuscitated rather than an in-depth, open-ended conversation. As mentioned earlier, this approach is suboptimal. So why does it persist?

Reimbursement

First, physicians are not financially incentivized to discuss patients' end-of-life wishes (e.g., advance directives). Because U.S. health care has historically followed a fee-for-service model, physicians are compensated more for volume of patients seen than time spent seeing them. In 2009, the Affordable Care Act proposed paying physicians for providing voluntary counseling to Medicare patients about advance directives, living wills, and end-of-life care options. However, critics politicized the concept, claiming it would give rise to judgmental "death panels" that could decide who was "worthy" enough to receive care. These political efforts were successful and the proposal was withdrawn. Because end-of-life discussions are typically time-consuming, it is difficult for physicians to find the time during an already busy schedule to initiate them, especially without compensation.

Role Confusion

Exactly who is responsible for initiating discussions of end-of-life care wishes remains ambiguous. It may often be assumed that a patient's primary care physician (PCP) should have these discussions. While reasonable, since often it is the PCP who has had a long-term relationship and is most familiar with the patient, there are several barriers – both practical (e.g., time, lack of compensation) and psychological (difficulty contemplating the death of patients long cared for). Further, chronically ill patients often fall into a cycle of being transferred back and forth between the hospital and nursing home, effectively preventing patients from seeing their PCP, especially when PCPs do not follow them in these facilities.

Some assume that the specialists taking care of the patient's terminal illness should have the conversation – e.g., oncologists should discuss the wishes of their patients with cancer. But often in practice, patients and families grapple with end-of-life decisions when patients are acutely hospitalized, thus obligating a new care team, often hospitalists, to discuss these intimate issues the very first time they meet them. These physicians may feel uncomfortable having such an intense and emotionally taxing conversation with patients and families whom they do not know well. As mentioned earlier, physician discomfort and anxiety may often lead to deferring the conversation.

PERCEPTIONS

Shifting family dynamics contribute to misperceptions about the dying process. The daily struggles of geriatric patients often go unrecognized by their loved ones since only a minority of elderly patients live with their families. In 1850, 70% of white elderly adults lived with their children, but in 2010, only 16% of the general population reported living in multigenerational homes (Pew Research Center, 2014). Family members are generally protected from seeing firsthand the increasing struggles and suffering a loved one might endure. If an elderly person is living with some family members while others live at a distance, it often seems that the local family is more accepting of their loved one's death. Whether it is because they cannot appreciate the decline or because of misplaced guilt, geographically remote family members may feel that in order to demonstrate their love for a frail loved one, they must "do everything possible," which can translate into more tests, more procedures, and more time in the hospital. In fact, any family member, whether close or distant, may feel a sense of powerlessness or panic as death nears, triggering the same reflex to ask for more invasive care.

Modern U.S. society insulates most people from death. Images are often based on media portrayals that perpetuate the concept of avoidable death. Television and movies commonly depict a comforting image of gravely ill patients who, once resuscitated, appear as good as new. When being revived appears so simple, death can seem optional. But reality is much harsher. While only about 17% of resuscitated patients survive to hospital discharge, patients estimate their own chances of survival at about 60% (Peberdy et al., 2003). Some data show that education about actual chances of survival can lead nearly half of patients who said they wanted CPR in the event of cardiac arrest to change their code status to allow natural death (Kaldjian et al., 2009). Tragically, this education is generally not a standard part of CPR discussion.

As alluded to previously, the perception of death as optional has led to growing frustration within medicine about patient and family demands for "futile" care. There is generally more tension over the right to demand care than to withdraw it. Clinicians are often dismayed by what they perceive as invasive, burdensome "care" and prolonged suffering of frail elders whose families struggle to accept their imminent death. As one retired nurse wrote, "I am so glad I don't have to hurt old people any more" (Bowron, 2012).

In these challenging cases, without a forum to discuss and process the emotions accompanying intense pressure and feeling forced to prolong – or increase – a patient's suffering, clinicians, consciously or not, often turn against patients and families. When working with patients and families in an end-of-life context, it can be difficult to differentiate between "desperate requests" and "insistent demands." This subtle difference may be largely in the eye of the beholder, but for clinicians, responding with empathy as opposed to blame can be vital to providing quality care and avoiding professional burnout.

EMPATHY VS BLAME

What is "normal" behavior at the end of life? Swiss psychiatrist Elizabeth Kubler-Ross described five normative stages of grief faced by someone who is dying: denial, anger, bargaining, depression, and acceptance (Kubler-Ross, 1969). However, neither patients with end-stage illness nor their families necessarily experience these stages sequentially or one by one, and they may experience myriad related emotions including guilt, desperation, hope, powerlessness, and despair. The current health care system often provides inadequate time and space to acknowledge or validate these emotions. As a frequent consequence, "normal" responses tragically become distorted as inappropriate or even annoying. It is not uncommon for patients and families to never reach the last stage (acceptance), which robs them of an opportunity to take advantage of their final moments with a loved one in a peaceful, dignified way. Because patients and families have not thought about or discussed death, they are ill-equipped to manage it.

In many ways, the health care system places unfair demands on patients and families. Society lulls the public into believing death is optional. Having never planned for the dying process, families are asked to make time-pressured decisions regarding artificial nutrition and hydration, intubation, and withdrawal of life support. Not wanting their loved one to die and saddled with feelings of powerlessness and desperation, families often assume "doing everything" is the appropriate course of action. Again, this can lead to care demands that physicians, given their medical knowledge, training, and experience deem futile. Health care professionals may even become angered by requests they perceive as placing undue burden on patients and prolonging suffering (and, in fact, it may actually be doing so). Frustration is often part of this decision-making process and may lead to disagreement and dissatisfaction with the health care professionals involved (Baker et al., 2000).

What must be remembered is that patients and families, by definition, are vulnerable. They may never have considered these issues before, and even if they have, they may not have discussed them with their physicians or each other. They are often unfamiliar with the medical literature regarding the treatments they are choosing, and may never have been asked to make such life and death decisions about their treatment plans. Navigating the medical system is often intimidating for patients and families, especially the frail elderly for whom chronic illness can be confusing and frightening. Further, many patients have limited insight into their disease processes. When hospitalized, patients are often made to feel marginalized. They are given tests, procedures, and treatments they may not understand. The flow of information tends to be impersonal and either inadequate or unidirectional, i.e., from practitioner to patient.

Though ethically obliged to avoid being judgmental, medical team members may view family members' decisions for terminally ill loved ones as selfish or even cruel. But some families may not even understand the concept of advance directives. The fact that decisions by surrogates are not supposed to be what they want for the patient but rather what the patient would want for him or herself is a subtle but important distinction that clinicians must make clear.

In other cases, family members may be well aware that they are acting in their own best interests, such as when a wife refused withdrawal of her husband's life support and stated, "I know it's not what he wants but it's what I want!" Since this decision violated the patient's living will, it was easy to be appalled by her apparent disregard of the patient's wishes. However, it was also important to consider her perspective, even though she technically was not the patient. Suppose no one had ever addressed with her (or her husband) the inevitable worsening of his chronic disease and its prognosis. Suppose he had made his living will many years before his illness and the couple never had a meaningful discussion about it. Even if they had discussed it and knew prognosis was poor, the "death is optional" belief may still have been ingrained in their minds. This case exemplifies the limbo where an acutely ill patient winds up on a ventilator and family is forced to make an immediate decision, often over the course of merely hours or days, about how to handle the situation. In medicine, critics might dismiss the patient's wife as irrational and carried away by her emotions. But rarely do physicians criticize patients or family for being carried away by reason. Emotion cannot be separated from end-of-life care. Yet many physicians and the very design of U.S. health care delivery function as though they can.

Recognizing and validating emotion fosters trust and can often resolve conflicts within a decision-maker's own mind, between family members, and between families and the health care team. Due to the current system-level inadequacies, care teams often struggle against time constraints and their own emotions as they seek to do "the right thing" for patients. Clinical psychologists could be a great asset in maintaining clarity. Interventions could target patients and families on one end and health care professionals on the other, helping both understand each other's motivations, ideally reducing the communication gap and increasing the synergy between them.

Every patient–family dyad interacts differently with the health care system and some feel more empowered or engaged than others. In fact the public is often instructed to be "informed consumers" of care, especially by the pharmaceutical industry through direct-to-consumer television advertising, a controversial and influential practice illegal in every other nation except New Zealand (Donohue, Cevasco, & Rosenthal, 2007). While patient and family empowerment is ostensibly positive, physicians are often chagrined by the onslaught of online articles eager families and patients print and bring to physicians, with hope that they have somehow found a cure for their illness. If handled poorly, communication can break down, which can ultimately lead to poor preparation for the end of life. In one study, 40% of informal caregivers of hospice patients reported never receiving information about life expectancy and 21% reported never being told their loved one's illness was incurable (Hebert et al., 2008). Not surprisingly, roughly 20–25% of caregivers say they were not prepared for the death.

Current health care reform and policymakers are turning to quality metrics and further implementation of electronic medical records as possible methods to enhance patient care. However, such transitions are difficult, and recent changes have spurred patients and physicians alike to feel more time is spent on paperwork and interfacing with a computer screen than with each other (Ogden et al., 2004; Rouf, Whittle, Lu, & Schwartz, 2007). Clinical psychologists could be enormously helpful members of the health care team but they are rarely found in the inpatient setting where much of end-of-life care currently takes place. As noted, better integration could bridge divides, bolster communication, and offer emotional support to patients, families, and health care team members.

As illustrated in this chapter, high quality care provision at the end of life is challenged by medical, societal, and systemic barriers. Underlying these obstacles is the profound, uniquely human, psychological discomfort of confronting mortality. This chronic symptom of the human condition is unlikely to abate. Therefore, integration with those most trained to understand and manage these concerns certainly seems indicated.

References

Back, A. L., & Arnold, R. M. (2005). Dealing with conflict in caring for the seriously ill: It was just out of the question. *Journal of the American Medical Association*, 293, 1374–1381.

Baker, D. W., Einstadter, D., Husak, S., & Cebul, R. D. (2003). Changes in the use of do-not-resuscitate orders after the implementation of the Patient Self-Determination Act. *Journal of General Internal Medicine*, 18, 343–349.

Baker, R., Wu, A. W., Teno, J. M., Kreling, B., Damiano, A. M., Rubin, H. R., et al. (2000). Family satisfaction with end-of-life care in seriously ill hospitalized adults. *Journal of the American Geriatrics Society, 48*(5), S61–S69.

Barnato, A. E., & Arnold, R. M. (2013). The effect of emotion and physician communication behaviors on surrogates' life-sustaining treatment decisions: A randomized simulation experiment. *Critical Care Medicine, 41*(7), 1686–1691.

Beecher, H. K. (1955). The powerful placebo. *Journal of the American Medical Association, 159*, 1602–1606.

Bendaly, E. A., Groves, J., Juliar, B., & Gramelspacher, G. P. (2008). Financial impact of palliative care consultation in a public hospital. *Journal of Palliative Medicine, 11*, 1304–1308.

Bensadon, B. A., & Odenheimer, G. L. (2014). Listening to our elders: A story of resilience and recovery. *Patient Education and Counseling, 95*(3), 433–434.

Bickel-Swenson, D. (2007). End-of-life training in US medical schools: A systematic literature review. *Journal of Palliative Medicine, 10*(1), 229–235.

Bowron, Craig. Opinions: Our unrealistic views of death, through a doctor's eyes. The Washington Post, February 17, 2012.

Brown, K. W., & Ryan, R. M. (2003). The benefits of being present: Mindfulness and its role in psychological well-being. *Journal of Personality & Social Psychology, 84*(4), 822–848.

California Health Care Foundation (2012). Poll finds wide gap between the care patients want and receive at end of life. Available at: <http://www.chcf.org/media/press-releases/2012/end-of-life-care>.

Center to Advance Palliative Care (2013). Website available at: <http://www.capc.org/>.

Centers for Disease Control and Prevention (CDC) (2005). Website available at: <www.cdc.org>.

Christakis, N. A., & Iwashyna, T. J. (2000). Impact of individual and market factors on the timing of initiation of hospice terminal care. *Medical Care, 38*, 528–541.

Christakis, N. A., & Lamont, E. B. (2000). Extent and determinants of error in doctor's prognoses in terminally ill patients: Prospective cohort study. *BMJ, 320*, 469–472.

Ciemens, E. L., Blum, L., Nunley, M., Lasher, A., & Newman, J. M. (2007). The economic and clinical impact of an inpatient palliative care consultation service: A multifaceted approach. *Journal of Palliative Medicine, 10*, 1347–1355.

Connor, S. R., Teno, J., Spence, C., & Smith, N. (2005). Family evaluation of hospice care: Results from voluntary submission of data via website. *Journal of Pain and Symptom Management, 30*(1), 9–17.

Connors, A. F., Jr, et al., Dawson, N. V., Desbiens, N. A., Fulkerson, W. J., Goldman, L., Knaus, W. A., et al. (1995). A controlled trial to improve care for seriously ill hospitalized patients: The study to understand prognoses and preferences for outcomes and risks of treatments (SUPPORT). *Journal of the American Medical Association, 274*(20), 1591–1598.

Danis, M. (1998). Improving end-of-life care in the intensive care unit: What's to be learned from outcomes research? *New Horizons, 6*(1), 110–118.

Danis, M., Southerland, L. I., Garrett, J. M., Smith, J. L., Hielema, F., Pickard, C., et al. (1991). A prospective study of advance directives for life-sustaining care. *New England Journal of Medicine, 324*, 882–888.

Dawson, N. (1991). Need satisfaction in terminal care settings. *Social Science & Medicine, 32*, 83–87.

DeBakey, L. (1966). Language and the physician. *Archives of Surgery, 92*(6), 964–972.

Detering, K. M., Hancock, A. D., Reade, M. C., & Sylvester, W. (2010). The impact of advance care planning on end of life care in elderly patients: Randomised controlled trial. *British Medical Journal, 340*, c1345.

Ditto, P. H., Danks, J. H., Smucker, W. D., Bookwala, J., Coppola, K. M., Dresser, R., et al. (2001). Advance directives as acts of communication: A randomized controlled trial. *Archives of Internal Medicine, 161*, 421–430.

Donohue, J. M., Cevasco, M., & Rosenthal, M. B. (2007). A decade of direct-to-consumer advertising of prescription drugs. *New England Journal of Medicine, 357,* 673–681.

Fagerlin, A., Ditto, P. H., Hawkins, N. A., Schneider, C. E., & Smucker, W. D. (2002). The Use of Advance Directives in End-of-life Decision Making: Problems and Possibilities. *American Behavioral Scientist, 46*(2), 268–283.

Fagerlin, A., & Schneider, C. E. (2004). Enough: The failure of the living will. *Hastings Center Report, 34*(2), 30–42.

Freud, A. (1936). The ego and the mechanisms of defence. London.

Friedman, E. (1990). The perils of detachment. *The Health care Forum Journal, 33,* 9–10.

Frost, D. W., Cook, D. J., Heyland, D. K., & Fowler, R. A. (2011). Patient and health care professional factors influencing end-of-life decision-making during critical illness: A systematic review. *Critical Care Medicine, 39*(5), 1174–1189.

Gade, G., Venohr, I., Conner, D., McGrady, K., Beane, J., Richardson, R. H., et al. (2008). Impact of an inpatient palliative care team: A randomized controlled trial. *Journal of Palliative Medicine, 11,* 180–190.

Gallo, J. J., Straton, J. B., Klag, M. J., Meoni, L. A., Sulmasy, D. P., Wang, N. Y., et al. (2003). Life-sustaining treatments: What do physicians want and do they express their wishes to others? *Journal of the American Geriatrics Society, 51*(7), 961–969.

Gawande, A. (2014). *Being mortal: medicine and what matters in the end.* Canada: Doubleday.

Goldstein, N. E., Cohen, L. M., Arnold, R. M., Goy, E., Arons, S., & Ganzini, L. (2012). Prevalence of formal accusations of murder and euthanasia against physicians. *Journal of Palliative Medicine, 15*(3), 334–339.

Goodman, D.C., Esty, A.R., Fisher, E.S., & Chang, C.-H. (2011). Trends and variation in end-of-life care for Medicare beneficiaries with severe chronic illness. Dartmouth Atlas of Health Care. Available from: <http://www.dartmouthatlas.org/downloads/reports/EOL_Trend_Report_0411.pdf>.

Gramelspacher, G. P., Zhou, X. H., Hanna, M. P., & Tierney, W. M. (1997). Preferences of physicians and their patients for end-of-life care. *Journal of General Internal Medicine, 12*(6), 346–351.

Hanson, L., Tulsky, J., & Danis, M. (1997b). Can clinical interventions change care at the end of life? *Annals of Internal Medicine, 126,* 381–388.

Hanson, L. C., Danis, M., & Garrett, J. (1997a). What is wrong with end-of-life care? Opinions of bereaved family members. *Journal of the American Geriatrics Society, 45*(11), 1339–1344.

Haskard, K. B., Williams, S. L., DiMatteo, M. R., Rosenthal, R., White, M. K., & Goldstein, M. G. (2008). Physician and patient communication training in primary care: Effects on participation and satisfaction. *Health Psychology, 27*(5), 513.

Hebert, R. S., Schulz, R., Copeland, V., & Arnold, R. M. (2008). What questions do family caregivers want to discuss with health care providers in order to prepare for the death of a loved one? An ethnographic study of caregivers of patients at end of life. *Journal of Palliative Medicine, 11*(3), 476–483.

Hillier, T. A., Patterson, J. R., Hodges, M. O., & Rosenberg, M. R. (1995). Physicians as patients: Choices regarding their own resuscitation. *Archives of internal Medicine, 155*(12), 1289–1293.

Hogan, C., Lynn, J., Gabel, J., Lunney, J., O'Mara, A., & Wilkinson, A. (2000). *Medicare beneficiaries' costs and use of care in the last year of life. Final Report to MedPAC.* Washington (DC): Medicare Payment Advisory Commission.

Kaldjian, L. C., Erekson, Z. D., Haberle, T. H., Curtis, A. E., Shinkunas, L. A., Cannon, K. T., et al. (2009). Code status discussions and goals of care among hospitalised adults. *Journal of Medical Ethics, 35*(6), 338–342.

Knox, S., Hess, S. A., Petersen, D. A., & Hill, C. E. (1997). A qualitative analysis of client perceptions of the effects of helpful therapist self-disclosure in long-term therapy. *Journal of Counseling Psychology, 44*(3), 274–283.

Korsch, B. M., Gozzi, E. K., & Francis, V. (1968). Gaps in doctor–patient communication I. Doctor–patient interaction and patient satisfaction. *Pediatrics, 42*(5), 855–871.

Kubler-Ross, E. (1969). *On death and dying.* New York: Macmillan.

Luther, V. P., & Crandall, S. J. (2011). Ambiguity and uncertainty: Neglected elements of medical education curricula? *Academic Medicine, 86*(7), 799–800.

Lynn, J. (2001). Serving patients who may die soon and their families. *Journal of the American Medical Association, 285*(7), 925–932.

Lynn, J., Schall, M. W., Milne, C., Nolan, K. M., & Kabcenell, A. (2000). Quality improvements in end of life care: Insights from two collaboratives. *Joint Commission Journal on Quality Improvement, 26*(5), 254–267.

Maguire, P. (1999). Improving communication with cancer patients. *European Journal of Cancer, 35*(14), 2058–2065.

May, R. (1961). *Existential psychology.* New York: Crown Publishing Group/Random House.

Meier, D. E. (2014). 'I don't want jenny to think I'm abandoning her': Views On overtreatment. *Health Affairs, 33*(5), 895–898.

Meier, D. E., Back, A. L., & Morrison, R. S. (2001). The inner life of physicians and care of the seriously ill. *Journal of the American Medical Association, 286*(23), 3007–3014.

Molloy, D. W., Guyatt, G. H., Russo, R., Goeree, R., O'Brien, B. J., Bédard, M., et al. (2000). Systematic implementation of an advance directive program in nursing homes: A randomized controlled trial. *Journal of the American Medical Association, 283*, 1437–1444.

Morrison, R. S., Penrod, J. D., Cassel, J. B., Caust-Ellenbogen, M., Litke, A., Spragens, L., et al. (2008). Cost savings associated with U.S. hospital palliative care consultation programs. *Archives of Internal Medicine., 168*, 1783–1790.

National Hospice and Palliative Care Organization (2006). Facts and figures: Hospice care in America. Website of the National Hospice and Palliative Care Organization. Available at: <www.nhpco.org/sites/default/files/public/Statistics_Research/2012_Facts_Figures.pdf>. Accessed 20.09.14.

National Hospice and Palliative Care Organization, (2012). *Facts and figures: Hospice care in America, 2012 edition.* Alexandria, PA: NHPCO.

National Hospice and Palliative Care Organization National Data Set: National Trend Study. (2004). Website of the National Hospice and Palliative Care Organization. Available from: <www.nhpco.org/performance-measures/national-data-set-nds>. Accessed 20.09.14.

Nolen-Hoeksema, S., Larson, J., & Bishop, M. (2000). Predictors of family members' satisfaction with hospice. *The Hospice Journal, 15*, 29–48.

Novack, D. H., Suchman, A. L., Clark, W., Epstein, R. M., Najberg, E., & Kaplan, C. (1997). Calibrating the physician: Personal awareness and effective patient care. *Journal of the American Medical Association, 278*(6), 502–509.

Ogden, J., Bavalia, K., Bull, M., Frankum, S., Goldie, C., Gosslau, M., et al. (2004). "I want more time with my doctor": a quantitative study of time and the consultation. *Family Practice, 21*(5), 479–483.

Ogden, J., Fuks, K., Gardner, M., Johnson, S., McLean, M., Martin, P., et al. (2002). Doctors expressions of uncertainty and patient confidence. *Patient Education & Counseling, 48*(2), 171–176.

Ouslander, J. G., Lamb, G., Perloe, M., Givens, J. H., Kluge, L., Rutland, T., et al. (2010). Potentially avoidable hospitalizations of nursing home residents: Frequency, causes, and costs. *Journal of the American Geriatrics Society, 58*(4), 627–635.

Peberdy, M. A., Kaye, W., Ornato, J. P., Larkin, G. L., Nadkarni, V., Mancini, M. E., et al. (2003). Cardiopulmonary resuscitation of adults in the hospital: A report of 14720 cardiac arrests from the National Registry of Cardiopulmonary Resuscitation. *Resuscitation, 58*(3), 297–308.

Penrod, J. D., Deb, P., Dellenbaugh, C., Burgess, J. F., Jr., et al., Zhu, C. W., Christiansen, C. L., et al. (2010). Hospital-based palliative care consultation: Effects on hospital cost. *Journal of Palliative Medicine, 13*, 973–979.

Periyakoil, V. S., Neri, E., Fong, A., & Kraemer, H. (2014). Do unto others: Doctors' personal end-of- life resuscitation preferences and their attitudes toward advance directives. *PLoS ONE* http://dx.doi.org/10.1371/journal.pone.0098246.

Pew Research Center (2014). Website available at: <http://www.pewsocialtrends.org/>.

Rabow, M. W., Hardie, G. E., Fair, J. M., & McPhee, S. J. (2000). End-of-life care content in 50 textbooks from multiple specialties. *Journal of the American Medical Association, 283,* 771–778.

Ramirez, A. J., Graham, J., Richards, M. A., Cull, A., & Gregory, W. M. (1996). Mental health of consultants: The effects of stress and satisfaction at work. *Lancet, 347,* 724–728.

Rao, J. K., Anderson, L. A., Inui, T. S., & Frankel, R. M. (2007). Communication interventions make a difference in conversations between physicians and patients: A systematic review of the evidence. *Medical Care, 45*(4), 340–349.

Ravakkah, K., Chideme-Munodawafa, A., & Nakagawa, S. (2010). Financial outcomes of palliative care services in an intensive care unit. *Journal of Palliative Medicine, 13,* 7.

Rouf, E., Whittle, J., Lu, N., & Schwartz, M. D. (2007). Computers in the exam room: Differences in physician–patient interaction may be due to physician experience. *Journal of General Internal Medicine, 22*(1), 43–48.

Schaefer, K. G., Chittenden, E. H., Sullivan, A. M., Periyakoil, V. S., Morrison, L. J., Carey, E. C., et al. (2014). Raising the bar for the care of seriously ill patients: Results of a national survey to define essential palliative care competencies for medical students and residents. *Academic Medicine, 89,* 1024–1031.

Smith, T. J., Dow, L. A., Virago, E., Khatcheressian, J., Lyckholm, L., & Matsuyama, R. (2010). Giving honest information to patients with advanced cancer maintains hope. *Oncology, 24,* 521–525.

Smith, T. J., Dow, L. A., Virago, E., Khatcheressian, J., Lyckholm, L., & Matsuyama, R. (2011). A pilot trial of truthful decision aid for patients with metastatic advanced cancer. *Journal of Supportive Oncology, 9,* 79–86.

Smucker, W. D., Ditto, P. H., Moore, K. A., Druley, J. A., Danks, J. H., & Townsend, A. (1993). Elderly outpatients respond favorably to a physician-initiated advance directive discussion. *Journal of the American Board of Family Practice, 6*(5), 473–482.

Steinhauser, K. E., Christakis, N. A., Clipp, E. C., McNeilly, M., McIntyre, L., & Tulsky, J. A. (2000). Factors considered important at the end of life by patients, family, physicians, and other care providers. *Journal of the American Medical Association, 284,* 2476–2482.

Studdert, D. M., Mello, M. M., Burns, J. P., Puopolo, A. L., Galper, B. Z., Truog, R. D., et al. (2003). Conflict in the care of patients with prolonged stay in the ICU: Types, sources, and predictors. *Intensive Care Medicine, 29,* 1489–1497.

Temel, J. S., Greer, J. A., Muzikansky, A., Gallagher, E. R., Admane, S., Jackson, V. A., et al. (2010). Early palliative care for patients with metastatic non-small cell lung cancer. *New England Journal of Medicine, 363,* 733–742.

Teno, J., Lynn, J., Wenger, N., Phillips, R. S., Murphy, D. P., Connors, A. F., Jr., et al. (1997). Advance Directives for seriously ill hospitalized patients: effectiveness with the patient self-determination act and the SUPPORT intervention. *Journal of the American Geriatrics Society, 45,* 500–507.

Teno, J. M., Clarridge, B., Welch, L., Wetle, T., Shield, R., & Mor, V. (2004). Family perspectives on end-of-life care at the last place of care. *Journal of the American Medical Association, 291,* 88–93.

Teno, J. M., Fisher, E., Hamel, M. B., Wu, A. W., Murphy, D. J., Wenger, N. S., et al. (2000). Decision-making and outcomes of prolonged ICU stays in seriously ill patients. *Journal of the American Geriatrics Society, 48,* S70–S74.

Teno, J. M., Gozalo, P. L., Bynum, J. P. W., Leland, N. E., Miller, S. C., Morden, N. E., et al. (2013). Change in end-of-life care for Medicare beneficiaries: Site of death, place of care, and health care transitions in 2000, 2005, and 2009. *Journal of the American Medical Association, 309,* 470–477.

Teno, J. M., Stevens, M., Spernak, S., & Lynn, J. (1998). Role of written advance directives in decision making. *Journal of General Internal Medicine, 13,* 439–446.

Tulsky, J. A. (2005). Beyond advance directives: Importance of communication skills at the end of life. *Journal of the American Medical Association, 294*(3), 359–365.

Tulsky, J. A., Fischer, G. S., Rose, M. R., & Arnold, R. M. (1998). Opening the black box: How do physicians communicate about advance directives? *Annals of Internal Medicine, 129*, 441–449.

Ury, W. A., Berkman, C. S., Weber, C. M., Pignotti, M. G., & Leipzig, R. M. (2003). Assessing medical students' training in end-of-life communication: A survey of interns at one urban teaching hospital. *Academic Medicine, 78*(5), 530–537.

Wright, A. A., Zhang, B., Ray, A., Mack, J. W., Trice, E., Balboni, T., et al. (2008). Associations between end-of-life discussions, patient mental health, medical care near death, and caregiver bereavement adjustment. *Journal of the American Medical Association, 300*, 1665–1673.

Yates, J. L., & Glick, H. R. (1997). The failed Patient Self-Determination Act and policy alternatives for the right to die. *Journal of Aging & Social Policy, 9*, 29–50.

Zinn, W. M. (1988). Doctors have feelings too. *Journal of the American Medical Association, 259*, 3296–3298.

10

Experiential Learning and "Selling" Geriatrics

Jonathan M. Flacker

Emory University School of Medicine, Atlanta, Georgia, USA

INTRODUCTION

Experiential learning takes trainees out of the classroom and provides real-life experience in their field of study. As defined by Shea and colleagues (1996), it is "an activity in which a student observes and directly participates in a quality learning experience external to the classroom setting which is structured to complement the students' major field of study or reflect interdisciplinary goals that enhance his or her engagement and understanding of career opportunities in a diverse and ever changing world".

Most medical and health sciences education is experiential. However, the first two years of medical school are traditionally spent in a classroom setting with mostly didactic, lecture-style teaching methodology. The anatomy lab is the lone exception during this classroom-based education. But even in that setting, where students perform dissections to gain a better understanding of the human body, the learning is highly directed and structured. It is usually not until the third year of medical school that trainees begin their clinical experience. Even then, specific exposure to geriatric medical practice is limited. Examples may include medical students taking a history from caregivers of patients with advanced dementia; observing emergency medicine residents evaluating older adults with abdominal pain; and seeing cardiology Fellows master the techniques of heart catheterization for frail elders, all under the watchful eye of experienced clinicians. Each of these activities occurs outside of the traditional classroom. In fact the majority of medical training occurs in the context

B. Bensadon (Ed): Psychology and Geriatrics.
DOI: http://dx.doi.org/10.1016/B978-0-12-420123-1.00010-1

of real-world patients and health care delivery. This approach is best described as a modification of the traditional apprenticeship model of education.

Yet, despite the experiential contact learners might have with older adults, a diminishing number of medical graduates are choosing to specialize in the care of the older population. According to the American Geriatrics Society, in 2000 there were 7,762 geriatricians in the United States for 16.6 million people aged 75 and older. This translates to 2,127 older adults for each geriatrician in the US. If present trends continue, by 2050 this will decline to an estimated 7,264 geriatricians for the estimated 48.4 million adults aged 75 and older. Such a demographic shift would reduce that ratio to only 1 geriatrician for every 6,700 adults at or above age 75. The shortage of graduates choosing to care for older adults is as much due to qualitative aspects of their training experiences as it is the more commonly cited financial pressures. So we must ask ourselves two questions – why is this happening and what can be done?

Many factors contribute to the declining popularity of geriatric medicine. These include professional, personal, and training factors. Professional factors are those related to practice, such as job satisfaction, prestige, lifestyle, and income. Personal factors are those related to the trainee, such as background, culture, socioeconomic class, and predisposition toward certain areas of medicine. Training factors are those related to learners' exposure, to explicit and implicit priorities of training programs, and faculty role modeling. Psychologically, experiential learning interacts with each of these factors in ways that ultimately shape trainees' perceptions of geriatric care.

PROFESSIONAL FACTORS

Economics is among the most commonly cited barriers to choosing a career in primary care, including geriatric medicine. The average medical student in 2010 graduated with $157,944 of debt. Choosing a primary care specialty extends the time necessary to pay that debt off. What's more, post-residency fellowship training in geriatrics not only requires additional training time, but actually results in a pay cut (Bensadon, Teasdale, & Odenheimer, 2013). Though economics offers an intuitively clear rationale for career choices, studies indicate very little relation between level of debt and choice of a primary care career. A 2002 study of medical graduates found those with higher debt were actually more likely to be planning to eventually work in underserved areas (Rosenblatt & Andrilla, 2005). Nonetheless, those with debt greater than $250,000 and those expecting a higher income were less likely to choose primary care. It appears then that salary, while a motivating factor, is not the only one.

EARLY EXPOSURE

There is some question as to how early medical trainees should gain experience with older adults. At Emory School of Medicine, our outpatient experience (OPEX) pairs first-year medical students with physicians in a primary care outpatient clinic that includes some geriatrics exposure for half a day every two weeks for a year. This program affords students the opportunity to experience relationship-oriented aspects of what primary care providers really do, and understand the personal and professional reward of this career choice.

Some suggest instituting experiential programs to proactively target the predisposed undergraduate is a useful strategy. In fact, several notable premedical programs do introduce learners to elder care even before medical school begins.

The University of Pittsburgh Health Career Scholars Academy hosts a summer program for students interested in learning more about careers in health care (Health Career Scholars Academy, 2014). Students enroll in one of four concentration areas, including geriatrics. The program includes a variety of 90-minute, interactive, case-based sessions on topics relevant to elder health care. Students also visit and interview older adults, shadow health care professionals, and visit various research settings.

At the University of Texas Health Sciences Center in San Antonio, the Positively Aging® Curriculum targets both teachers and students. Primary and secondary school teachers from the San Antonio area collaborate with university scientists to create interdisciplinary lessons and learning activities. Teaching materials are written by teachers for teachers, and have resulted in nearly 350 educational activities designed to create not only factual knowledge but also empathy towards older adults.

UCLA offers a freshman course on "Frontiers in Human Aging: Biomedical, Social and Policy Perspectives." Students attend two weekly lectures that present key concepts and content and are augmented by weekly two-hour small-group discussions, an elder-interview project, film review, and a career panel to provide students with the opportunity to explore a multitude of aging-related career paths. In addition, each student completes 20 hours of structured "Service Learning" with the ethnically diverse older Los Angeles community.

The Adulthood and Aging seminar for undergraduates at Lyndon State University in Vermont includes students "adopting" a nursing home resident for the semester, visiting a local day care center, and having lunch at a senior meal site. Such programs demonstrate the perception that graduate medical education is far too late to be influencing geriatrics-related attitudes, knowledge, and skills. To maximize impact, training should begin well before what is usually considered the formal beginning of medical education.

BIAS

Geriatrics is often perceived to be low in prestige, particularly in comparison to interventional specialties. As a trainee I was encouraged to consider oncology by an oncologist. I still recall his surprise when I expressed my interest in geriatrics and he replied "Why? That's so depressing." (He could have said, "Great, that might be challenging but will likely be a gratifying choice.") Unfortunately, this perception, shaped in part by strong and enduring stereotypes, is fairly common and pervasive both within and outside medicine (Bensadon et al., 2013). In medical training, learners are exposed to a range of negative ageist labels such as "social admission," "bed-blocker," and "GOMER," ("Get Out of My Emergency Room," medical slang for a patient who, due to infirmity, is considered by some clinicians a "difficult," unwelcome and/or hopeless patient).

Care of older patients is often referred to as "baby sitting" or "gardening." All too frequently, when faculty role models demonstrate their own lack of interest or even disdain for geriatrics, students internalize the message that older patients are somehow less interesting and important than others. This can lead trainees to ask themselves why they would go to medical school to become a babysitter or gardener.

Interestingly, the possible downside of becoming ultraspecialized practitioners in high-tech, low-touch fields, who rarely if ever develop personal connections with patients and may eventually regard themselves as glorified technicians, goes largely undiscussed. In a health care training environment enamored with "gizmo idolatry" (Leff & Finucane, 2008), it should not be surprising that psychological and social determinants of health are undervalued and mistakenly viewed as fuzzy topics of little relevance to the physician's professional domain.

Though daunting and discouraging, this negative description is hard to reconcile with physician job satisfaction data that repeatedly demonstrate the opposite (e.g., Leigh, Tancredi & Kravitz, 2009). In fact, in a recent nationally representative sample of physicians from 33 different specialties, geriatrics was ranked first in job satisfaction, a finding consistent with prior studies. How can this be explained?

At its core, geriatrics is about life experience. Patient stories, society's stories, and our own stories, spun together in a fashion that creates connection, communicates caring and aids in healing. These stories flow from our patients and develop into meaningful relationships. They emanate from caregivers in the context of a loved one's complicated medical, psychological, and social problems. Geriatrics practice is holistic, transdisciplinary, and systems-based. The frequent but inadequately publicized result for physicians is a daily sense of making an important, positive impact in the lives of others.

An important challenge lies in creating an optimal educational approach that effectively allows learners to appreciate and understand these fulfilling aspects of providing geriatric care. If our current training continues to be based on an acute rather than chronic care model, learners will not be encouraged or exposed to longitudinal relationships that can be built and maintained, and this reality will remain hidden.

THE ALLURE OF CURE

Impeding the shift toward teaching about chronic disease management is medicine's relatively recent emphasis on cure. This has fundamentally changed the expectations of physicians and modern medicine. *Success* is often equated with *cure*, and *failure* with its absence, which can often result in "resorting" to palliative care. This is understandable to some degree, given the inherently human discomfort with death. But much of this is also rooted in marketing and perception. Medical school applicants generally want to become physicians to heal people. In fact, the motto at the Association of American Medical Colleges, the primary organizing body of medical education, is "tomorrow's doctors, tomorrow's cures." The *lure of cure* is understandable, but the truth is humbler. What beginning medical students may not realize is that many, if not most, will spend the majority of their professional lives managing patients for whom cure is not possible. Frankly, most patient care is disease management, not cure. This can often be experienced as a harsh reality across specialties and patient populations. Indeed, the difference between expectation and reality can be detrimental to physician and patient alike. Psychologically, clinicians may feel inadequate or, worse, resentful when faced with patients for whom cure is not possible. Interactions with these physicians can become impersonal, terse, or insensitive. Physicians themselves may manage this experience by employing unconscious defense mechanisms to cope with the difference between their own expectations of the physician's role and the reality of medicine's limitations.

BUILDING RELATIONSHIPS

Central to effective chronic disease management is a therapeutic patient–physician relationship. However, the treatment of chronic disease conflicts so fundamentally with deeply held expectations of curative health care that it tends to be neglected. When surveyed, practicing physicians from both surgical and nonsurgical specialties report they are inadequately trained to care for chronic illness (Darer, Hwang, Pham,

Bass, & Anderson, 2004). In contemporary medical training, students typically have monthly rotations in which they rarely see the same patient twice. Even over the course of a three-year, internal medicine, resident continuity clinic, seeing the same patient more than six times is atypical. Such an impersonal training approach does not lend itself to cultivating an appreciation for the ongoing challenges of chronic multimorbidity seen in geriatric medicine. Nor does it allow trainees to experience the therapeutic value, healing power, and professional fulfillment of a caring patient–physician relationship.

Creating an environment where job satisfaction derives from effectively managing rather than curing illness entails reshaping trainee perceptions of what it means to be a physician. But if not made explicit in the curriculum, this difficult transition is one that some learners will never make. Programs that teach students to explore both physical and emotional burdens of suffering; to assist patients in formulating and adhering to self-management programs; and to participate on interprofessional health care teams are strategically sound approaches to both developing skills and adjusting expectations that will lead to job satisfaction later on (e.g., Dent, Mathis, Outland, Thomas, & Industrious, 2010).

PERSONAL FACTORS

Students enter medical school with a variety of beliefs, prior experiences, and predispositions. Generally, though, their previous exposure to older adults outside of their families is limited. Fitzgerald and colleagues (2003) found that 61% of first-year medical students felt "close" or "very close" to their grandparents and 69% reported that they had an "important" relationship with an older person who was not a relative. However, 70% reported that they had "little" or no experience actually providing care to older adults. While this lack of personal experience may result in first-year students being particularly open to learning, the practice of medicine is becoming impersonal, making it increasingly difficult to showcase the powerful and important human elements of the patient–physician relationship.

Block and colleagues (2013) conducted a time-motion study of internal medicine residents and found that in their first year, residents spent only 12% of their time in direct patient care, while computer use occupied 40% of their time. Per shift, these residents were with each patient for an average of 7.7 minutes (Block et al., 2013). Ironically, the recently coined term "personalized medicine" has nothing to do with knowing the individual receiving care, but refers instead to understanding the unique, genetic, health and disease susceptibility profile of each patient in order to customize and target medical therapy.

MEDICAL CULTURE

As described elsewhere in this publication, the culture of medicine and medical training can be insensitive and numbing. It is not uncommon to hear patients remembered and referred to by their diseases such as "that gallbladder in 205" or "the lung mass in 328." Medical schools may try to identify and combat this unwanted and unwritten (i.e., "hidden") curriculum but the practice persists nonetheless. Trainees learn that disrespectful behavior is not only acceptable but routine (Leape et al., 2012). The clinical value of patients' personal stories, often the key to creating the human connectedness that enables true empathy, has been distorted and deemphasized in the new age of the electronic medical record. Stories are not easy to put into a point-and-click record with a cut-and-paste culture. In this model, stories become stagnant and impersonal. Medical charts are filled with more data and less information. Under the pressure of time constraints, documentation requirements, and conflicting priorities, stories are often misperceived by learners and providers as inefficient and distracting.

Though perhaps less powerfully than physicians may believe, economic factors also influence career choice. A recent study examined the relationships between academic performance, specialty choice, and accumulated educational debt in relation to parental income of 1,464 graduates over 10 years (Cooter, Erdmann, & Gonnella, 2004). During the basic science years, the high-income group performed better, but this difference vanished in the clinical years. Those in the high-income group tended to pursue surgery, while those in the low-income group tended towards family medicine. Mean debt was significantly higher for the low-income group. Once again, while relevant, it appears economics are not the only driver of specialty choice. If we as a society want to produce more primary care physicians and geriatricians, we must stop focusing solely on reimbursement and rethink the medical training experience, starting with the medical school admission process.

TRAINING FACTORS

The lens through which trainees first experience the care of older adults may be part of the problem. The acute care training environment, which emphasizes rapid diagnosis and even more rapid discharge, is antithetical to developing an appreciation for multimorbidity and chronic disease management. Again, perception is key. Complex patients may be perceived by trainees as "problems" because of either behavioral issues or iatrogenic complications, the blame for which might be projected onto the patients themselves. Other patients may be considered boring due to medical conditions some perceive as straightforward (e.g., pneumonia, waiting for placement once acute issues are resolved). How faculty present these issues matters.

The message trainees receive regarding which areas of medicine are important is, in part, created by national and institutional training requirements. For example, the Residency Review Committee, the organization that determines residency requirements in the United States, has no geriatric medicine requirement for internal medicine residents beyond 1) Demonstrating a qualified individual exists to act as a geriatric medicine subspecialty coordinator, 2) The residents' patient population includes geriatric patients, and 3) That there be an "assignment" in geriatric medicine. This lack of specificity leads to inconsistent quality of geriatrics exposure across institutions.

While some training programs in both family and internal medicine do maintain their own month-long, geriatrics-specific rotations, the importance of geriatrics nationally is determined by individual programs and is subject to related politics and pressures. Changing this landscape will be difficult without fundamentally revamping residency training. The University of Pittsburgh and the Medical College of Wisconsin are two examples of positive change. Each has a specific "geriatrics track" in their internal medicine residency program and each provides in-depth experience by increasing clinic time and structuring geriatric patient care experiences longitudinally.

ROLE MODELING

Psychologists described the important links between modeling and imitation in behavior acquisition more than a half-century ago (e.g., Bandura & Huston, 1961). It follows that many practicing physicians attribute their choice of specialty to connections with faculty role models. Geriatric medicine not only suffers from fewer practitioners, but also from an unwritten but common thread of advice that suggests geriatrics is not a good career choice for smart, talented trainees. Had I not been exposed to several geriatricians during medical school, and not been given the opportunity to work with several inspiring role models, I may not have known geriatrics existed, let alone have practiced it today.

Trainees must be offered sufficient opportunities for longitudinal experiences not only with older patients, but also with those who love practicing geriatrics. This can highlight the humanistic elements of such work and, while not all trainees will choose such a career, the option and experience will be presented favorably.

TIME AND MONEY

Nationally, the explosion in scope of medical knowledge has led to high levels of specialization. This results in medical training that is less cohesive, with a broad range of professional role models of varying quality. Trainees see patients of lower socioeconomic status since wealthier patients can choose not to be treated by them. While this may not matter much to the trainees, it does skew their experiences, and likely their attitudes, toward people with limited abilities and resources.

For educators, the number of learners has increased, while contact time has decreased, leading to less individual connection and instruction. Due to a variety of factors, including duty hour limits for residents and clinical productivity expectations for faculty, traditional bedside teaching is waning (Ramani, Orlander, Strunin, & Barber, 2003). Limited duty hours and sites for clinical training may also lead to an inability to assure that learners have a sufficient number of patient encounters to achieve mastery of desired skills, though the overall impact on care quality is unclear (Moonesinghe, Lowery, Shahi, Millen, & Beard, 2011). Increasingly, learners are encouraged to focus on in-depth knowledge in a few areas rather than a wide breadth of knowledge in many. While we may be providing some opportunities for experiential learning, these experiences may not show geriatrics in its best light.

Effective geriatric care requires much more than learning to make diagnoses and provide appropriate patient management. Medical providers must skillfully and empathically help patients and families understand and accept diagnoses, become motivated to work together, implement significant lifestyle changes, and understand a growing range of social and cultural contexts of care. Yet all too often, when older patients' nonbiomedical concerns are raised, such as isolation, finances, bereavement, and life role adjustments, the modeled response is a refocusing on the biomedical realm while avoiding underlying social and psychological issues. This may be a natural reaction to feeling ill-prepared to address these matters, or feeling powerless at the lack of resources to help. Clinical psychologist integration can help both.

Teaching physicians to identify and manage clinically relevant psychosocial issues can be difficult in a classroom setting. Further, these considerations may be overlooked if available role models have never been appropriately trained to recognize and address them. As a result, learners may view nonbiomedical aspects of care as "fluff" or somehow peripheral to what a medical provider's knowledge and scope of practice should include. Even if faculty members mention the importance of teamwork and collaboration, unless learners actually see teamwork and collaboration occur, and even participate in it themselves, the concept remains abstract.

Faculty should model for learners how to request help and seek appropriate psychological and other professional consultation. Notably, the use of interdisciplinary health care teams, traditionally at the core of the geriatrics model, continues to garner support across contemporary medical practice. However, to trainees engaged in monthly rotations often at multiple sites, the term "team" often means students, attending physician, and resident. Sometimes this can be expanded to hospitalists, cardiologists, nephrologists, endocrinologists, and possibly nurses. Rarely are trainees exposed to a truly integrated, interprofessional team that includes clinical psychologists, pharmacists, and physical therapists. Without such exposure learners are trained to work *alongside* rather than *with* allied health professionals in what is essentially parallel rather than collaborative work. Increasingly, teaching rounds on intensive care units do include multiple disciplines along with patients and their families. If done effectively, this experience can help learners appreciate the multidimensional experience of aging, illness, and related biopsychosocial care needs.

EDUCATIONAL INTERVENTIONS

Knowledge-building exercises and activities are inadequate to positively shape trainee attitudes and perceptions of geriatric patients (Samra, Griffiths, Cox, Conroy, & Knight, 2013). Direct interaction with older adults and targeted empathy-building interventions are more effective at challenging bias and stereotypes (e.g., Bensadon & Odenheimer, 2014a). One increasingly popular example is healthy senior mentorship programs, in which students are matched with community dwelling older adults whom they befriend and visit on an ongoing basis. Reflective journaling is a promising approach in which trainees can develop insight through narrative by expressing their thoughts about aging-related content and experiences (Farrell, Campbell, Nanda, Shield, & Wetle, 2008; Farrell, Shield, Wetle, Nanda, & Campbell, 2013; Goldenhar, Margolin, & Warshaw, 2008; Shield, Farrell, Nanda, Campbell, & Wetle, 2012; Shield, Tong, Tomas, & Besdine, 2011).

The "aging game" is a form of simulation that attempts to sensitize trainees to commonly experienced physical challenges of aging through the use of special maladaptive devices, such as ear plugs, obscuring glasses, and other equipment that compromises physical ability and restricts agility. Formal debriefing usually follows the activity, and trainees are encouraged to reveal how the experience of being impaired actually felt. Evidence in support of this intervention and its lasting positive impact on trainee attitudes spans decades (McVey, Davis, & Cohen, 1989; Pacala, Boult, & Hepburn, 2006; Pacala, Boult, Bland, & O'Brien, 1995; Varkey, Chutka, & Lesnick, 2006). Examples of related educational "products" include the

University of Oklahoma ASiST (Aging Simulation Sensitivity Training) Kit (University of Oklahoma, 2014), and the SECURE Aging Sensitivity Training Program from the Lee Memorial Health System in Florida (Lee Memorial Health System, 2014). While these products provide structure, generally the effectiveness of such interventions is determined by the psychological insight of faculty facilitators.

SUPPORT GROUPS

Patients managing multiple comorbid conditions require unwavering emotional support. Data documenting the benefits of group psychotherapy span multiple decades and patient populations (Abbass, Kisely, & Kroenke, 2009; Fawzy et al., 1993; Krishna et al., 2011; Ornish et al., 1990; Spiegel, Kraemer, Bloom, & Gottheil, 1989), including those diagnosed with dementia (Haslam et al., 2010; Hsieh et al., 2010). Support groups, though typically less intensive, can serve a similar function, particularly in light of members' shared narrative and social identity (e.g., Rappaport, 1993; Yalom, 1995). While methodological challenges such as member self-selection make it difficult to measure support group impact and use (e.g., Hornillos & Crespo, 2012; Lieberman & Snowden, 1993), some have suggested their value can be measured by attendance. In other words, support group participants "vote with their feet" (e.g., Davison, Pennebaker, & Dickerson, 2000).

More formal measures have demonstrated psychosocial and medical benefits of group participation across a variety of chronic conditions, including cancer, epilepsy, rheumatoid arthritis, and heart disease, as compared to nonparticipation (e.g., Bradley et al., 1987; Dracup, 1985; Droge, Arnston, & Norton, 1986; Sorensen, Pinquart, & Duberstein, 2002; Telch & Telch, 1986). Similar outcomes have been reported in studies evaluating groups targeting dementia patients and their caregivers (e.g., Ballard et al., 2009; Barnes, Raskind, Scott, & Murphy, 1981; Caserta, Lund, Wright, & Redburn, 1987; Chien et al., 2011; Gitlin, Winter, Dennis, Hodgson, & Hauck, 2010; Lawton, Brody, & Saperstein,1989; Logsdon, Pike, & McCurry, 2010; Pinquart & Sorensen, 2006).

Despite evidence of clinical value, support group exposure and adequate consideration of the caregiver are rarely included in medical training. Psychiatry is a notable exception, yet as mentioned elsewhere in this publication, time and financial constraints have increasingly led psychiatrists to rely on psychopharmacology at the exclusion of "talk therapy," a controversial shift whose origins have been questioned (Cosgrove, Krimsky, Vijayaraghavan, & Schneider, 2006) and shortcomings well-documented (e.g., Carlat, 2010; Kirsch, 2010).

Evidence of the educational benefit and training impact of support groups is also emerging (e.g., Bensadon & Odenheimer, 2014b). In many ways, learner exposure to this setting is the quintessential example of experiential learning. Observers can experience daily life with chronic disease directly through the eyes, words, emotions, and other behaviors, of support group members themselves. Impact can reach learners on both emotional and cognitive levels, that is, in both their head and their gut. Because of this "dual impact," the effects may endure. Such benefit is not limited to any one specific disease. Support group exposure offers the most authentic experience of coping with chronic disease short of being chronically ill or caring for someone else who is.

SUMMARY

Experiential learning continues to evolve. This modality is especially vital to teaching geriatrics, a medical subspecialty that does not sell itself. Aging remains psychologically threatening to all – patients, faculty, and learners alike. Learners' perceptions of a geriatrics career hinge on qualitative aspects of their training experience. While economic disincentives posed by procedure-based healthcare reimbursement are challenging, it is unknown whether these factors are on the minds of learners as they begin training. Debt is a legitimate concern for trainees, but financial incentives aimed at increasing the nonphysician geriatric workforce have yielded very limited success. This suggests there are other influences. So do consistent physician satisfaction data revealing those who choose geriatrics are glad they did. Educators must increase their own awareness of why this finding persists, and make this explicit when delivering curricular content. Experiential learning provides a compelling format by which to do so.

References

Abbass, A., Kisely, S., & Kroenke, K. (2009). Short-term psychodynamic psychotherapy for somatic disorders. *Psychotherapy & Psychosomatics, 78*(5), 265–274.

Ballard, G., Gauthier, S., Cummings, J. L., Brodaty, H., Grossberg, G. T., Robert, P., et al. (2009). Management of agitation and aggression associated with Alzheimer disease. *Nature Reviews Neurology, 5,* 245–255.

Bandura, A., & Huston, A. C. (1961). Identification as a process of incidental learning. *Journal of Abnormal and Social Psychology, 63*(2), 311–318.

Barnes, R. F., Raskind, M. A., Scott, M., & Murphy, C. (1981). Problems of families caring for Alzheimer patients: Use of a support group. *Journal of the American Geriatrics Society, 29*(2), 80–85.

Bensadon, B. A., & Odenheimer, G. L. (2014a). Listening to our elders: A story of resilience and recovery. *Patient Education and Counseling, 95*(3), 433–434.

Bensadon, B. A., & Odenheimer, G. L. (2014b). Understanding chronic disease: Student exposure to support groups. *Medical Education, 48*(5), 526–527.

Bensadon, B. A., Teasdale, T. A., & Odenheimer, G. L. (2013). Attitude adjustment: Shaping medical students' perceptions of older patients with a geriatrics curriculum. *Academic Medicine, 88*(11), 1630–1634.

Block, L., Habicht, R., Wu, A. W., Desai, S. V., Wang, K., Silva, K. N., et al. (2013). In the wake of the 2003 and 2011 duty hours regulations, how do internal medicine interns spend their time? *Journal of General Internal Medicine, 28*(8), 1042–1047.

Bradley, L. A., Young, L. D., Anderson, K. O., Turner, R. A., Agudelo, C. A., McDaniel, L., et al. (1987). Effects of psychological therapy on pain behavior of rheumatoid arthritis patients. Treatment outcome and six-month followup. *Arthritis & Rheumatism, 30*(10), 1105–1114.

Carlat, D. J. (2010). *Unhinged – The trouble with psychiatry – A doctor's revelations about a profession in crisis.* London, UK: Simon & Schuster.

Caserta, M. S., Lund, D. A., Wright, S. D., & Redburn, D. E. (1987). Caregivers to dementia patients: The utilization of community services. *Gerontologist, 27*(2), 209–214.

Chien, L. Y., Chu, H., Guo, J. L., Liao, Y., Chang, L., Chen, C., et al. (2011). Caregiver support groups in patients with dementia: a meta-analysis. *International Journal of Geriatric Psychiatry, 26*(10), 1089–1098.

Cooter, R., Erdmann, J. B., & Gonnella, J. S. (2004). Economic diversity in medical education: The relationship between students' family income and academic performance, career choice, and student debt. *Evaluation & the Health Professions, 27*(3), 252–264.

Cosgrove, L., Krimsky, S., Vijayaraghavan, M., & Schneider, L. (2006). Financial ties between DSM-IV panel members and the pharmaceutical industry. *Psychotherapy & Psychosomatics, 75*, 154–160.

Darer, J. D., Hwang, W., Pham, H. H., Bass, E. B., & Anderson, G. (2004). More training needed in chronic care: A survey of U.S. physicians. *Academic Medicine, 79*(6), 541–548.

Davison, K. P., Pennebaker, J. W., & Dickerson, S. S. (2000). Who talks? The social psychology of illness support groups. *American Psychologist, 55*(2), 205–217.

Dent, M. M., Mathis, M. W., Outland, M., Thomas, M., & Industrious, D. (2010). Chronic disease management: Teaching medical students to incorporate community. *Family Medicine, 42*(10), 736–740.

Dracup, K. (1985). A controlled trial of couples group counseling in cardiac rehabilitation. *Journal of Cardiopulmonary Rehabilitation, 5*(9), 436–442.

Droge, D., Arnston, P., & Norton, R. (1986). The social support function in epilepsy self-help groups. *Small Group Research, 17*(2), 139–163.

Farrell, T., Campbell, S., Nanda, A., Shield, R., & Wetle, T. (2008). Evaluating geriatrics in the medical school curriculum: Using student journals. *Medicine & Health/Rhode Island, 91*, 378–381.

Farrell, T. W., Shield, R. R., Wetle, T., Nanda, A., & Campbell, S. (2013). Preparing to care for an aging population: Medical student reflections on their clinical mentors within a new geriatrics curriculum. *Gerontology and Geriatrics Education, 34*(4), 393–408.

Fawzy, F. I., Fawzy, N. W., Hyun, C. S., Elashoff, R., Guthrie, D., Fahey, J. L., et al. (1993). Malignant melanoma: Effects of an early structured psychiatric intervention, coping, and affective state on recurrence and survival 6 years later. *Archives of General Psychiatry, 50*(9), 681–689.

Fitzgerald, J. T., Wray, L. A., Halter, J. B., Williams, B.C., & Supiano, M. A. (2003). Relating medical students' knowledge, attitudes, and experience to an interest in geriatric medicine. *The Gerontologist, 43*(6), 849–855.

Gitlin, L. N., Winter, L., Dennis, M. P., Hodgson, N., & Hauck, W. W. (2010). A biobehavioral home-based intervention and the well-being of patients with dementia and their caregivers:The COPE randomized trial. *Journal of the American Medical Association, 304*(9), 983–991.

Goldenhar, L. M., Margolin, E. G., & Warshaw, G. (2008). Effect of extracurricular geriatric medicine training: A model based on student reflections on healthcare delivery to elderly people. *Journal of the American Geriatrics Society, 56*(3), 548–552.

Haslam, C., Haslam, A. S., Jetten, J., Bevins, A., Ravenscroft, S., & Tonks, J. (2010). The social treatment: The benefits of group interventions in residential care settings. *Psychology & Aging, 25*(1), 157–167.

Health Career Scholars Academy (2014). University of Pittsburgh. Website available at: <http://www.hcsa.pitt.edu>.

Hornillos, C., & Crespo, M. (2012). Support groups for caregivers of Alzheimer patients: A historical review. *Dementia, 11*(2), 155–169.

Hsieh, C., Chang, C., Su, S., Hsiao, Y., Shih, Y., Han, W., et al. (2010). Reminiscence group therapy on depression and apathy in nursing home residents with mild-to-moderate dementia. *Journal of Experimental & Clinical Medicine, 2*(2), 72–78.

Kirsch, I. (2010). *The emperor's new drugs: Exploding the antidepressant myth.* New York, NY: Basic Books.

Krishna, M., Jauhari, A., Lepping, P., Turner, J., Crossley, D., & Krishnamoorthy, A. (2011). Is group psychotherapy effective in older adults with depression? A systematic review. *International Journal of Geriatric Psychiatry, 26*(4), 331–340.

Lawton, M. P., Brody, E. M., & Saperstein, A. R. (1989). A controlled study of respite service for caregivers of Alzheimer's patients. *Gerontologist, 29*(1), 8–16.

Leape, L. L., Shore, M. F., Dienstag, J. L., Mayer, R. J., Edgman-Levitan, S., Meyer, G. S., et al. (2012). Perspective: A culture of respect, part 1: The nature and causes of disrespectful behavior by physicians. *Academic Medicine, 87*(7), 845–852.

Lee Memorial Health System (2014). SECURE Aging Sensitivity Training Program. Available at: <http://www.leememorial.org/shareclub/secure.asp>.

Leff, B., & Finucane, T. E. (2008). Gizmo idolatry. *Journal of the American Medical Association, 299*(15), 1830–1832.

Leigh, J. P., Tancredi, D. J., & Kravitz, R. L. (2009). Physician career satisfaction within specialties. *BMC Health Services Research, 9,* 166.

Lieberman, M. A., & Snowden, L. R. (1993). Problems in assessing prevalence and membership characteristics of self-help group participants. *Journal of Applied Behavioral Sciences, 29*(2), 166–180.

Logsdon, R. G., Pike, K. C., & McCurry, S. M. (2010). Early-stage memory loss support groups: Outcomes from a randomized controlled clinical trial. *Journals of Gerontology B: Psychological Sciences & Social Sciences, 65B*(6), 691–697.

McVey, L. J., Davis, D. E., & Cohen, H. J. (1989). The "aging game": An approach to education in geriatrics. *Journal of the American Medical Association, 262*(11), 1507–1509.

Moonesinghe, S. R., Lowery, J., Shahi, N., Millen, A., & Beard, J. D. (2011). Impact of reduction in working hours for doctors in training on postgraduate medical education and patients' outcomes: Systematic review. *British Medical Journal, 342,* d1580.

Ornish, D., Brown, S. E., Scherwitz, L. W., Billings, J. H., Armstrong, W. T., Ports, T. A., et al. (1990). Can lifestyle changes reverse coronary heart disease?: The lifestyle heart trial. *Lancet, 336*(8708), 129–133.

Pacala, J. T., Boult, C., Bland, C., & O'Brien, J. (1995). Aging game improves medical students' attitudes toward caring for elders. *Gerontology & Geriatrics Education, 15*(4), 45–57.

Pacala, J. T., Boult, C., & Hepburn, K. (2006). Ten years' experience conducting the aging game workshop: Was it worth it? *Journal of the American Geriatrics Society, 54*(1), 144–149.

Pinquart, M., & Sorensen, S. (2006). Helping caregivers of persons with dementia: Which interventions work and how large are their effects? *International Psychogeriatrics, 18*(4), 577–595.

Ramani, S., Orlander, J. D., Strunin, L., & Barber, T. W. (2003). Whither bedside teaching? A focus-group study of clinical teachers. *Academic Medicine, 78,* 384–390.

Rappaport, J. (1993). Narrative studies, personal stories, and identity transformation in the mutual help context. *Journal of Applied Behavioral Sciences, 29*(2), 239–256.

Rosenblatt, R., & Andrilla, C. (2005). The impact of U.S. medical students' debt on their choice of primary care careers: An analysis of data from the 2002 Medical School Graduation Questionnaire. *Academic Medicine, 80*(9), 815–819.

Samra, R., Griffiths, A., Cox, T., Conroy, S., & Knight, A. (2013). Changes in medical student and doctor attitudes toward older adults after an intervention: A systematic review. *Journal of the American Geriatrics Society, 61*(7), 1188–1196.

Shea, (Smith) D., & Associates, (1996). *University of North Carolina Experiential Learning Council Report and Recommendations.* Wilmington, NC: UNC Charlotte.

Shield, R., Tong, I., Tomas, M., & Besdine, R. (2011). Teaching communication and compassionate care skills: An innovative curriculum for pre-clerkship medical students. *Medical Teacher, 33*(8), e408–e416.

Shield, R. R., Farrell, T. W., Nanda, A., Campbell, S. E., & Wetle, T. (2012). Integrating geriatrics into medical school: Student journaling as an innovative strategy for evaluating curriculum. *Gerontologist, 52*(1), 98–110.

Sorensen, S., Pinquart, M., & Duberstein, P. (2002). How effective are interventions with caregivers? An updated meta-analysis. *Gerontologist, 42*, 356–372.

Spiegel, D., Kraemer, H. C., Bloom, J. R., & Gottheil, E. (1989). Effect of psychosocial treatment on survival of patients with metastatic breast cancer. *Lancet, 334*(8668), 888–891.

Telch, C. F., & Telch, M. J. (1986). Group coping skills instruction and supportive group therapy for cancer patients: A comparison of strategies. *Journal of Consulting & Clinical Psychology, 54*(6), 802–808.

University of Oklahoma (2014). Aging Simulation Sensitivity Training (ASiST) Kit. Available at: <http://www.ouhsc.edu/okgec/ASiSTKits.asp>.

Varkey, P., Chutka, D. S., & Lesnick, T. G. (2006). The aging game: Improving medical students' attitudes toward caring for the elderly. *Journal of the American Medical Directors Association, 7*(4), 224–229.

Yalom, I. D. (1995). *The theory and practice of group psychotherapy.* New York, NY: Basic Books.

Simulation Education

Benjamin A. Bensadon

Charles E. Schmidt College of Medicine, Florida Atlantic University,
Boca Raton, Florida, USA

INTRODUCTION

Video technology has long been used in applied psychology doctoral training (e.g., Ivey, Normington, Miller, Morrill, & Haase, 1968). Though specific approaches vary by program, generally, psychologists in training independently review their recorded sessions (self-assessment) to identify specific areas that can be analyzed and critiqued during clinical supervision with a licensed psychologist. Accreditation standards require a minimum of 2 hours of such supervision per week. Weekly group supervision, also required, often includes the use of trainees' personal videos as well.

Ethical protocol requires consenting patients about videotaping their sessions primarily for training purposes. While patients may ask questions about related paperwork (e.g., consent forms), they rarely refuse. In fact, discussion that takes place at the beginning of intake (i.e., initial) encounters is itself an effective learning opportunity to establish rapport while educating about the sensitive area of patient confidentiality and its limits. Generally, patients are comforted by three important assurances:

1. The video will not leave the facility or be viewed by anyone externally.
2. The video will be erased at the end of the academic semester or earlier.
3. The primary purpose and focus of the video is recording trainee – not patient – behavior.

In medicine, psychiatry residency training has included a similar approach to education, using videotaped encounters, for half a century (Abbass, 2004). Gradually, as patient safety has become a national priority, many other areas of academic medicine are following suit. In 2000, the

B. Bensadon (Ed): Psychology and Geriatrics.
DOI: http://dx.doi.org/10.1016/B978-0-12-420123-1.00011-3

Institute of Medicine (IOM) released a report, *To Err Is Human* (Kohn, Corrigan, & Donaldson, 2000), linking patient safety with avoidable medical error. Evidence was clear and compelling. Data included estimates of 44,000–98,000 annual iatrogenic (i.e., medically caused) deaths and associated economic costs of $17–29 billion in hospitals nationally. While some physicians may continue to view ethics of patient safety and medical error as a "soft" aspect of medical training (e.g., Leape & Berwick, 2005), many continue to reiterate its importance and advocate full disclosure of error in what has become a national movement.

Consistent with this trend, simulation education has gained in popularity. The greatest advantage of this training method is that it closely approximates actual clinical work, but in a controlled setting with minimal potential for harm. Simulation centers have become ubiquitous on health sciences campuses across the nation. These facilities are designed like medical settings (e.g., hospitals, clinics), replete with exam rooms, gurneys, and related equipment (e.g., nasal cannulas, portable oxygen tanks). Technologically sophisticated mannequins function as "simulated patients." They are programmed to blink, bleed, and breathe. Faculty provide human voice and sounds (e.g., pain, anger), as they read standardized scripts, usually from an office out of sight or behind a one-way mirror. Although the mannequins are not alive, if trainees administer the wrong medication or wrong dosage, they can "die." Though of great appeal to the human fascination with technology, and a safe "body" on which to perform physical exams or related procedures, simulated patients do not fully replace people. Bluntly, the realism of talking to dummies is limited.

To complement this training, a human version has emerged. Actors (professional or not) serving as "standardized patients" (SPs) help teach and evaluate trainees' clinical examination skills. Evaluated skills include both routine technical behaviors, such as *inspection, auscultation* of the lungs, *palpation* to assess tenderness or pain, and *percussion* of the thorax or abdomen, and "inquiry" behaviors, encompassing the subtler, psychosocially relevant communication and interpersonal skills of diagnostic interviewing and patient history-taking. Faculty and students can review the videos to ensure technical aspects of these behaviors are performed correctly, such as placing one's hands or equipment (e.g., stethoscope) appropriately. The videos also reveal key aspects of communication quality, such as interruption patterns and body language.

The use of SPs allows medical trainees to not only practice *what* to do, but also receive direct feedback from SPs themselves about *how* their actions are perceived. This type of learning allows these subtle but vital aspects of care, frequently referred to as the "art" of medicine, to be taught, modeled, documented, and measured, in a systematic and rigorous fashion. In addition to training, SPs enable assessment based on competency, not merely knowledge. This is rapidly becoming the evaluation method of choice in medicine (e.g., Batalden et al., 2002), geriatric medicine (e.g., Leipzig et al., 2009), professional psychology (Belar, 2009; Kaslow, 2004; Kenkel & Peterson, 2009; Rubin et al., 2007), and geropsychology (Karel, Emery, & Molinari, 2010b; Karel, Knight, Duffy, Hinrichsen, & Zeiss, 2010a; Knight, Karel, Hinrichsen, Qualls & Duffy 2009).

OBJECTIVE STRUCTURED CLINICAL EXAMINATION

Objective Structured Clinical Examination (OSCE) is the gold standard of such assessments. This format generally includes a videotaped encounter in which trainee performance is observed by faculty, and skill level is rated by the SPs against a list of behaviors (i.e., benchmarks). Medical schools pattern these exams after the clinical skills component of the national board examination (USMLE Clinical Skills Step 2) that all medical graduates must pass prior to beginning residency training.

Specific OSCE focus and stations (i.e., case scenarios/objectives) vary by institution and discipline. Disease types, patient populations, and constellations of psychosocial, cultural, and behavioral factors are as varied as actual patients themselves. OSCE is currently not a standard component of doctoral training in applied psychology though some suggest it should be (e.g., Cramer, Johnson, McLaughlin, Rausch, & Conroy, 2013).

In medicine, myriad OSCE examples have been published. Some focus explicitly on patient safety (Singh et al., 2009). Others include appropriate prescribing and administering of medications (Scobie et al., 2003); documentation, coding, and billing (Sarzynski, Wagner, & Noel, 2013); women's health (Schillerstrom, Lutz, Ferguson, Nelson, & Parker, 2013); and interprofessional collaboration and team-based care (Solomon et al., 2011). Many have been designed specifically for geriatric care (Fabiny, McArdle, Perls, Inui, & Sheehan, 1998; O'Sullivan, Chao, Russell, Levine, & Fabiny, 2008), targeting challenges prevalent in the geriatric patient population. Examples include falls and polypharmacy (Martinez & Mora, 2012), obtaining informed consent (Shah et al., 2011), and leading difficult conversations during family conferences (Chipman, Beilman, Schmitz, & Seatter, 2007). Suffice it to say, the popularity of these educational methods will likely continue to grow. As elucidated below, this educational approach represents important opportunities to incorporate psychological insight into medical training and care, and clinical psychologists could be a uniquely valuable contributor to these efforts.

MECHANISM OF ACTION

The inherent "threat" of observing oneself is an unparalleled learning tool. Videotaped self-assessment can facilitate – at times painfully – increased self-awareness. Frequently, trainees complete an encounter with an idea of what transpired, only to realize upon video review that their subjective memory differs from the objective evidence. Though surprising (to the trainee), it should not be. For decades psychologists have theorized (Brewer, 1986; Johnson, Hashtroudi, Lindsay, 1993) and demonstrated memory to be a reconstructive process (James, Thompson, & Baldwin, 1973; Schacter, 1999), influenced (i.e., distorted) by emotional and other factors (e.g., Kennedy et al., 2004; Schmidt, 2004), especially when remembering one's own performance (e.g., Gramzow & Willard, 2006). A recent study found those with objectively superior memory ability were no more immune to this inaccuracy than others (Patihis et al., 2013). In terms of developing trainees' insight into their own clinical behavior, this discrepancy is vital. Video review not only enhances self-awareness but can also be humbling and upsetting, especially when the evidence conflicts with the trainees' original perceptions of their behavior and, frankly, themselves. Learners who are subjectively convinced they are caring, warm, active listeners, are often shocked to learn via video review that they can come across as detached, inattentive, frequent interrupters. Similarly, students confident that they are comfortable using expressive touch with patients are surprised to discover, when reviewing simulated encounters, they did not touch the SP once.

Stanford psychologist Leon Festinger first addressed humans' need for consistency, especially between their beliefs and behaviors, in his theory of *cognitive dissonance* (Festinger, 1962). [*According to Google Scholar, this original work has since been cited more than 25,000 times.*] In essence, the theory suggests psychological discomfort caused by conflicting beliefs drives behavior change if we cannot readily justify the inconsistency (i.e., dissonance). Common resistance to watching one's own performance, be it alone, with a supervisor, or especially in a group of peers such as other doctoral trainees, underscores the threat and utility of this training method (e.g., Goldberg, 1983).

VIDEO: NECESSARY BUT INSUFFICIENT

A central barrier to viewing psychology as a science and clinical psychologists as health care providers has been the claim that much of this work and skill set is subjective and unobservable. With video, this is not the case. It is observable. Subtle behavioral aspects of care, such as body language, silence, interruption patterns, and tone of voice, all communication skills relevant to clinical care (Ambady et al., 2002; Collins, Schrimmer, Diamond, & Burke, 2011; DiMatteo, Taranta, Friedman, & Prince, 1980; Hall, Roter, & Katz, 1988; Ong, de Haes, Hoos, & Lammes, 1995; Stewart, 1995; Waitzkin, 1984; Zolnierek & DiMatteo, 2009), are captured objectively.

Of course, disagreement about interpretation and meaning of such factors may still occur. For example, some may view quiet trainees as attentively listening while others may perceive them as not paying close enough attention. Some may view avoidance of touching the SP as problematic while others will see it as benign. Interpretive complexity is difficult to reconcile with video alone. Trainee and SP behavior, including their respective reactions to each other, are captured. But technology is not sufficiently sensitive to name and recognize these behaviors, nor to decode subtle emotional and affective cues that may be present. Nor can it "read" trainees who, while watching their video, may show signs of confusion, anger, fear, and uncertainty. Effective faculty can identify these subtle signs in "real time," and encourage trainee introspection about potential links to their own attitudes, beliefs, and emotional response to the SP during the encounter. Acute sensitivity to these dynamics offers something the video alone does not. In short, optimal training requires knowing what to look for. Clinical psychologists are likely to be most qualified and equipped to provide such behavioral analyses of these SP encounters. Here are several reasons why:

> Clinical psychologists are accustomed to similar, though more intensive, self-assessment methods from their own training. Weekly video review on a one-to-one basis with a licensed clinical supervisor sensitizes psychology trainees to their own behavior and its impact on others (i.e., patients). Cumulatively, this knowledge guides them in what to look and strive for in trainees. In addition, the experience of having one's performance acutely scrutinized often facilitates empathy with trainees. Ideally this insight enables clinical psychologists to provide delicate feedback in a palatable fashion. In medical training such interpersonal sensitivity is not always a point of emphasis and has often been negatively referred to as "touchy feely" (Thomas, 2013).

While physicians and psychologists may both recognize the importance and therapeutic impact of their relationship with patients, generally speaking, there are also important differences. Unlike physicians, whose daily healing practices can include ordering tests, prescribing medications, performing operative procedures, and using tools (e.g., stethoscope, oscilloscope), practicing clinical psychologists provide therapy that is usually the encounter itself, i.e., the behavior and communication (much of which is nonverbal) that transpires during the session. In simple terms, a major difference in perception about the respective healing traditions has been:

- Physicians heal by doing something *to* patients.
- Psychologists heal by doing something *with* patients, who can ultimately *heal themselves*.

Generally, clinical psychologists in training spend 2–4 years conducting weekly psychotherapy, the content of which, as mentioned, is recorded for analysis with faculty. This "clinical practicum" experience usually cannot begin until after several years of didactic coursework, including in-depth review of prominent explanatory theories of human behavior and development. In most PhD programs, an additional prerequisite is research experience that involves testing hypotheses generated by these theories. This blend of clinical and research skills is of paramount importance, given the modern day emphasis on evidence-based practice. The following paragraph illustrates the relevance of these skills to video review.

It is one thing to point out a trainee's interruption patterns on video, which many health care professionals may be able to do. It is another, however, to identify the trainee's behavior, recognize and call attention to the subsequent behavioral response in the SP, name and explain psychological theory and/or terms that have described this relationship, and cite empirical evidence where a similar behavioral link has been demonstrated. By definition, this sensitizing approach requires a unique skill set that clinical psychologists are equipped to offer. And, perhaps most importantly, given the personally sensitive nature of behavioral feedback, the manner in which this is done should at once:

- accurately and supportively recognize, validate, and normalize trainees' discomfort
- help trainees identify and reflect about whether issues are really within patients or themselves
- offer clear strategies and phrases trainees can use clinically going forward.

Clinical acumen is subtle but critical. As graphically illustrated by the literature describing academic medicine's "hidden curriculum" (e.g., D'eon, Lear, Turner, & Jones, 2007; Gaufberg, Sands, & Bell, 2010; Hafferty, 1998), too often learners' initial exposure to the actual practice of patient care includes professional behavior that is antithetical to what they've been taught. Exposure to death and terminal illness are challenging in their own right. But they are exacerbated when the modeled professional response is jaded insensitivity, burnout, cynicism, and disrespectful communication, be it directed toward other clinicians, trainees, or the patients themselves. Not coincidentally, studies have shown these behaviors are adopted by trainees (e.g., Billings, Lazarus, Wenrich, Curtis, & Engelberg, 2011) and that "empathy erosion" begins in year 3 of medical school, precisely when actual patient contact increases (Hojat et al., 2009; Neumann et al., 2011). Of course, with appropriate support and intervention from positive models, such behavior need not become normalized. Multiple studies aimed at building or preserving empathy in medical students and residents have been successful (see review by Batt-Rawden, Chisolm, Anton, and Flickinger, 2013), including a randomized controlled trial by Riess and colleagues that showed empathy could be increased during residency, the greatest increases occurring among women (e.g., Riess,

Kelley, Bailey, Dunn, & Phillips, 2012). Again, these concepts are nothing new. For more than 50 years, psychologist Albert Bandura has theorized and subsequently demonstrated in his comprehensive social learning theory (Bandura, 1977) that imitation and modeling are among the most common and powerful ways people acquire and modify their behavior (Bandura, 1965; Bandura, Ross, & Ross, 1961, 1963). Other psychologists have also examined influences on empathy, including sex differences, and published similar results for just as long (e.g., Cowden, 1955; Eisenberg & Lennon, 1983; Hoffman, 1977).

Videotaped simulation allows trainees and faculty to identify any negative habits that may have been absorbed from faulty professional models. Without video and related insight into themselves, trainees may learn to justify their behavior at all costs, avoiding responsibility by attributing negative behaviors to external causes. In addition, medical trainees may explain away their avoidance of personally uncomfortable (often psychosocial) areas of medical care by deflecting attention away from their own discomfort. They may instead criticize the quality of SP training or the artificial quality of simulation; other times, they may frame their behavior as reflecting a desire to "protect" the SP, to make sure they're not misinterpreted or seen as insensitive or offensive. These very same anxieties have been documented among practicing physicians (Cocksedge, George, Renwick, & Chew-Graham, 2013; Meier, 2014; Meier, Back, & Morrison, 2001; Miles, 1994). While in professional psychology training and practice, clinicians are expected to process, explore, and better understand personally generated barriers, traditionally this has not been emphasized in medicine. However, this philosophy may now be changing due to a growing shift away from what has historically been termed medical paternalism (Bassford, 1982; McKinstry, 1992; Siegler, 1985) toward greater transparency and shared clinical decision-making (Charles, Gafni, & Whelan, 1997).

THE FAU EXPERIENCE

Every week at our institution, Florida Atlantic University, a 91-year-old volunteer SP and I serve as patient and brother during a 15-minute standardized encounter for third-year medical students addressing end-of-life (EoL) communication. See Box 11.1 for the actual scenario given to the students beforehand.

Core to this scenario are conflicting care preferences between the SP and her brother, who is also her attorney and health care proxy. The SP is tired of fighting her chronic lung disease and her recent fall has left her in pain and frightened about the future. In some ways, she thinks death might be the ideal next step. Conversely, her brother is adamant that she regain her strength and attend his son's graduation from a nearby medical

BOX 11.1

MEDICAL/SOCIAL HX

Ms. G is an 85-year-old white female residing in Jacksonville, FL. She has been living with chronic obstructive pulmonary disease (COPD) for 7 years. Exacerbations have worsened and are more frequent. She tells you they scare her and she feels she's at "death's door" each time they occur. She was found to have a large lung mass 6 months ago. She was too frail to tolerate treatment. The biopsy confirmed small cell cancer. Last week, she developed back pain. MRI confirms metastatic disease. Your pulmonologist colleagues describe Ms. G's prior pulmonary rehabilitation as successful though increasing weakness makes it difficult for her to ambulate w/ her 8 lb oxygen tank. As a result, she has rarely left her home in the last few months. There is consensus among your colleagues that her disease has reached "end stage."

Ms. G is unmarried, with no children, one younger brother (Ron) and many friends. Though she has no children of her own, she is very close to her nephew, Chris (Ron's son), who attends UCF medical school in Orlando, and for whom she has filled the role of surrogate mother after Ron's wife died unexpectedly. Ron believes Ms. G's memory is "not so sharp." Chart review shows neurology has diagnosed her w/ mild cognitive impairment (MCI), though she carries on conversation w/ ease and her decision-making capacity is intact. Dementia has been ruled out. As her health has deteriorated, so has her mood. She reports minimal benefit from her daily antidepressant medication, and Ron insists the solution is to try a different medication, based on TV commercials he has seen.

Reason for Admission

Recently Ms. G fell at home and was unable to get back up. Luckily her brother was with her. But when he was unable to lift her back to her feet, he called 911. The two were subsequently transported by ambulance to the local hospital emergency department where you are now meeting with them.

Your Task

At this point your medical knowledge of this case suggests there is little reason to believe Ms. G will survive more than the next 4 months. Ron is adamant she must "stick around" for his only child's medical school graduation (in 6 months). This is particularly important since no one in the family has ever gone beyond high school; it was Ms. G who paid for Chris to attend medical school; and as Ron has explained to you, Chris is "like her son." At this point, Chris is unaware of the fall and hospitalization.

continued

BOX 11.1   *(Cont'd)*

Using the Advance Care Planning (ACP) Communication Guide to help you, you must address Ms. G's current medical status and likely prognosis, care goals (of both Ms. G and Ron), and various advance care options.

Learning Objectives
Develop comfort and experience in empathically addressing and managing:

- EoL decision-making
- Family conflict
- Care preferences vs. limited curative treatment options.

---

school in 6 months. After reviewing the "chart" (i.e., scenario), students must also consider recent imaging findings suggesting cancer and comorbid conditions of mild cognitive impairment and depression. Based on these data, consensus suggests a prognosis of 4 months' survival, which students must convey to patient and brother.

Whenever the patient expresses concern or lack of confidence, the brother abruptly takes over and reiterates the important goal of attending graduation. Though this goal is really his, he makes it sound as if it is hers, adding whenever possible that it would hurt the patient if she had to let down her nephew by not attending, especially since she raised him like her son. Throughout this conflict, the medical student must remain focused on the patient and her wishes, while attempting to empathize with the brother to the extent possible. This includes attempting to maintain eye contact with both parties, interrupting the louder, more demonstrative brother when necessary, and checking in with both to see how they are coping with what is being discussed. Students must also decide whether to use expressive touch with the SP and gauge when to allow for silence as well, so that the impact of conversation can be absorbed.

Predictably, student performance has varied more than their level of discomfort has. Most have been anxious and have felt challenged, though not all have admitted this. One broke into a rash. Another had a panic attack. After the encounter, the students, SP, and I debrief to discuss the experience. Our initial questioning aims to elicit students' perspectives of the experience (e.g., "How do you think it went?"). Most admit it was difficult but only a few elaborate in more detail. Some remain quiet, apart from repeatedly commenting, "It's hard." Almost all report having hospice in mind but virtually none mentions it by name during the encounter. When asked why, many say they didn't know how to raise the subject or were worried about the patient and brother's reaction. A few expressed concern that the SP and brother weren't ready to discuss it. But when asked what could be done to indicate readiness, no answer was given. Instead, we use this teaching moment to invite the students to reflect on their own readiness to explicitly introduce and guide such a conversation, and later provide evidence from medical journals of related psychosocial challenges facing physicians (e.g., Novack et al., 1997; Kaplan, 1997; Meier et al., 2001).

Another of our examples addresses cross-cultural communication. In response to well-documented health care disparities in the United States, academic medicine has formally recognized the need to train culturally competent physicians. As mentioned previously, OSCEs are widely used in medical training but OSCEs of cultural competence (ccOSCE) are rare. Collins and colleagues (2011), including researchers from both medical and psychology disciplines, analyzed verbal and nonverbal communication during ethnogeriatric OSCE interviews conducted by medical students, residents, and fellows. Results suggested the nonverbal behaviors had a significant positive effect on perceived quality of cultural competence and the interview overall.

Our own ccOSCE, also with third-year medical students, targets poor medication adherence and health literacy (Bensadon & Servoss, 2014). Ethnically diverse, dark-skinned, bilingual SPs are recruited and trained to evaluate students postencounter in the exam room. Ten standardized clinical benchmarks are used as performance criteria. Case scenario was adapted from an extant ccOSCE (Green et al., 2007) and, to maximize realism, SP personal experience. Following the encounters, learners review their videos and select two excerpts (<60 seconds each) for presentation and self-assessment in small groups facilitated by medical school faculty.

Virtually all students satisfactorily elicit the chief complaint, attempt to build trust/establish rapport, and end the encounter with a summary/recap of an agreed-upon plan. Conversely, very few assess patient understanding and motivation for adopting treatment recommendations or barriers to accepting them, and few students explore and document relevant social history or understand patient comprehension of the medication regimen, lapses documented in actual practice (e.g., Schillinger et al., 2003). In addition, many students complain that the SPs are reluctant to disclose information. Small group discussion centers on health literacy, linguistic competence, and patients' potential distrust and/or shame. While students seem to understand these factors rationally, frustration is common, as are feelings of discomfort and inadequacy when forced to sit with a patient, armed with no equipment other than their communication skills. Learners sometimes blame the SP for not divulging information when asked. Again, future physicians may accept the logic behind the need to earn trust and speak without jargon; however, once they feel they have adequately done this, if it does not automatically yield the information they need, frustration is expressed by blaming the patient, a behavioral pattern also documented among practicing physicians (Levinson, Stiles, Inui, & Engle, 1993). Our format allows learners to better understand their own practice behavior, identify specific areas for skills improvement, and discuss alternative strategies to maximize their clinical effectiveness.

BARRIERS

As mentioned earlier, some may point out that while the video is objective, interpretation is not. This is a valid criticism. But this challenge is no more complex or problematic than analogous disagreement among physicians reading diagnostic imaging. CT, PET, and MRI are all "objective" technologies. But interpreting their findings and clinical implications can lead to similar disagreements. And even when physicians agree with each other, they may not agree with the technology (O'Laughlin et al., 2013).

As shown throughout this publication, subjective human judgment is an inevitable part of both medical and clinical psychology practice. The aspirational goal of medical science to remove bias is a good one, but must be balanced against psychological harm resulting from well-documented trends toward overscreening (e.g., Cassels, 2012; Stewart-Brown & Farmer, 1997), overdiagnosing (e.g., Welch & Black, 2010), and their relationship to each other (e.g., Esserman, Thompson, & Reid, 2013), also known as "surveillance bias" (Haut & Pronovost, 2011).

Simulation education, especially with SPs, minimizes harm and maximizes authenticity. Video technology transforms even the subtlest elements of therapeutic encounters into observable, behavioral data. Clinically relevant interpersonal competencies, therefore, can be assessed objectively. And for trainees, video review is an unparalleled learning tool. Given simulation's precise fit with clinical psychologists' training, better integration of psychology and medicine can uniquely sensitize learners and cultivate their self-awareness and insight, in a manner that no other modality can.

References

Abbass, A. (2004). Small-group videotape training for psychotherapy skills development. *Academic Psychiatry, 28*(2), 151–155.

Ambady, N., LaPlante, D., Nguyen, T., Rosenthal, R., Chaumeton, N., & Levinson, W. (2002). Surgeons' tone of voice: A clue to malpractice history. *Surgery, 132*(1), 5–9.

Bandura, A. (1965). Influence of models' reinforcement contingencies on the acquisition of imitative responses. *Journal of personality and social psychology, 1*(6), 589–595.

Bandura, A. (1977). *Social learning theory*. Oxford, England: Prentice-Hall.

Bandura, A., Ross, D., & Ross, S. A. (1961). Transmission of aggression through imitation of aggressive models. *The Journal of Abnormal and Social Psychology, 63*(3), 575–582.

Bandura, A., Ross, D., & Ross, S. A. (1963). Imitation of film-mediated aggressive models. *The Journal of Abnormal and Social Psychology, 66*(1), 3–11.

Bassford, H. A. (1982). The justification of medical paternalism. *Social Science and Medicine.*, *16*(6), 731–739.

Batalden, P. (2002). General competencies and accreditation in graduate medical education. *Health Affairs*, *21*(5), 103–111.

Batt-Rawden, S. A., Chisolm, M. S., Anton, B., & Flickinger, T. E. (2013). Teaching empathy to medical students: An updated, systematic review. *Academic Medicine*, *88*(8), 1171–1177.

Belar, C. D. (2009). Advancing the culture of competence. *Training and Education in Professional Psychology*, *3*, S63–S65.

Bensadon, B. A. & Servoss, J. C. (2014). Training culturally competent physicians via simulation. Poster session presented at the annual meeting of the Association of American Medical Colleges, Chicago, IL.

Billings, M. E., Lazarus, M. E., Wenrich, M., Curtis, J. R., & Engelberg, R. A. (2011). The effect of the hidden curriculum on resident burnout and cynicism. *Journal of Graduate Medical Education*, *3*(4), 503–510.

Brewer, W. F. (1986). What is autobiographical memory? In D. C. Rubin (Ed.), *Autobiographical memory* (pp. 25–49). New York: Cambridge University Press.

Cassels, A. (2012). *Seeking sickness*. Vancouver: Greystone Books.

Charles, C., Gafni, A., & Whelan, T. (1997). Shared decision-making in the medical encounter: What does it mean? (or it takes at least two to tango). *Social Science & Medicine*, *44*(5), 681–692.

Chipman, J. G., Beilman, G. J., Schitz, C. C., & Seatter, S. C. (2007). Development and pilot testing of an OSCE for difficult conversations in surgical intensive care. *Journal of Surgical Education*, *64*(2), 79–87.

Cocksedge, S., George, B., Renwick, S., & Chew-Graham, C. A. (2013). Touch in primary care consultations: Qualitative investigation of doctors' and patients' perceptions. *British Journal of General Practice*, *63*(609), e283–e290.

Collins, L. G., Schrimmer, A., Diamond, A., & Burke, J. (2011). Evaluating verbal and non-verbal communication skills in an ethnogeriatric OSCE. *Patient Education and Counseling*, *83*(2), 158–162.

Cowden, R. C. (1955). Empathy or projection? *Journal of Clinical Psychology*, *11*, 188–190.

Cramer, R. J., Johnson, S. M., McLaughlin, J., Rausch, E. M., & Conroy, M. A. (2013). Suicide risk assessment training for psychology doctoral programs: Core competencies and a framework for training. *Training and Education in Professional Psychology*, *7*(1), 1–11.

D'eon, M., Lear, N., Turner, M., & Jones, C. (2007). Perils of the hidden curriculum revisited. *Medical Teacher*, *29*(4), 295–296.

DiMatteo, M. R., Taranta, A., Friedman, H. S., & Prince, L. M. (1980). Predicting patient satisfaction from physicians' nonverbal communication skills. *Medical Care*, 376–387.

Eisenberg, N., & Lennon, R. (1983). Sex differences in empathy and related capacities. *Psychological Bullletin*, *94*(1), 100–131.

Esserman, L. J., Thompson, I. M., & Reid, B. (2013). Overdiagnosis and overtreatment in cancer: An opportunity for improvement. *Journal of the American Medical Association*, *310*(8), 797–798.

Fabiny, A., McArdle, P., Perls, T., Inui, T., & Sheehan, M. (1998). The geriatric objective structured clinical exercise. *Gerontology & Geriatrics Education*, *18*(4), 63–70.

Festinger, L. (1962). *A theory of cognitive dissonance* (Vol. 2). Stanford, CA: Stanford University Press.

Gaufberg, E. H., Batalden, M., Sands, R., & Bell, S. K. (2010). The hidden curriculum: What can we learn from third-year medical student narrative reflections? *Academic Medicine*, *85*(11), 1709–1716.

Goldberg, D. A. (1983). Resistance to the use of video in individual psychotherapy training. *The American Journal of Psychiatry*, *140*(9), 1172–1176.

Gramzow, R. H., & Willard, G. (2006). Exaggerating current and past performance: Motivated self-enhancement versus reconstructive memory. *Personality & Social Psychology Bulletin*, *32*(8), 1114–1125.

Green, A. R., Miller, E., Krupat, E., White, A., Taylor, W. C., Hirsh, D. A., et al. (2007). Designing and implementing a cultural competence OSCE: Lessons learned from interviews with medical students. *Ethnicity & Disease, 17*(2), 344–350.

Hafferty, F. (1998). Beyond curriculum reform: Confronting medicine's hidden curriculum. *Academic Medicine, 73*(4), 403–407.

Hall, J. A., Roter, D. L., & Katz, N. R. (1988). Meta-analysis of correlates of provider behavior in medical encounters. *Medical Care, 26*(7), 657–675.

Haut, E. R., & Pronovost, P. J. (2011). Surveillance bias in outcomes reporting. *Journal of the American Medical Association, 305*(23), 2462–2463.

Hoffman, M. L. (1977). Sex differences in empathy and related behaviors. *Psychological Bulletin, 84*(4), 712–722.

Hojat, M., Vergare, M. J., Maxwell, K., Brainard, G., Herine, S. K., Isenberg, G. A., et al. (2009). The devil is in the third year: A longitudinal study of erosion of empathy in medical school. *Academic Medicine, 84*(9), 1182–1191.

Ivey, A. E., Normington, C. J., Miller, C. D., Morrill, W. H., & Haase, R. F. (1968). Microcounseling and attending behavior: An approach to prepracticum counselor training. *Journal of Counseling Psychology, 15*(5 pt 2), 1–12.

James, C. T., Thompson, J. G., & Baldwin, J. M. (1973). The reconstructive process in sentence memory. *Journal of Verbal Learning & Verbal Behavior, 12*(1), 51–63.

Johnson, M. K., Hashtroudi, S., & Lindsay, D. S. (1993). Source monitoring. *Psychology Bulletin, 114*(1), 3–28.

Karel, M. J., Emery, E. E., & Molinari, V. (2010b). Development of a tool to evaluate geropsychology knowledge and skill competencies. *International Psychogeriatrics, 22*(06), 886–896.

Karel, M. J., Knight, B. G., Duffy, M., Hinrichsen, G. A., & Zeiss, A. M. (2010a). Attitude, knowledge, and skill competencies for practice in professional geropsychology: Implications for training and building a geropsychology workforce. *Training and Education in Professional Psychology, 4*(2), 75–84.

Kaslow, N. J. (2004). Competencies in professional psychology. *American Psychologist, 59*(8), 774–781.

Kenkel, M. B., & Peterson, R. L. (2009). *Competency-based education in professional psychology.* Washington, DC: American Psychological Association.

Kennedy, Q., Mather, M., & Carstensen, L. L. (2004). The role of motivation in the age-related positivity effect in autobiographical memory. *Psychological Science, 15*(3), 208–214.

Knight, B. G., Karel, M. J., Hinrichsen, G. A., Qualls, S. H., & Duffy, M. (2009). Pikes Peak model for training in professional geropsychology. *American Psychologist, 64*(3), 205–214.

Kohn, L. T., Corrigan, J. M., & Donaldson, , & M. S. (Eds.), (2000). *To err is human: Building a safer health system* (Vol. 627). Washington, DC: National Academies Press.

Leape, L. L., & Berwick, D. M. (2005). Five years after to err is human: What have we learned? *JAMA, 293*(19), 2384–2390.

Leipzig, R. M., Granville, L., Simpson, D., Anderson, B., Sauvigne, K., & Soriano, R. (2009). Keeping Granny safe on July 1: A consensus on geriatric competencies for graduating medical students. *Academic Medicine, 84,* 604–610.

Levinson, W., Stiles, W. B., Inui, T. S., & Engle, R. (1993). Physician frustration in communicating with patients. *Medical Care, 31*(4), 285–295.

Martinez, I. L., & Mora, J. C. (2012). A community-based approach for integrating geriatrics and gerontology into undergraduate medical education. *Gerontology and Geriatrics Education, 1*(1), 2152–2165.

McKinstry, B. (1992). Paternalism and the doctor–patient relationship in general practice. *British Journal of General Practice., 42*(361), 340–342.

Meier, D. E. (2014). I don't want Jenny to think I'm abandoning her: Views on overtreatment. *Health Affairs, 33*(5), 895–898.

Meier, D. E., Back, A. L., & Morrison, R. S. (2001). The inner life of physicians and care of the seriously ill. *Journal of the American Medical Association, 286*(23), 3007–3014.

Miles, S. H. (1994). Physicians and their patients' suicides. *Journal of the American Medical Association, 271*(22), 1786–1788.

Neumann, M., Edelhäuser, F., Tauschel, D., Fischer, M. R., Wirtz, M., & Woopen, C., et al. (2011). Empathy decline and its reasons: A systematic review of studies with medical students and residents. *Academic Medicine, 86*(8), 996–1009.

Novack, D. H., Suchman, A. L., Clark, W., Epstein, R. M., Najberg, E., & Kaplan, C. (1997). Calibrating the physician: Personal awareness and effective patient care. *Journal of the American Medical Association, 278*(6), 502–509.

Ong, L. M., De Haes, J. C., Hoos, A. M., & Lammes, F. B. (1995). Doctor–patient communication: A review of the literature. *Social Science & Medicine, 40*(7), 903–918.

O'Laughlin, K. N., Hoffman, J. R., Go, S., Gabayan, G. Z., Iqbal, E., Merchant, G., et al. (2013). Nonconcordance between clinical and head CT findings: The specter of overdiagnosis. *Emergency Medicine International, 2013*(314948).

O'Sullivan, P., Chao, S., Russell, M., Levine, S., & Fabiny, A. (2008). Development and implementation of an objective structured clinical examination to provide formative feedback on communication and interpersonal skills in geriatric training. *Journal of the American Geriatrics Society, 56*(9), 1730–1735.

Patihis, L., Frenda, S. J., LePort, A. K. R., Petersen, N., Nichols, R. M., Stark, C. E. L., et al. (2013). False memories in highly superior autobiographical memory individuals. *Proceedings of the National Academy of Sciences, 110*(52), 20947–20952.

Riess, H., Kelley, J. M., Bailey, R. W., Dunn, E. J., & Phillips, M. (2012). Empathy training for resident physicians: A randomized controlled trial of a neuroscience-informed curriculum. *Journal of General Internal Medicine, 27*(10), 1280–1286.

Rubin, N. J., Bebeau, M., Leigh, I. W., Lichtenberg, J. W., Nelson, P. D., & Portnoy, S. (2007). The competency movement within psychology: An historical perspective. *Professional Psychology: Research and Practice, 38*(5), 452–462.

Sarzynski, E., Wagner, D., & Noel, M. (2013). Expanding the objective structured clinical examination (OSCE) to teach documentation, coding and billing. *Medical Teacher, 35*(8), 699–700.

Schacter, D. L. (1999). The seven sins of memory: Insights from psychology and cognitive neuroscience. *American Psychologist, 54*(3), 182–203.

Schillerstrom, J. E., Lutz, M. L., Ferguson, D. M., Nelson, E. L., & Parker, J. A. (2013). The women's health objective structured clinical exam: A multidisciplinary collaboration. *Journal of Psychosomatic Obstetrics & Gynecology, 34*(4), 145–149.

Schillinger, D., Piette, J., Grumbach, K., Wang, F., Wilson, C., Daher, C., et al. (2003). Closing the loop: physician communication with diabetic patients who have low health literacy. *Archives of Internal Medicine, 163*(1), 83–90.

Schmidt, S. R. (2004). Autobiographical memories for the September 11th attacks: Reconstructive errors and emotional impairment. *Memory & Cognition, 32*(3), 443–454.

Scobie, S. D., Lawson, M., Cavell, G., Taylor, K., Jackson, S. H. D., & Robert, T. E. (2003). Meeting the challenge of prescribing and administering medicines safely: structured teaching and assessment for final year medical students. *Medical Education, 37*(5), 434–437.

Shah, B., Miler, R., Poles, M., Zabar, S., Gillespie, C., Weinshel, E., et al. (2011). Informed consent in the older adult: OSCEs for assessing fellows' ACGME and geriatric gastroenterology competencies. *The American Journal of Gastroenterology, 106*, 1575–1579.

Siegler, M. (1985). The progression of medicine: From physician paternalism to patient autonomy to bureaucratic parsimony. *Archives of Internal Medicine, 145*(4), 713–715.

Singh, R., Singh, A., Fish, R., McLean, D., Anderson, D., & Singh, G. (2009). A patient safety objective structured clinical examination. *Journal of Patient Safety, 5*(2), 55–60.

Solomon, P., Marshall, D., Boyle, A., Burns, S., Casimiro, L. M., Hall, P., et al. (2011). Establishing face and content validity of the McMaster-Ottawa Team Observed Structured Clinical Encounter (TOSCE). *Journal of Interprofessional Care, 25*(4), 302–304.

Stewart, M. A. (1995). Effective physician–patient communication and health outcomes: A review. *Canadian Medical Association Journal, 15*(9), 1423–1433.

Stewart-Brown, S., & Farmer, A. (1997). Screening could seriously damage your health. *British Medical Journal, 314*(7080), 533.

Thomas, H. (2013). From the trainee. *InnnovAiT: Education and Inspiration for General Practice, 6*(12), 772–773.

Waitzkin, H. (1984). Doctor–patient communication: Clinical implications of social scientific research. *Journal of the American Medical Association, 252*(17), 2441–2446.

Welch, H. G., & Black, W. C. (2010). Overdiagnosis in cancer. *Journal of the National Cancer Institute, 102*(9), 605–613.

Zolnierek, K. B. H., & DiMatteo, M. R. (2009). Physician communication and patient adherence to treatment: A meta-analysis. *Medical Care, 47*(8), 826–834.

Index

Note: Page numbers followed by "*b*," "*f*," and "*t*" refer to boxes, figures, and tables, respectively.

Printed in the United States
By Bookmasters